T0264331

Ruminant Parasitology

Editor

RAY M. KAPLAN

VETERINARY CLINICS OF NORTH AMERICA: FOOD ANIMAL PRACTICE

www.vetfood.theclinics.com

Consulting Editor
ROBERT A. SMITH

March 2020 • Volume 36 • Number 1

ELSEVIER

1600 John F. Kennedy Boulevard • Suite 1800 • Philadelphia, Pennsylvania, 19103-2899

http://www.vetfood.theclinics.com

VETERINARY CLINICS OF NORTH AMERICA: FOOD ANIMAL PRACTICE Volume 36, Number 1
March 2020 ISSN 0749-0720, ISBN-13: 978-0-323-69598-5

Editor: Colleen Dietzler
Developmental Editor: Laura Kavanaugh

Veterinary Clinics of North America: Food Animal Practice (ISSN 0749-0720) is published in March, July, and November by Elsevier Inc., 360 Park Avenue South, New York, NY 10010-1710. Subscription prices are $259.00 per year (domestic individuals), $456.00 per year (domestic institutions), $100.00 per year (domestic students/residents), $283.00 per year (Canadian individuals), $601.00 per year (Canadian institutions), $335.00 per year (international individuals), $601.00 per year (international institutions), $100.00 per year (Canadian students), and $165.00 (international students). To receive student/resident rate, orders must be accompanied by name of affiliated institution, date of term, and the signature of program/residency coordinator on institution letterhead. *Clinics* subscription prices. All prices are subject to change without notice. **POSTMASTER:** Send address changes to *Veterinary Clinics of North America: Food Animal Practice*, Elsevier Health Sciences Division, Subscription Customer Service, 3251 Riverport Lane, Maryland Heights, MO 63043. Customer Service (orders, claims, online, change of address): Elsevier Health Sciences Division, Subscription **Customer Service, 3251 Riverport Lane, Maryland Heights, MO 63043. Tel: 1-800-654-2452 (U.S. and Canada); 314-447-8871 (ouside U.S. and Canada). Fax: 314-447-8029. E-mail: journalscustomerservice-usa@elsevier.com (for print support); journalsonlinesupport-usa@elsevier.com (for online support).**

Reprints. For copies of 100 or more, of articles in this publication, please contact the Commercial Reprints Department, Elsevier Inc., 360 Park Avenue South, New York, NY 10010-1710. Tel.: 212-633-3874; Fax: 212-633-3820; E-mail: reprints@elsevier.com.

Veterinary Clinics of North America: Food Animal Practice is covered in *Current Contents/Agriculture, Biology and Environmental Sciences, MEDLINE/PubMed (Index Medicus), and Excerpta Medica.*

Contributors

CONSULTING EDITOR

ROBERT A. SMITH, DVM, MS
Diplomate, American Board of Veterinary Practitioners; Veterinary Research and Consulting Services, LLC, Greeley, Colorado, USA

EDITOR

RAY M. KAPLAN, DVM, PhD
Diplomate, American College of Veterinary Microbiologists; Diplomate, European Veterinary Parasitology College; Professor of Parasitology, Department of Infectious Diseases, College of Veterinary Medicine, University of Georgia, Athens, Georgia, USA

AUTHORS

BERIT BANGOURA, DVM, PhD
EBVS European Veterinary Specialist in Parasitology, Department of Veterinary Sciences, University of Wyoming, Laramie, Wyoming, USA

KATHERINE D. BARDSLEY, MS
Department of Veterinary Sciences, University of Wyoming, Laramie, Wyoming, USA

JOAN M. BURKE, PhD
Research Animal Scientist, USDA ARS Dale Bumpers Small Farms Research Center, Booneville, Arkansas, USA

CHARLES BYARUHANGA, PhD
Department of Veterinary Tropical Diseases, Faculty of Veterinary Science, University of Pretoria, Onderstepoort, South Africa

JOHANNES CHARLIER, DVM, PhD
Diplomate, European Veterinary Parasitology College; Kreavet, Kruibeke, Belgium

UMER N. CHAUDHRY, DVM, MSc, PhD
Research Scientist, University of Edinburgh Royal (Dick) School of Veterinary Studies, The Roslin Institute, Easter Bush Veterinary Centre, Midlothian, Scotland

EDWIN CLAEREBOUT, DVM, PhD
Diplomate, European Veterinary Parasitology College; Faculty of Veterinary Medicine, Laboratory of Parasitology, Ghent University, Merelbeke, Belgium

J.P. DUBEY, MVSc, PhD
Senior Scientist, United States Department of Agriculture, Agricultural Research Service, Beltsville Agricultural Research Center, Beltsville, Maryland, USA

JAVIER GARZA, PhD
Leica Biosystems, Buffalo Grove, Illinois, USA

PETER GELDHOF, PhD
Faculty of Veterinary Medicine, Laboratory of Parasitology, Ghent University, Merelbeke, Belgium

ANDREW W. GREER, PhD
Faculty of Agriculture and Life Sciences, Lincoln University, Christchurch, Canterbury, New Zealand

JOSEPH C. HAMIE, PhD
Faculty of Agriculture and Life Sciences, Lincoln University, Christchurch, Canterbury, New Zealand; Department of Agricultural Research Services, Lunyangwa Agricultural Research Station, Mzuzu, Malawi

MICHAEL B. HILDRETH, PhD
Professor, Department of Biology and Microbiology, South Dakota State University, Brookings, South Dakota, USA

JOHAN HÖGLUND, MSc, PhD
Diplomate, European Veterinary Parasitology College; Swedish University of Agricultural Sciences, Department of Biomedical Sciences and Veterinary Public Health, Section for Parasitology, Uppsala, Sweden

ALISON K. HOWELL, BVSc, MSc, MRes, PhD, MRCVS
Postdoctoral Research Associate, Institute of Infection and Global Health, University of Liverpool, Leahurst Campus, Neston, United Kingdom

RAY M. KAPLAN, DVM, PhD
Diplomate, American College of Veterinary Microbiologists; Diplomate, European Veterinary Parasitology College; Professor of Parasitology, Department of Infectious Diseases, College of Veterinary Medicine, University of Georgia, Athens, Georgia, USA

FIONA KENYON, PhD
Disease Control, Moredun Research Institute, Pentlands Science Park, Midlothian, Scotland

MANIGANDAN LEJEUNE, BVSc, MSc, PhD
Diplomate, American College of Veterinary Microbiologists (Parasitology); Senior Extension Associate and Director, Clinical Parasitology, Department of Population Medicine and Diagnostic Sciences, Cornell University, College of Veterinary Medicine, Animal Health Diagnostic Center, Ithaca, New York, USA

DAVID S. LINDSAY, PhD
Professor, Department of Biomedical Sciences and Pathobiology, Center for One Health Research, Virginia Maryland College of Veterinary Medicine, Virginia Tech, Blacksburg, Virginia, USA

JOHN B. McKENZIE, BS
Graduate Student, Department of Biology and Microbiology, South Dakota State University, Brookings, South Dakota, USA

JAMES E. MILLER, DVM, MPVM, PhD
Diplomate, American College of Veterinary Pathologists; Department of Pathobiological Sciences, School of Veterinary Medicine, Louisiana State University, Baton Rouge, Louisiana, USA

ROBERT D. MITCHELL III, MS, PhD
Postdoctoral Researcher, United States Department of Agriculture – Agricultural Research Service, Knipling-Bushland U.S. Livestock Insects Research Laboratory and Veterinary Pest Genomics Center, Kerrville, Texas, USA

ERIC R. MORGAN, MA, VetMB, PhD, MRCVS
Diplomate, European Veterinary Parasitology College; Biological Sciences, Queen's University of Belfast, Belfast, United Kingdom

CHRISTINE B. NAVARRE, DVM, MS
Diplomate, American College of Veterinary Internal Medicine (Large Animal); Professor, School of Animal Sciences, Louisiana State University Agricultural Center, Louisiana State University, Baton Rouge, Louisiana, USA

ADALBERTO A. PÉREZ DE LEÓN, DVM, MS, PhD
Director and Research Leader, United States Department of Agriculture – Agricultural Research Service, Knipling-Bushland U.S. Livestock Insects Research Laboratory and Veterinary Pest Genomics Center, Kerrville, Texas, USA

HANNAH ROSE VINEER, BSc (Hons) Zoology, PhD Veterinary Parasitology
Veterinary Parasitology, Department of Infection Biology, Institute of Infection and Global Health, University of Liverpool, Institute of Veterinary Science, Neston, United Kingdom

MONICA SANTIN, DVM, PhD
Environmental Microbial and Food Safety Laboratory, Beltsville Agricultural Research Center, Agricultural Research Service, US Department of Agriculture, Beltsville, Maryland, USA

JAN A. VAN WYK, PhD
Department of Veterinary Tropical Diseases, Faculty of Veterinary Science, University of Pretoria, Onderstepoort, South Africa

JOZEF VERCRUYSSE, DVM
Diplomate, European Veterinary Parasitology College; Faculty of Veterinary Medicine, Laboratory of Parasitology, Ghent University, Merelbeke, Belgium

GUILHERME G. VEROCAI, DVM, MSc, PhD
Diplomate, American College of Veterinary Microbiologists (Parasitology); Clinical Assistant Professor and Director, Parasitology Diagnostic Laboratory, Department of Veterinary Pathobiology, Texas A&M University, College of Veterinary Medicine and Biomedical Sciences, College Station, Texas, USA

DAVID W. WATSON, MS, PhD
Professor and Associate Department Head, Entomology and Plant Pathology Department, North Carolina State University, Raleigh, North Carolina, USA

DIANA J.L. WILLIAMS, BSc, PhD
Professor, Institute of Infection and Global Health, University of Liverpool, Leahurst Campus, Neston, United Kingdom

ANNE M. ZAJAC, DVM, PhD
Diplomate, American College of Veterinary Microbiology (Parasitology Specialty); Professor, Department of Biomedical Sciences and Pathobiology, Virginia/Maryland College of Veterinary Medicine, Virginia Tech, Blacksburg, Virginia, USA

Contents

Johannes Charlier, Johan Höglund, Eric R. Morgan, Peter Geldhof, Jozef Vercruysse, and Edwin Claerebout

This article reviews the basics of gastrointestinal nematode biology and pathophysiology in cattle and describes how gastrointestinal nematode epidemiology is driven by environmental, host, and farm economic determinants. Adverse effects from gastrointestinal nematodes on their hosts are caused by tissue damage, nutrient absorption, immunopathologic effects, and reduced food intake induced by hormonal changes. Weather and microenvironmental factors influence the development and survival of free-living parasitic stages. A holistic control approach entails the consideration of environmental, immunologic, and socioeconomic aspects of nematode epidemiology and is key for the development and communication of sustainable control strategies.

Ray M. Kaplan

Gastrointestinal nematode parasites of ruminants have many biologic and genetic features that favor the development of drug resistance, which has led to the worldwide development of high levels of anthelmintic resistance. The rate of resistance development is affected by a number of controllable factors, thus there is an urgent need to change the paradigm of control in order to reduce the rate with which resistance develops. This article reviews the biology and prevalence of anthelmintic resistance, and provides recommendations for diagnosing resistance and for strategies that should be implemented to reduce the development of resistance.

Andrew W. Greer, Jan A. Van Wyk, Joseph C. Hamie, Charles Byaruhanga, and Fiona Kenyon

Refugia-based strategies are intended to help slow the development of anthelmintic resistance by providing a population of parasites that are not exposed to the treatment. Evidence from field studies is lacking. There is no single way to incorporate refugia into a parasite control program. There are many options available varying greatly in complexity and practicality, and none are suitable for all situations. Incorporating refugia into production systems typically requires a change in farmer mindset and greater input of time, labor, and/or technology, but is necessary to help preserve anthelmintic efficacy and promote sustainable animal production systems.

livestock species. In addition, and perhaps most importantly, genetic selection focuses on parasite resistance. Producers should use as many tools as possible to minimize the need for pharmaceutical interventions and optimize animal production.

Fasciola hepatica, Fasciola gigantica, and Fascioloides magna are liver flukes causing disease in cattle and sheep. Damage to the liver due to F hepatica and F gigantica results in clinical disease and/or production losses. F magna seems to have little effect in cattle but causes high mortality in sheep. The fluke life cycle involves an aquatic or amphibious snail intermediate host and thus requires suitable moisture and temperature conditions. F magna requires the presence of deer. Drug treatment is the mainstay of control and needs to be applied considering the life cycle and epidemiology of the parasite.

Internal parasites are a major concern in livestock production because they can impact the health and well-being of animals clinically and subclinically, and ultimately cause significant production loss. Among these internal parasites are nematodes, tapeworms, flukes, and coccidian protozoans. This review focuses on the diagnostic tests that are routinely performed by veterinarians and diagnostic laboratories, but also highlights recently developed tools that may improve diagnostic capabilities, including molecular and immunodiagnostic tests. Overall, diagnostic tests for parasites of livestock are an integral part of health management practices, and for assessing individual animal and herd health.

Veterinarians and farmers must contend with the development of drug resistance and climate variability, which threaten the sustainability of current parasite control practices. Field trials evaluating competing strategies for controlling parasites while simultaneously slowing the development of resistance are time consuming and expensive. In contrast, modelling studies can rapidly explore a wide range of scenarios and have generated an array of decision support tools for veterinarians and farmers such as real-time weather-dependent infection risk alerts. Models have also been valuable for predicting the development of anthelmintic resistance, evaluating the sustainability of current parasite control practices and promoting the responsible use of novel anthelmintics.

This article summarizes the state of the art in vaccine research against parasitic helminths in sheep and cattle. Optimization of antigen production (eg, recombinant expression) and antigen delivery, followed by extensive field testing, is still required for further development of vaccines. Helminth vaccines should sufficiently reduce parasite transmission to protect vaccinated animals against parasite-induced disorders and production loss. Vaccine efficacy requirements depend on the parasite's epidemiology and farm management, both of which vary in different geographic regions and are influenced by climate. Vaccination is likely to be part of integrated worm control, together with other worm control measures.

Diverse groups of ectoparasitic arthropods cause significant morbidity and mortality in most of the approximately 1.49 billion head of cattle worldwide. Hematophagous ectoparasites (ie, blood-feeding flies, myiasis-causing flies, lice, mites, ticks) are the most important in cattle. Intense use of synthetic ectoparasiticides to treat infestations can result in ectoparasite populations becoming resistant to this treatment method. Approaches integrating the use of different technologies are required to manage cattle ectoparasites effectively while addressing societal expectations regarding food safety and environmental health. Assessing the status of coparasitism with ectoparasites and endoparasites in cattle across agroecosystems is critical in advancing integrated parasite management.

Ruminant coccidiosis, caused by *Eimeria* species, is a significant and widespread enteric disease in young livestock worldwide. High morbidities and significant mortalities may be observed. For disease diagnosis, fecal samples from clinically ill animals should be analyzed for both, identity (ie, pathogenicity) of *Eimeria* species and excreted oocyst amount. To prevent coccidiosis-related economic losses, management measures to reduce infection pressure and improve general animal health are crucial. Anticoccidial drugs are widely used to control clinical and subclinical disease. Treatment is most efficient when applied prophylactically or metaphylactically. To avoid development of parasite drug resistance, drugs should be used sustainably.

Neospora caninum, *Toxoplasma gondii*, and *Sarcocystis* spp. are related Apicomplexan parasites that have 2 hosts in their life cycles. The definitive hosts excrete unsporulated (*Neospora caninum*, *T gondii*) or sporulated (*Sarcocystis* spp.) oocysts in their feces after ingesting tissue cysts from the tissues of ruminant intermediate hosts. These coccidians can cause abortion and neonatal mortality in ruminants. *T gondii* and *Sarcocystis hominis* (from cattle) are zoonotic. This article reviews information on the etiology, life cycle, diagnosis, control and prevention of these parasites and the diseases they cause in ruminants.

Cryptosporidium and *Giardia* are ubiquitous protozoan parasites that infect a broad range of vertebrate hosts, including domestic and wild animals as well as humans. Both parasites are of medical and veterinary importance. Infections with *Cryptosporidium* and *Giardia* in ruminants are associated with diarrhea outbreaks, mainly in young animals. Ruminants are potential sources of infection for humans because some species of *Cryptosporidium* and assemblages of *Giardia duodenalis* have been isolated from both ruminants and humans. Knowledge of these parasites has greatly expanded in the last 2 decades from simple microscopic observations of organisms to the knowledge acquired from molecular tools.

VETERINARY CLINICS OF NORTH AMERICA: FOOD ANIMAL PRACTICE

SERIES OF RELATED INTEREST

Veterinary Clinics of North America: Equine Practice

THE CLINICS ARE NOW AVAILABLE ONLINE!
Access your subscription at:
www.theclinics.com

Preface

Ruminations on Parasite Control

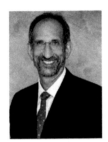

Ray M. Kaplan, DVM, PhD
Editor

Recommendations and strategies for the control of gastrointestinal nematode (GIN) parasites in ruminants have undergone major changes since the last *Veterinary Clinics of North America: Food Animal Practice* issue on Ruminant Parasitology was published 14 years ago. Key to these changes is the escalation of anthelmintic resistance, which is now a major problem not only in small ruminants but also in cattle. The problem of anthelmintic resistance is further magnified as no new drug classes have been introduced for ruminants in the United States, and no new drug classes have been introduced for cattle anywhere in the world since the avermectin/milbemycins (macrocyclic lactones) almost 40 years ago. On many goat and sheep farms, resistance in *Haemonchus contortus* to all available anthelmintics now exists, and on cattle farms, anthelmintic resistance in multiple parasite species, including *Ostertagia ostertagi*, is an increasing problem. As a result, parasite control practices of the past based almost exclusively on relatively frequent whole-herd anthelmintic treatments are no longer viable or sustainable. Consequently, recommendations for parasite control have evolved from those of the past, and in many respects are fundamentally different from those that served as the basis for parasite control for the past few decades. In addition, new technologies have advanced the development of parasite vaccines and the capabilities of computer modeling. Computer modeling now allows long-term field experiments to be performed in silico; thus, multiple different control strategies can be compared under multiple climatic conditions for their ability to control parasites and reduce the development of resistance. A vaccine for *H contortus* is now available in some countries, and advances are being made in vaccines for other important nematode species.

To address these many changes, this new issue provides updates of article topics present in the previous issue as well as new articles on topics that have recently gained increasing importance. We include an updated article on anthelmintic resistance with recommendations for diagnosing resistance using the fecal egg count reduction test,

Vet Clin Food Anim 36 (2020) xiii–xiv
https://doi.org/10.1016/j.cvfa.2019.12.007
0749-0720/20/© 2019 Published by Elsevier Inc.

vetfood.theclinics.com

and the use of anthelmintic combinations to improve treatment efficacy while also reducing the development of resistance. Updated articles are also provided for the control of GIN, ectoparasites, and protozoan parasites in both small ruminants and cattle. Furthermore, new articles are included on refugia-based strategies, novel nonchemical approaches, parasite vaccines, computer modeling, and liver flukes.

Finally, this new issue of *Veterinary Clinics of North America: Food Animal Practice* was only made possible by the hard work of many people. I would like to thank all of the authors and reviewers for contributing their valuable time, energy, and commitment to making this issue a relevant and valuable new addition to the veterinary literature.

Ray M. Kaplan, DVM, PhD
Department of Infectious Diseases
College of Veterinary Medicine
University of Georgia
501 DW Brooks Drive
Athens, GA 30602, USA

E-mail address:
rkaplan@uga.edu

Biology and Epidemiology of Gastrointestinal Nematodes in Cattle

Johannes Charlier, DVM, PhD[a],*, Johan Höglund, MSc, PhD[b],
Eric R. Morgan, MA, VetMB, PhD, MRCVS[c], Peter Geldhof, PhD[d],
Jozef Vercruysse, DVM[d], Edwin Claerebout, DVM, PhD[d]

KEYWORDS

- Gastrointestinal nematodes • *Ostertagia* • *Cooperia* • Epidemiology • Environment
- Immunity • Pathophysiology

KEY POINTS

- Gastrointestinal nematode epidemiology is determined by climatic factors, environmental conditions, host susceptibility, and management systems that characterize cattle production globally.
- Gastrointestinal nematodes occur usually in mixed infections of several species. More than 20 different species are known, but the relative importance differs in different climatic regions and according to host age because of acquired immunity.
- The influence of weather and microenvironmental factors on the development and survival of free-living stages is increasingly understood and is modeled to study the effects of climate change and adapted control approaches.
- Human behavior and social epidemiology are increasingly used to improve the communication of control strategies.

INTRODUCTION

Gastrointestinal nematodes (GINs) of livestock have a direct life cycle and infection takes place during pasture grazing. In temperate areas with cold winters, cattle deposit parasite eggs in the beginning of the pasture season in the spring, and larval pasture contamination typically builds up during the summer until early autumn. During winter and early spring, pastures are ungrazed and the pasture contamination

[a] Kreavet, Hendrik Mertensstraat 17, Kruibeke 9150, Belgium; [b] Swedish University of Agricultural Sciences, Department of Biomedical Sciences and Veterinary Public Health, Section for Parasitology, Box 7036, Uppsala 75007, Sweden; [c] Biological Sciences, Queen's University of Belfast, 19 Chlorine Gardens, Belfast BT9 5DL, UK; [d] Faculty of Veterinary Medicine, Laboratory of Parasitology, Ghent University, Salisburylaan 133, Merelbeke 9820, Belgium
* Corresponding author.
E-mail address: jcharlier@kreavet.be
Twitter: @charlierjo (J.C.)

Vet Clin Food Anim 36 (2020) 1–15
https://doi.org/10.1016/j.cvfa.2019.11.001
0749-0720/20/© 2019 Elsevier Inc. All rights reserved.

reaches its minimal levels.[1] This repeating annual pattern allowed the development of standard or calendar-based control approaches that minimize pasture contamination and thus animal infection levels. These control approaches were mostly based on anthelmintics with persistent efficacy, were highly effective, and were easily communicable to and applied by farmers.[2] However. GIN epidemiology is determined by differing environmental conditions and management systems that characterize cattle production globally. In addition, the emergence of anthelmintic resistance has necessitated that these previous approaches be modified. Factors that influence the epidemiology of GINs, and optimal approaches for control, are under constant change, and, now and in the future, climate change, anthelmintic resistance, and consumer influence on production methods will further alter GIN epidemiology and thus provoke the need to adapt sustainable control strategies. Moreover, control regimens developed in temperate areas will be poorly adapted to other climatic zones Christine B. Navarre's article, "Epidemiology and Control of Gastrointestinal Nematodes of Cattle in Southern Climates", Michael B. Hildreth and John B. McKenzie's article, "Epidemiology and Control of Gastrointestinal Nematodes of Cattle in Northern Climates", (more specific issues relating to control of GINs in cattle in warm and cold climates are discussed elsewhere in this issue).

This article focuses on common GINs of cattle, excluding threadworms (*Strongyloides* spp) and ascarids (*Toxocara* sp) and reviews the basics of their biology and pathophysiology. Next, it describes how GIN epidemiology is driven by environmental (pillar I) and host (pillar II) determinants and how GINs adapt to new constraints in their development. In addition, it explores how human behavior (pillar III) acting to optimize farm economic returns or driven by seemingly irrational motives may be a third and often overlooked factor determining GIN epidemiology. Understanding these determinants help clinicians to predict parasite epidemiology under future change scenarios and to design adapted control approaches.

POPULATION BIOLOGY

All cattle GINs have a direct life cycle (**Fig. 1**). The eggs, which are typical for the order Strongylida, are passed in the feces and develop in the fecal pat on pasture. Development occurs through successive molts from the first-stage larva (L1) to the infective third stage (L3). This process takes 1 to 2 weeks if temperature and humidity are optimal. When moist conditions prevail, the L3 migrate from the feces on to the herbage (also called translation). L3 maintain the cuticle of L2, making them more resistant to harsh environmental conditions and allowing survival for months up to more than a year on pasture. After ingestion by a suitable host, the L3 exsheath in the rumen and further development takes place in the mucosa of the abomasum or the intestine, depending on the species. After 2 additional molts, adults emerge on the surface of the mucosa, around 3 weeks after infection. Besides knowing the life cycle, several other concepts are important to understand how nematode populations behave (**Box 1**).

GINs occur usually in mixed infections of several species. More than 20 different species are described, but the relative importance and prevalence differ in different climatic regions and according to host age because of acquired immunity. The most common and important species in temperate climate zones are *Ostertagia ostertagi* and *Cooperia oncophora*, but different species may be predominant in other regions. Automated polymerase chain reaction platforms and DNA sequencing technologies (metabarcoding) now allow detailed studies into GIN species diversity.[3,4] A study conducted across Australia, Belgium, and Scotland confirmed *O ostertagi* and

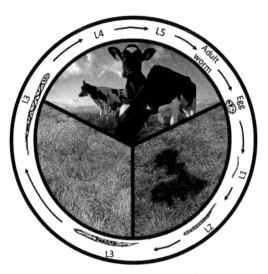

Fig. 1. Life cycle of GINs in cattle. (*From* Charlier J, Claerebout E, Vercruysse J. Gastrointestinal nematode infections in adult dairy cattle. Reference Module in Food Science. 2016; with permission.)

Box 1
Phenomena observed in gastrointestinal nematode population behavior

Overdispersion: GINs tend to be unevenly distributed among hosts, with few of the animals in a group carrying more of the parasites. This distribution can be related to variation in host exposure (eg, different grazing behavior) and parasite establishment or survival (eg, immunocompetence of the host)[82] and has important implications for transmission, diagnosis, and control (eg, group-level control by targeting the most infected animals).

Hypobiosis: under certain conditions and for several nematode species (eg, *Ostertagia ostertagi*, *Cooperia oncophora*), a proportion of the ingested L3 becomes arrested in their development at the early fourth stage (EL4). This strategy can overcome harsh climatic conditions. It can also trigger severe disease, when many larvae resume their development at the same time (ostertagiosis type II), but in recent decades this is rarely seen (drug resistance to macrocyclic lactone anthelmintics could change this in the future; Ray M. Kaplan's article, "Biology, Epidemiology, Diagnosis, and Management of Anthelmintic Resistance in Gastrointestinal Nematodes of Livestock", more details on anthelmintic resistance are given elsewhere in this issue). Recent meta-analyses found average hypobiosis rates of 4% and 0.7% for *O ostertagi* and *C oncophora*, with ranges between 0% and 31% between experiments.[83,84] The triggers for entering or leaving the hypobiotic state are only partially understood: host immune status (more hypobiotic stages in older animals) and exposure of free-living stages to colder temperatures, warmer temperatures, or drought conditions and density dependence effects all play a role.

Density dependence: when cattle ingest large numbers of larvae, the acquired worm burden is higher, but the proportion of larvae succeeding to establish and reproduce is lower. Many nematodes in the same location lead to competition between worms of the same as well as other species. This competition is shown by lower establishment rates, smaller worm lengths, lower fecundity, and increased worm mortality. Density dependence, along with hypobiosis, is also one of the reasons why there is often a poor correlation between fecal egg counts and worm burden.

C oncophora as the most prevalent species, with important presence of other species in specific regions.[4] An initial study in North America revealed overall low GIN species diversity in commercial cow-calf beef herds in Canada, with most parasite communities consisting of only 2 species.[5] More species diversity was present in central/southeastern United States and Sao Paulo State, Brazil. In these regions, *Cooperia punctata* and *Haemonchus placei* were the main species present.[5] Different GIN species, along with their distribution and other characteristics, are summarized in **Table 1**.

PATHOGENESIS

Adverse effects from GINs on their hosts are caused by (1) direct effects from the parasites that depend on host nutrients for their metabolic requirements and that may cause physical organ damage; (2) indirect effects that stem from the host's response to parasite invasion; and (3) reduced food intake, which is linked to parasite-induced hormonal changes in the host.[1,6] Because disease is commonly the result of mixed infections of nematodes invading both the abomasum and the intestine, this is referred to as parasitic gastroenteritis (PGE). Severe PGE can lead to mortality and important animal welfare issues. Clinical PGE is characterized by watery diarrhea, dull hair coat, anorexia, and general loss of body condition. However, this level of clinical severity is uncommon; more often, the effects of GINs are subclinical, affecting production parameters without causing overt clinical signs of disease.

In the case of infection with *O ostertagi*, detrimental effects are induced by destruction of the function of the abomasum when the developing larvae invade the fundic glands. The parasite damages the glandular tissue, causing the mucus cells and the pepsinogen-releasing zymogen cells to be replaced by undifferentiated cells.[7] Severe damage is also attributed to the emergence of adult worms on the mucosal surface, when the submucosa becomes infiltrated with mononuclear inflammatory cells and eosinophils. Inflammatory factors, combined with excretory-secretory products from adult worms inhibit parietal cell function.[8] Combined, this leads to impaired gastric function and an increase of the pH of abomasal contents from 2 to 7.[9] The net effect

Table 1
Characteristics of some gastrointestinal nematodes in cattle

Species	Distribution (Climate)	Localization	Prepatent Period (d)	Pathologic Importance
O ostertagi	Temperate	Abomasum	21	+++
H placei and *Haemonchus* spp	(Sub)tropical	Abomasum	18–21	+++
Mecistocirrus digitatus	Tropical	Abomasum	54–72	++
Trichostrongylus axei	Worldwide	Abomasum	15–23	+
C oncophora	Temperate	Small intestine	12–15	++
C punctata and *Cooperia pectinata*	Worldwide	Small intestine	14–21	++ (+)
Trichostrongylus colubriformis, *Trichostrongylus vitrinus*	Temperate	Small intestine	15–23	++
Nematodirus helvetianus	Temperate	Small intestine	21	++
Bunostomum phlebotomum	(Sub)tropical	Small intestine	40–70	++
Capillaria bovis	Worldwide	Small intestine	40	+
Oesophagostomum radiatum	Worldwide	Large intestine	40–45	++
Trichuris discolor	Worldwide	Large intestine	50–90	+(+)

is that pepsinogen released from zymogen cells is not converted to pepsin, the active digestive proteolytic enzyme that breaks down proteins into smaller peptides. Pepsinogen is accumulated and, because of increased vascular permeability, plasma pepsinogen concentrations increase. In addition, a loss of tight junctions allows leakage of macromolecules leading to hypoalbuminemia.[10] At necropsy, severe PGE can be observed by the naked eye and is characterized by a thickened, hyperplastic abomasal submucosa with raised nodules elevating the overlying epithelium (**Fig. 2**).

Cooperia spp are located in the first segments (duodenum and jejunum) of the small intestine, where infection may lead to villous atrophy, mucosal thickening, and hypersecretion of mucus. The disorder resulting from *Cooperia* spp monoinfection is less obvious than that for *O ostertagi*. However, *Cooperia* spp infection alone can lead to reduced weight gains in infected calves.[11] It can also be imagined that animals with massive worm burdens and mucoid enteritis cannot compensate for the poor protein digestion caused by the parasitized abomasum. GIN species that are direct blood feeders (eg *H placei*[12] and *Mecistocirrus digitatus*[13]) cause anemia along with mucosal damage and protein-losing gastroenteritis.

In temperate climate regions, clinical signs of PGE are most frequently observed in first-season grazing (FSG) cattle after some months on pasture and before the onset of immunity.[14] Type I disease from *O ostertagi* refers to the damage usually observed in FSG cattle and is a result of ingested third-stage larvae (L3) beginning 3 to 4 weeks earlier.[14] Type II disease from *O ostertagi* typically occurs in yearlings housed after their first grazing season and is related to the massive emergence of inhibited stages from the mucosa.[15] However, in cattle operations with good nutritional and herd health standards and equipped with broad-spectrum anthelmintics, clinical PGE has become rare and subclinical infections are now the most abundant.[16] Subclinical infections may lead to reduced growth, milk yield, and carcass conformation.[17,18] These effects may be largely explained by parasite-induced anorexia[19] as well as the cost of the immune response, although the latter has only been shown in sheep.[20]

A recent area of research is the mutual interaction between metazoan parasites and the gastrointestinal microbiome. Nematode infections affect microbiota compositions in the gut, and this may contribute to gastric or intestinal function loss.[21] However, the causal mechanisms of the interactions are poorly understood and require further research.[22]

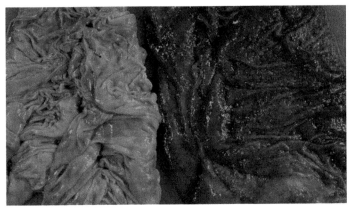

Fig. 2. Opened abomasa of an infected (*right*) and uninfected (*left*) calf, showing the general abomasal enlargement as well as the inflammation of the mucosa in the infected calf.

Given the pathology described earlier, serum or plasma pepsinogen is considered one of the best biomarkers to evaluate infection levels with *O ostertagi*.[23] In a European multicountry study, most calves in their FSG season had a low (<1 U Tyr) or intermediate serum pepsinogen concentration (1–3 U Tyr) and only 2% to 6% of the calves had serum pepsinogen concentrations at levels that are associated with important production losses (>3 U Tyr).[24] In contrast, economically relevant subclinical infections in adult cattle occur more commonly, with 30% to 50% of the herds having anti–*O ostertagi* antibody levels that indicate potential production losses in many regions across Europe[25,26] and in Mexico.[27] Reported levels of infection in Canada are considerably lower,[28,29] whereas no data are currently available for the United States.

DEVELOPMENT, TRANSLATION, AND SURVIVAL OF FREE-LIVING STAGES

The survival of free-living stages, and the development from eggs to larvae, are strongly affected by environmental conditions. The processes in this part of the life cycle and factors influencing them have been subject to detailed experimental work, as well as to observations of infection patterns in experimental and commercial cattle herds. Most work has focused on the nematode species dominant in temperate areas, *O ostertagi* and *C oncophora*, and detailed information on other species, such as *C punctata* and *H placei*, is more scarce. Some processes are quantified only for GINs in sheep, with extrapolation to the related species in cattle.

Development of eggs to L3 accelerates with increasing temperature, but so does mortality, such that maximum yield of L3 from a given number of eggs is optimal at an intermediate temperature, which differs between species and tends to decrease between 20°C and 30°C.[30] Development at temperatures less than 5°C is negligible. In general, there is sufficient moisture present in the dung to permit development to L3, although in warm climates and sunny conditions feces can dry quickly enough to slow or stop development.[30]

Translation of L3 onto pasture depends heavily on moisture, with larvae appearing on pastures following rainfall. High humidity and free water enhanced the ability of mixed GIN L3 populations to climb onto grass,[31] and more L3 were recovered from fields irrigated by spraying than by flooding, although flooding allowed L3 to migrate into soil.[32] Using cylindrical guards, Krecek and Murrell[33] showed that *O ostertagi* larvae could migrate vertically from dung pats into the soil and then onto herbage, leading to delayed but successful translation onto herbage. Allied to findings that L3 move into soil in dry conditions and survive better there than on grass,[34] this suggests that soil can act as a reservoir of larvae during adverse environmental conditions. Fecal consistency[35] and the activity of dung beetles[36] can affect the timing and extent of L3 appearance on pasture.

Mortality of infective L3 of *O ostertagi* and *C oncophora* increases at both high and low temperatures and is lowest between 1°C and 4°C, and increases in dry conditions.[37] On grass, sunlight is also likely to increase L3 mortality, as shown for sheep GIN species,[38] although simultaneously dry conditions might lead them to seek refuge lower in the sward or in the soil.

The outcome of these complex interacting processes on L3 availability on pasture has been studied in a wide range of environments. In general, in temperate climates, L3 are best able to develop and move onto pasture in the warmer summer months; favorable conditions in hot environments are limited by moisture, and L3 therefore appear in periods with rain. Persistence of pasture infectivity then depends on effects of climate on L3 mortality. In cool-temperate areas (eg, in Argentina and northern Europe), L3 of *Ostertagia*, *Trichostrongylus*, and *Cooperia* develop in dung within 1 to 2 weeks after deposition of infected feces in summer, and 6 weeks in winter, but their appearance on pasture can be delayed 2 months or more, depending on rainfall; L3 persist on pasture for up to 1 year.[39] Mortality of L3 during temperate winters is very low.[39] In humid subtropical climates, including the southeastern United States, conditions for L3 development and translation are optimal in spring and fall (eg, Ref.[40]), when temperatures are close to optimal for L3 yield and moisture is not limiting to translation. Elsewhere, peak L3 levels also tend to follow conditions suitable for L3 development and translation (ie, fall in temperate dry areas,[41] and toward the end of the rains in tropical areas). In unfavorable conditions, GIN larvae often undergo seasonal hypobiotic arrest in the mucosa and delay egg production until a more suitable time (eg, Ref.[42]) (see **Box 1**).

Knowledge of climatic effects on L3 translation and survival can guide planned grazing of lower-risk pasture; for example, through rotational livestock movements[43] or transhumance.[44] However, because the timing of L3 appearance and survival is so variable in different climates and weather, such planning relies on good empirical evidence from the region and system in question. In order to generalize insights gained from diverse regional studies, attempts have been made to formalize understanding of the underlying processes governing L3 availability, and their climatic dependence, into predictive models.[45] These models can be applied to optimize livestock movements, to enhance control, as well as to explore likely changes in seasonal patterns of challenge under climate change scenarios. Such models have shown that prolonged grazing seasons in warmer spring and autumn conditions present new opportunities for transmission of parasites, whereas hot, dry summers can drive biphasic peaks in infective-stage development and shift the seasonality of infection[46] (Hannah Rose Vineer's article, "What Modeling Parasites, Transmission, and Resistance Can Teach Us", more details on parasite transmission models are provided elsewhere in this issue).

In reality, direct effects of climate on larval dynamics is just 1 of several drivers of seasonal infection patterns, and are modified by hypobiosis, housing and calving periods, and other management factors. Changes in these factors can be at least as important as climate in explaining altering epidemiologic patterns.[47] Seasonal exposure of cattle of different age classes to L3 also drives immunologic responses, which in turn determine onward pasture contamination.

DEVELOPMENT OF IMMUNITY AND ITS INFLUENCES ON GASTROINTESTINAL NEMATODE EPIDEMIOLOGY

The development of immunity against GINs in ruminants depends on host factors, parasite factors, and factors influencing host-parasite contact, such as grazing management and anthelmintic treatments.

Host factors include the genetic constitution, sex, age, and nutritional status of the animals. Frequency distributions of worm burdens in cattle are typically overdispersed (see **Box 1**). This wide variation in worm burdens is partly caused by individual genetic differences in susceptibility between animals. The most important phenotypic trait associated with genetic resistance to GINs is reduction in fecal egg output.[48] According to Gasbarre and colleagues,[49] calves can be divided into 3 phenotypes, based on egg output: type I, which never shows high fecal egg counts (FECs); type II, which shows increases in FECs through the first 2 months on pasture, which then decrease and remain at levels associated with type I calves; and type III calves, which maintain high FECs.

Bulls are generally more susceptible than females to GIN infections.[50] Cows are more susceptible to infection around parturition and during early lactation.[51,52] This phenomenon is best known in sheep ewes (resulting in a periparturient increase in FECs), in which the effect is of much greater epidemiologic importance. An age effect, with resistance developing more rapidly in older cattle than in calves, has been shown for *C oncophora* but not for *O ostertagi*.[53] Nutrition also has an effect on the host's resilience and resistance against GINs. Protein supplementation results in an increased rate of immunity development and resistance to reinfection.[54]

Apart from host-related factors, the immune response to GINs is strongly influenced by the site of infection. In cattle, protective immunity against the abomasal parasites *O ostertagi*, *Trichostrongylus axei*, and *H placei* develops more slowly than immunity against the intestinal-dwelling genera such as *Cooperia* and *Nematodirus*.[53,55]

Ultimately, the development of immunity depends on the duration and level of infection.[56,57] Consequently, interventions or circumstances that reduce the amount of host-parasite contact, such as mowing, reduction of grazing time, (preventive) anthelmintic treatments, and periods of drought and housing diminish host immunity.[58,59] Therefore, to avoid underprotection or overprotection, (preventive) anthelmintic treatments and grazing management should be integrated rather than superimposed. In France, the time of effective contact (TEC) with nematodes at cow or herd level was used as a proxy for immunity development.[60,61] TEC is calculated based on grazing and treatment history of heifers and used as a proxy for immunity development. Ravinet and colleagues[61] found that cows or herds[60] with a TEC less than 8 months (considered as nonimmune) benefitted most from anthelmintic treatment in terms of production response.

Development of immunity has a major effect on GIN epidemiology. Host immunity regulates worm establishment, development, fecundity, and survival. Immunity also contributes to arrested development (hypobiosis) of L4 (see **Box 1**). The overall result of all the manifestations of the immune response is a reduction in parasite transmission within the cattle herd.[49] These reductions can reach 50% to 90% in experimental settings[62] and are the reason why nematode vaccines are considered a promising control method if several research bottlenecks regarding understanding of immune effector mechanisms and production of recombinant protective antigens can be overcome.[63]

The first manifestations of acquired immunity to GINs is usually a stunting of worm growth and decreasing egg output, followed by arrested development (hypobiosis), and finally resistance to establishment of ingested larvae.[64] As a result, mean FECs in FSG calves typically peak around 2 months after turnout, followed by a gradual decrease.[65] Because immunity against some species (eg, *C oncophora*, *C punctata*) develops faster than against other species (eg, *O ostertagi*), the generic composition of the excreted eggs changes over time. Although *Cooperia* spp predominate in the first months of grazing, *O ostertagi* usually becomes the most prevalent GIN species thereafter. Cattle remain susceptible to infection by *Ostertagia* for many months, and immunity that reduces the development of newly acquired larvae is usually not evident until the animals are more than 2 years old.[49] As a consequence, the main GIN species in adult cows is *O ostertagi*, with prevalences of 80% to 100%.[66] GINs are known as successful modulators of the host immune response to favor their own survival,[67] but they may also suppress immune responses to bystander diseases, and this is particularly described in humans.[68] In cattle, suggestions have been made that nematode infection can alter vaccination responses to viral disease, but evidence for this so far is not convincing,[69] and more research in this area is needed.

Host immunity thus influences GIN epidemiology, which in turn influences animal productivity and farm economic performance. How (unconscious) human behavior to optimize farm economics is intrinsically linked with GIN epidemiology is discussed next.

SOCIOECONOMICS DRIVING GASTROINTESTINAL NEMATODE EPIDEMIOLOGY

The host, the pathogen, and the environment are the 3 traditional determinants of disease and are referred to as the epidemiologic triad. When epidemiology is used to provide health management and advice within the economic framework of a herd, the epidemiologic triad should be extended to include economic and social aspects as intrinsic elements of the environmental influence on disease.[70] Production impacts and the direct costs of GIN infections are increasingly described, especially for dairy herds. The costs can be attributed to prolonged heifer rearing, reduced carcass weight, milk yield and fertility, anthelmintic treatment, and labor. Because of general low infection levels in young stock in most herds, production losses in adult cows and treatment costs in adult and growing cattle represent the main components in the overall costs of infection.[71] Costs associated with retarded growth or reduced fertility in young stock represented only a small part of the overall costs in Belgian and German dairy herds.[71,72] The recoverable cost of infection after anthelmintic treatment may be in the magnitude of $60 to $70 per cow lactation in grazing dairy herds in temperate climate regions.[73] However, the impact of infection and control measures is always farm specific and depends on the farm infection level, management practices, input use, and external economic circumstances (eg, milk price). Economic impact assessments require careful veterinary advice that takes into account farm objectives and technicity and may in some cases lead clinicians to leave herds with significant levels of worm exposure untreated. van der Voort and colleagues[74,75] found different economic improvement paths depending on the farm's technical efficiency and input use. Technically inefficient farms with low use of concentrates were unlikely to benefit economically from nematode control even if levels of exposure to infection were high, but could increase economic returns by increasing concentrate use and improving feed efficiency. In contrast, on farms with a high technical efficiency and high or intermediate concentrate use, control of nematodes and other diseases was generally considered an important step to further increase efficiency.[74,75] Also, grazing management interventions to reduce worm exposure need to be evaluated at the individual farm level because gains through worm control and increased productivity are often offset by increased feed, maintenance, and cultivation costs.[76]

From a historical perspective, epidemiologists and veterinarians assumed that farmers' decisions were mainly based on rational, technical, and economic considerations. It has now become clear that the social environment and personal traits play a major role in farmers' decisions on disease control and thus disease epidemiology.[77] Most human behavior is based on intuition and unconscious paths[78] and therefore seemingly irrational farmer behavior may have a profound influence on GIN epidemiology. If the objective is to influence farmer behavior as an advisor, the method of choice remains the cognitive persuasion.[79] Low awareness of nematode infections compared with other health issues, previous experiences and attitude toward parasite diagnostics and anthelmintics, the behavior of peer farmers, and the opinion of veterinarians have been shown to be the key influencing factors determining GIN control practices, at least in Belgian dairy farms.[80,81] The investigators showed that different types of motivation influence GIN control practices: sustainable behavior, such as use of diagnostics, is influenced by moral motives, whereas management behavior, such as anthelmintic treatment, is primarily driven by economic motives.[79] The veterinarian was identified as the most important reference with regard to GIN control. However, farmers often also point to veterinarians to explain why new recommendations or practices are not implemented on their farms. As such, the farmers did not hold themselves responsible for implementing sustainable control strategies. Joint discussions and planning between vet and farmer are important to maintain a new behavior.[80] The factors discussed earlier should be used to improve and plan veterinary communication when advising on GIN nematode epidemiology and economic impact.

SUMMARY

GIN species occur mostly in mixed infections. More than 20 different species are described, but the relative importance and epidemiology are determined by the diversity of climates, environmental conditions, host susceptibility, and management systems that characterize cattle production globally. Adverse effects from GINs on their hosts are caused by tissue damage, nutrient absorption, immunopathologic effects, and reduced food intake induced by hormonal changes. The influence of weather and microenvironmental factors on the development and survival of free-living parasitic stages is increasingly understood and used to study the effects of climate change and adapted control approaches. Development of immunity regulates worm populations and thus has a major effect on GIN epidemiology. However, development of immunity is often slow and incomplete and therefore production losses can still occur in adult animals. Costs of GIN infections occur through prolonged heifer rearing; reduced carcass weight, milk yield, and fertility; anthelmintic treatment; and labor. Human behavior and social epidemiology are increasingly used to improve and communicate anthelmintic control strategies. A holistic approach thus entails the consideration of environmental, immunologic, and socioeconomic aspects of nematode epidemiology and is key for the development and communication of sustainable control strategies.

ACKNOWLEDGMENTS

This article is based upon work from COST Action COMBAR CA16230, supported by COST (European Cooperation in Science and Technology).

DISCLOSURE

The authors have nothing to disclose.

REFERENCES

1. Sutherland I, Scott I. Gastrointestinal nematodes of sheep and cattle - biology and control. Oxford (England): Wiley-Blackwell; 2010.
2. Vercruysse J, Rew RS. Macrocyclic lactones in antiparasitic therapy. Wallingford (England): CABI Publishing; 2002.
3. Avramenko RW, Redman EM, Lewis R, et al. Exploring the gastrointestinal "nemabiome": deep amplicon sequencing to quantify the species composition of parasitic nematode communities. PLoS One 2015;10(12):e0143559.
4. Roeber F, Hassan EB, Skuce P, et al. An automated, multiplex-tandem PCR platform for the diagnosis of gastrointestinal nematode infections in cattle: an Australian-European validation study. Vet Parasitol 2017;239:62–75.
5. Avramenko RW, Redman EM, Lewis R, et al. The use of nemabiome metabarcoding to explore gastro-intestinal nematode species diversity and anthelmintic treatment effectiveness in beef calves. Int J Parasitol 2017;47(13):893–902.
6. Charlier J, van der Voort M, Kenyon F, et al. Chasing helminths and their economic impact on farmed ruminants. Trends Parasitol 2014;30(7):361–7.
7. Taylor LM, Parkins JJ, Armour J, et al. Pathophysiological and parasitological studies on *Ostertagia ostertagi* infections in calves. Res Vet Sci 1989;46(2): 218–25.

8. Mihi B, Van Meulder F, Rinaldi M, et al. Analysis of cell hyperplasia and parietal cell dysfunction induced by *Ostertagia ostertagi* infection. Vet Res 2013;44:121.
9. Fox MT. Pathophysiology of infection with gastrointestinal nematodes in domestic ruminants: recent developments. Vet Parasitol 1997;72(3–4):285–97 [discussion: 297–308].
10. Anderson N, Armour J, Jennings FW, et al. The sequential development of naturally occurring ostertagiasis in calves. Res Vet Sci 1969;10(1):18–28.
11. Stromberg BE, Gasbarre LC, Waite A, et al. *Cooperia punctata*: effect on cattle productivity? Vet Parasitol 2012;183(3–4):284–91.
12. Gennari SM, Abdalla AL, Vitti DMSS, et al. *Haemonchus placei* in calves - Effects of dietary-protein and multiple experimental-infection on worm establishment and pathogenesis. Vet Parasitol 1995;59(2):119–26.
13. VanAken D, Vercruysse J, Dargantes AP, et al. Pathophysiological aspects of *Mecistocirrus digitatus* (Nematoda: trichostrongylidae) infection in calves. Vet Parasitol 1997;69(3–4):255–63.
14. Nansen P, Gronvold J, Jorgensen RJ, et al. Outbreaks of early-season trichostrongylosis in calves in Denmark. Vet Parasitol 1989;32(2–3):199–211.
15. Anderson N, Armour J, Jarrett WF, et al. A field study of parasitic gastritis in cattle. Vet Rec 1965;77(41):1196–204.
16. Vercruysse J, Claerebout E. Treatment vs non-treatment of helminth infections in cattle: defining the threshold. Vet Parasitol 2001;98(1–3):195–214.
17. Charlier J, De Cat A, Forbes A, et al. Measurement of antibodies to gastrointestinal nematodes and liver fluke in meat juice of beef cattle and associations with carcass parameters. Vet Parasitol 2009;166(3–4):235–40.
18. Charlier J, Hoglund J, von Samson-Himmelstjerna G, et al. Gastrointestinal nematode infections in adult dairy cattle: impact on production, diagnosis and control. Vet Parasitol 2009;164(1):70–9.
19. Forbes AB, Huckle CA, Gibb MJ. Evaluation of the effect of eprinomectin in young dairy heifers sub-clinically infected with gastrointestinal nematodes on grazing behavior and diet selection. Vet Parasitol 2007;150(4):321–32.
20. Greer AW. Trade-offs and benefits: implications of promoting a strong immunity to gastrointestinal parasites in sheep. Parasite Immunol 2008;30(2):123–32.
21. Li RW, Wu S, Li W, et al. Metagenome plasticity of the bovine abomasal microbiota in immune animals in response to *Ostertagia ostertagi* infection. PLoS One 2011;6(9):e24417.
22. Peachey LE, Jenkins TP, Cantacessi C. This gut ain't big enough for both of us. Or is it? Helminth-microbiota interactions in veterinary species. Trends Parasitol 2017;33(8):619–32.
23. Dorny P, Shaw DJ, Vercruysse J. The determination at housing of exposure to gastrointestinal nematode infections in first-grazing season calves. Vet Parasitol 1999;80(4):325–40.
24. Charlier J, Demeler J, Hoglund J, et al. *Ostertagia ostertagi* in first-season grazing cattle in Belgium, Germany and Sweden: general levels of infection and related management practices. Vet Parasitol 2010;171(1–2):91–8.
25. Forbes AB, Vercruysse J, Charlier J. A survey of the exposure to *Ostertagia ostertagi* in dairy cow herds in Europe through the measurement of antibodies in milk samples from the bulk tank. Vet Parasitol 2008;157(1–2):100–7.
26. Bennema SC, Vercruysse J, Morgan E, et al. Epidemiology and risk factors for exposure to gastrointestinal nematodes in dairy herds in northwestern Europe. Vet Parasitol 2010;173(3–4):247–54.

27. Villa-Mancera A, Pastelin-Rojas C, Olivares-Perez J, et al. Bulk tank milk preva-lence and production losses, spatial analysis, and predictive risk mapping of *Os-tertagia ostertagi* infections in Mexican cattle herds. Parasitol Res 2018;117(5): 1613–20.

28. Vanderstichel R, Dohoo I, Sanchez J, et al. Effects of farm management practices and environmental factors on bulk tank milk antibodies against gastrointestinal nematodes in dairy farms across Canada. Prev Vet Med 2012;104(1–2):53–64.

29. Colwell DD, Beck MA, Goater CP, et al. Annual variation in serum antibody con-centrations against gastrointestinal nematodes in beef calves from semi-arid ran-gelands of western Canada. Vet Parasitol 2014;205(1–2):169–74.

30. Rossanigo CE, Gruner L. Moisture and temperature requirements in faeces for the development of free-living stages of gastrointestinal nematodes of sheep, cattle and deer. J Helminthol 1995;69(4):357–62.

31. Silangwa SM, Todd AC. Vertical migration of trichostrongylid larvae on grasses. J Parasitol 1964;50(2):278–85.

32. Uriarte J, Gruner L. Development and distribution of bovine trichostrongyle infec-tive larvae on a pasture irrigated by flooding or by spraying. Parasitol Res 1994; 80(8):657–63.

33. Krecek RC, Murrell KD. Observations on the ability of Larval *Ostertagia ostertagi* to migrate through pasture soil. Proc Helminthol Soc Wash 1988;55(1):24–7.

34. Knapp-Lawitzke F, von Samson-Himmelstjerna G, Demeler J. Elevated tempera-tures and long drought periods have a negative impact on survival and fitness of strongylid third stage larvae. Int J Parasitol 2016;46(4):229–37.

35. Williams JC, Bilkovich FR. Development and survival of infective larvae of the cat-tle nematode, *Ostertagia ostertagi*. J Parasitol 1971;57(2):327–38.

36. Sands B, Wall R. Dung beetles reduce livestock gastrointestinal parasite avail-ability on pasture. J Appl Ecol 2017;54(4):1180–9.

37. Grenfell BT, Smith G, Anderson RM. Maximum-likelihood-estimates of the mortal-ity and migration rates of the infective larvae of *Ostertagia ostertagi* and *Cooperia oncophora*. Parasitology 1986;92:643–52.

38. van Dijk J, de Louw MDE, Kalis LPA, et al. Ultraviolet light increases mortality of nematode larvae and can explain patterns of larval availability at pasture. Int J Parasitol 2009;39(10):1151–6.

39. Fiel CA, Fernandez AS, Rodriguez EM, et al. Observations on the free-living stages of cattle gastrointestinal nematodes. Vet Parasitol 2012;187(1–2):217–26.

40. Couvillion CE, Siefker C, Evans RR. Epidemiological study of nematode infections in a grazing beef cow-calf herd in Mississippi. Vet Parasitol 1996;64(3):207–18.

41. Nogareda C, Mezo M, Uriarte J, et al. Dynamics of infestation of cattle and pasture by gastrointestinal nematodes in an Atlantic temperate environment. J Vet Med B Infect Dis Vet Public Health 2006;53(9):439–44.

42. Malczewski A, Jolley WR, Woodard LF. Prevalence and epidemiology of trichos-trongylids in Wyoming cattle with consideration of the inhibited development of *Ostertagia ostertagi*. Vet Parasitol 1996;64(4):285–97.

43. Eysker M, van der Aar WM, Boersema JH, et al. The effect of repeated moves to clean pasture on the build up of gastrointestinal nematode infections in calves. Vet Parasitol 1998;76(1–2):81–94.

44. Eckert J, Hertzberg H. Parasite control in transhumant situations. Vet Parasitol 1994;54(1–3):103–25.

45. Verschave SH, Charlier J, Rose H, et al. Cattle and nematodes under global chance: transmission models as an ally. Trends Parasitol 2016;32(9):724–38.

46. Rose H, Wang T, van Dijk J, et al. GLOWORM-FL: a simulation model of the effects of climate and climate change on the free-living stages of gastrointestinal nematode parasites of ruminants. Ecol Model 2015;297:232–45.
47. Morgan ER, Wall R. Climate change and parasitic disease: farmer mitigation? Trends Parasitol 2009;25(7):308–13.
48. Gasbarre LC, Leighton EA, Davies CJ. Genetic-control of immunity to gastrointestinal nematodes of cattle. Vet Parasitol 1990;37(3–4):257–72.
49. Gasbarre LC, Leighton EA, Sonstegard T. Role of the bovine immune system and genome in resistance to gastrointestinal nematodes. Vet Parasitol 2001;98(1–3):51–64.
50. Herd RP, Queen WG, Majewski GA. Sex-related susceptibility of bulls to gastrointestinal parasites. Vet Parasitol 1992;44(1–2):119–25.
51. Hammerberg B, Lamm WD. Changes in periparturient fecal egg counts in beef-cows calving in the spring. Am J Vet Res 1980;41(10):1686–9.
52. Michel JF, Lancaster MB, Hong C. Effect of age, acquired-resistance, pregnancy and lactation on some reactions of cattle to infection with *Ostertagia ostertagi*. Parasitology 1979;79(1):157–68.
53. Kloosterman A, Ploeger HW, Frankena K. Age resistance in calves to *Ostertagia ostertagi* and *Cooperia oncophora*. Vet Parasitol 1991;39(1–2):101–13.
54. Coop RL, Holmes PH. Nutrition and parasite interaction. Int J Parasitol 1996; 26(8–9):951–62.
55. Hilderson H, Vercruysse J, Claerebout E, et al. Interactions between *Ostertagia ostertagi* and *Cooperia oncophora* in calves. Vet Parasitol 1995;56(1–3):107–19.
56. Claerebout E, Vercruysse J, Dorny P, et al. The effect of different infection levels on acquired resistance to gastrointestinal nematodes in artificially infected cattle. Vet Parasitol 1998;75(2–3):153–67.
57. Ploeger HW, Kloosterman A, Rietveld FW. Acquired-immunity against *Cooperia* spp and *Ostertagia* spp in Calves - Effect of level of exposure and timing of the midsummer increase. Vet Parasitol 1995;58(1–2):61–74.
58. Claerebout E, Dorny P, Vercruysse J, et al. Effects of preventive anthelmintic treatment on acquired resistance to gastrointestinal nematodes in naturally infected cattle. Vet Parasitol 1998;76(4):287–303.
59. Ploeger HW, Eysker M, Borgsteede FHM, et al. Effect of nematode infections and management-practices on growth-performance of calves on commercial dairy farms. Vet Parasitol 1990;35(4):323–39.
60. Ravinet N, Bareille N, Lehebel A, et al. Change in milk production after treatment against gastrointestinal nematodes according to grazing history, parasitological and production-based indicators in adult dairy cows. Vet Parasitol 2014; 201(1–2):95–109.
61. Ravinet N, Lehebel A, Bareille N, et al. Design and evaluation of multi-indicator profiles for targeted-selective treatment against gastrointestinal nematodes at housing in adult dairy cows. Vet Parasitol 2017;237:17–29.
62. Matthews JB, Geldhof P, Tzelos T, et al. Progress in the development of subunit vaccines for gastrointestinal nematodes of ruminants. Parasite Immunol 2016; 38(12):744–53.
63. Charlier J, Thamsborg SM, Bartley DJ, et al. Mind the gaps in research on the control of gastrointestinal nematodes of farmed ruminants and pigs. Transbound Emerg Dis 2018;65:217–34.
64. Claerebout E, Vercruysse J. The immune response and the evaluation of acquired immunity against gastrointestinal nematodes in cattle: a review. Parasitology 2000;120:S25–42.

65. Shaw DJ, Vercruysse J, Claerebout E, et al. Gastrointestinal nematode infections of first-grazing season calves in western Europe: general patterns and the effect of chemoprophylaxis. Vet Parasitol 1998;75(2–3):115–31.

66. Agneessens J, Claerebout E, Dorny P, et al. Nematode parasitism in adult dairy cows in Belgium. Vet Parasitol 2000;90(1–2):83–92.

67. Mulcahy G, O'Neill S, Donnelly S, et al. Helminths at mucosal barriers - interaction with the immune system. Adv Drug Deliv Rev 2004;56(6):853–68.

68. van Riet E, Hartgers FC, Yazdanbakhsh M. Chronic helminth infections induce immuno-modulation: consequences and mechanisms. Immunobiology 2007;212(6):475–90.

69. Charlier J, Forbes A, Van Gucht S, et al. Serological evidence of *Ostertagia oster-tagi* infection in dairy cows does not impact the efficacy of rabies vaccination during the housing period. Res Vet Sci 2013;95(3):1055–8.

70. Charlier J, Velde FV, van der Voort M, et al. ECONOHEALTH: placing helminth infections of livestock in an economic and social context. Vet Parasitol 2015;212(1–2):62–7.

71. Fanke J, Charlier J, Steppin T, et al. Economic assessment of *Ostertagia ostertagi* and *Fasciola hepatica* infections in dairy cattle herds in Germany using Para-calc((R)). Vet Parasitol 2017;240:39–48.

72. Charlier J, Van der Voort M, Hogeveen H, et al. ParaCalc®-a novel tool to evaluate the economic importance of worm infections on the dairy farm. Vet Parasitol 2012;184(2–4):204–11.

73. Charlier J, Levecke B, Devleesschauwer B, et al. The economic effects of whole-herd versus selective anthelmintic treatment strategies in dairy cows. J Dairy Sci 2012;95(6):2977–87.

74. van der Voort M, Van Meensel J, Lauwers L, et al. The relation between input-output transformation and gastrointestinal nematode infections on dairy farms. Animal 2016;10(2):274–82.

75. van der Voort M, Van Meensel J, Lauwers L, et al. A stochastic frontier approach to study the relationship between gastrointestinal nematode infections and technical efficiency of dairy farms. J Dairy Sci 2014;97(6):3498–508.

76. van der Voort M, Van Meensel J, Lauwers L, et al. Economic modelling of grazing management against gastrointestinal nematodes in dairy cattle. Vet Parasitol 2017;236:68–75.

77. Ritter C, Jansen J, Roche S, et al. Invited review: determinants of farmers' adoption of management-based strategies for infectious disease prevention and control. J Dairy Sci 2017;100(5):3329–47.

78. Kahneman D, Tversky A. Prospect theory - Analysis of decision under risk. Econometrica 1979;47(2):263–91.

79. Vande Velde F, Charlier J, Claerebout E. Farmer behavior and gastrointestinal nematodes in ruminant livestock-uptake of sustainable control approaches. Front Vet Sci 2018;5:255.

80. Vande Velde F, Charlier J, Hudders L, et al. Beliefs, intentions, and beyond: a qualitative study on the adoption of sustainable gastrointestinal nematode control practices in Flanders' dairy industry. Prev Vet Med 2018;153:15–23.

81. Vande Velde F, Claerebout E, Cauberghe V, et al. Diagnosis before treatment: identifying dairy farmers' determinants for the adoption of sustainable practices in gastrointestinal nematode control. Vet Parasitol 2015;212(3–4):308–17.

82. Warburton EM, Vonhof MJ. From individual heterogeneity to population-level overdispersion: quantifying the relative roles of host exposure and parasite establishment in driving aggregated helminth distributions. Int J Parasitol 2018;48(3–4):309–18.

83. Verschave SH, Rose H, Morgan ER, et al. Modelling *Cooperia oncophora*: quantification of key parameters in the parasitic phase. Vet Parasitol 2016;223: 111–4.
84. Verschave SH, Vercruysse J, Claerebout E, et al. The parasitic phase of *Ostertagia ostertagi*: quantification of the main life history traits through systematic review and meta-analysis. Int J Parasitol 2014;44(14):1091–104.

Biology, Epidemiology, Diagnosis, and Management of Anthelmintic Resistance in Gastrointestinal Nematodes of Livestock

Ray M. Kaplan, DVM, PhD

KEYWORDS

- Anthelmintic resistance • Cattle • Sheep • Goats • Drug resistance • Combinations

KEY POINTS

- Anthelmintic resistance in gastrointestinal nematodes of livestock is a severe and worsening problem worldwide.
- Anthelmintic resistance is a natural evolutionary process that is impossible to prevent if anthelmintics are used on a farm; however, the rate can be substantially reduced by modifying strategies of anthelmintic use.
- The further development and spread of anthelmintic resistance will almost certainly outpace the introduction of new anthelmintic classes; active measures must be implemented to reduce the development of resistance.
- Fecal egg count reduction tests should be performed on every farm to determine the efficacy of anthelmintics being used.
- Refugia-based strategies and anthelmintic combinations must be implemented immediately across the livestock industry to reduce the development of resistance, and to preserve the efficacy of the few existing anthelmintics that remain effective.

INTRODUCTION

Beginning with phenothiazine in the 1950s, followed by the benzimidazoles (BZ) in the 1960s, the imidazothiazole/tetrahydropyrimidines in the 1970s and the avermectin/milbemycins (AM) in the 1980s, a new class of anthelmintics was introduced into the marketplace each decade.[1] This arsenal of highly effective and relatively inexpensive drugs led to recommendations for parasite control that were based almost solely

Department of Infectious Diseases, College of Veterinary Medicine, University of Georgia, 501 DW Brooks Drive, Athens, GA 30602, USA
E-mail address: rkaplan@uga.edu
Twitter: @ray_m_kaplan (R.M.K.)

Vet Clin Food Anim 36 (2020) 17–30
https://doi.org/10.1016/j.cvfa.2019.12.001
0749-0720/20/© 2019 Elsevier Inc. All rights reserved.

on the frequent and or strategic use of anthelmintics, the goals of which were to maximize livestock health, productivity, and profitability. Although this approach was highly successful for a number of decades, we are now experiencing ever-increasing levels of anthelmintic resistance in all drug classes, involving virtually all of the most economically important parasites of all livestock species.[1,2] Furthermore, no new classes of anthelmintic have been introduced for use in the United States for ruminants since ivermectin in 1981, almost 40 years ago. Other second-generation AM drugs have provided some improvements since then, but AM resistance demonstrates a class effect; resistance to any one AM drug tends to confer resistance to all AM drugs.[3] Additionally, no new novel classes of drugs have become available in the United States over this time. The new drug monepantel (an amino acetonitrile derivative) is sold throughout much of the world for sheep, but this drug has not yet been approved for use in the United States, and it is unknown when or even if it ever will be. A second new anthelmintic, derquantel (a spiroindole) is combined with abamectin and is sold as a product for sheep in several countries around the world, but it is not approved in the United States, and there is no evidence that it will be. Currently, there is no evidence that new anthelmintic prospects are in the late phase pipeline; thus, we are left in a situation where it could be many years before a new anthelmintic class is sold for ruminants in the United States. Additionally, the costs of performing research are ever increasing, and there are increased regulatory requirements for the health and safety of the environment, target and nontarget animals, and humans, as well as food residues. Thus, the time and cost required to bring an anthelmintic product to market has increased dramatically in recent decades. Consequently, the development and spread of anthelmintic resistance will almost certainly outpace the introduction of new anthelmintic classes, and in the future when a new anthelmintic is finally introduced for use in livestock, it will almost certainly be considerably more expensive than the most expensive of the current products. This reality makes it important that the efficacies of currently available products are protected as much as is reasonably possible, and this goal can only be achieved by changing the way we use these products.

Anthelmintic resistance is a heritable trait,[4] and is defined as occurring "when a greater frequency of individuals in a parasite population, usually affected by a dose or concentration of compound, are no longer affected, or a greater concentration of drug is required to reach a certain level of efficacy."[5] In practical terms, anthelmintic resistance is present in a population of worms when the efficacy of the drug falls below that which is historically expected, when other causes of reduced efficacy can be ruled out. Parasitic nematodes have many biologic and genetic features that favor the development of drug resistance. Short life cycles, high reproductive rates, rapid rates of evolution, and extremely large population sizes combine to give many parasitic worms an exceptionally high level of genetic diversity.[6] Thus, it is practically ensured that gene mutations that reduce the worm's susceptibility to a drug will occur. These resistant worms then have a tremendous reproductive advantage in the face of anthelmintic treatments, allowing them to increase in frequency when under drug selection. This process is occurring on every farm, although the rate of resistance development will be affected by a large number of variables including the host, the parasite species, the drug, the frequency of administration, and amount of refugia present at the time the treatments are administered.[7]

An increase in resistance within a worm population to levels that are clinically apparent is typically a slow and gradual process, requiring numerous generations under drug selection, and usually taking many years. Thus, from a practical perspective, the genetic phase of resistance develops slowly over time, during which it is impossible to detect, but then increases very rapidly in its later phase. Eventually, when a sufficient percentage of the worm population is resistant, the phenotype of reduced efficacy will finally be noticed clinically. Alternatively, resistant worms can be purchased, thus bypassing the many years of worm evolution and drug selection necessary to reach high levels. Depending on how many animals are purchased that harbor resistant worms and the worm burdens of those animals, and other management and pasture factors such as amount of refugia, treatment failures owing to drug resistance can occur practically instantly, or over a relatively short period.

This has great clinical relevance because, in either case, resistance can transition from undetectable to clinically important levels over a very short period of time. Consequently, unless a surveillance program is in place that closely monitors the effectiveness of drug treatments over time, resistance will not be noticed until levels of resistance are extremely high. In general, resistance to 1 drug in a class of anthelmintics confers resistance to all other drugs in that same class. However, drugs do differ in their potency; some drugs within a class are more effective than others in the early stages of resistance (eg, moxidectin vs ivermectin), but once resistance reaches high levels, it is unlikely that any drug in a given class would remain effective. There is also very strong evidence for the BZ and AM classes that once resistance is diagnosed as a clinical problem, reversion to susceptibility likely will never occur.[1,8,9] With levamisole, there is limited evidence of some degree of reversion back to susceptibility,[10] but any reversion is likely to be short lived and of little long-term practical benefit.

THE SCOPE AND PREVALENCE OF RESISTANCE ON SHEEP AND GOAT FARMS

For many years, worms were controlled in small ruminants by the frequent use of anthelmintics, and this approach was quite effective. However, we now know that this strategy has turned out to be shortsighted and unsustainable. During the period from 2002 to 2009, two studies were performed investigating the prevalence of anthelmintic resistance on 80 sheep and goat farms in the southern and mid-Atlantic states of the United States. In the southern states (2002–2006) Haemonchus contortus from 45 (98%), 25 (54%), 35 (76%), and 11 (24%) farms were resistant to BZ, levamisole, ivermectin, and moxidectin, respectively.[11] Resistance to all 3 classes of anthelmintics was detected on 22 farms (48%), and resistance to all 3 classes plus moxidectin was detected on 8 farms (17%). Thus, on almost 20% of all farms tested, resistance was detected to all available anthelmintics, a situation referred to as total anthelmintic failure. In the mid-Atlantic region study performed a few years later (2007–2009) the prevalence of moxidectin resistance was twice as high at 47% of farms.[12] Other (unpublished) data from The Kaplan Laboratory (R.M. Kaplan, personal communication, 2019) collected on 34 goat farms in the eastern United States from 2011 to 2016 found prevalences of resistance to H contortus of 100%, 44%, 94%, and 56% for BZ, levamisole, ivermectin, and moxidectin, respectively, with 30% of all the farms demonstrating total anthelmintic failure. The prevalences of resistance on sheep farms (n = 58) in the eastern United States were similar, although lower at 97%, 21%, 81%, and 40% for BZ, levamisole, ivermectin, and moxidectin, respectively. In contrast, resistance was less prevalent on sheep farms (n = 32) in the western United States, with prevalences of 91%, 13%, 38% and 3% for BZ, levamisole, ivermectin, and moxidectin, respectively (R.M. Kaplan, personal communication, 2019). These data indicate that a severe problem exists in the eastern United States on both sheep and goat farms, whereas differences in climate and management in the western United States have led to lower levels of resistance. It should be noted that most of these tests were performed more than 5 years ago, and our data collected over the past

20 years clearly demonstrate that resistance problems are worsening every year. Thus, the numbers reported here are almost certainly considerably lower than what would be found in 2020 and beyond. Elsewhere in the world, resistance is also very severe; however, those data will not be reviewed here. Studies performed over the past decade in Canada, Europe, Australia, and Brazil all reported high prevalences of resistance to multiple anthelmintics, including the newest drug, monepantel.[13–17]

THE SCOPE AND PREVALENCE OF RESISTANCE ON CATTLE FARMS

Resistance in parasites of cattle was slower to develop than in the small ruminant and equine sectors, but over the past decade we have seen a rapid escalation in the levels and distribution of anthelmintic resistance in gastrointestinal nematodes of cattle worldwide. Although there are some published case reports of resistance in parasites of cattle in the United States,[18,19] no studies have been performed to establish the national prevalence of resistance. Thus, we do not know how severe and widespread the problem is nationally. However, studies performed by the Kaplan Laboratory on a number of cow–calf farms in Georgia and on stocker cattle purchased at various stockyards in the southern region suggest that AM resistance in cattle is both common and widespread. More than 90% of farms tested by our laboratory in the last 5 years have AM-resistant *Cooperia*. More recently, we completed a study of resistance in weaned calves on 12 cow–calf farms in Georgia, and found resistance to AM drugs on 11 of the 12 farms (91.6%). Resistance in *Cooperia* spp. and *Haemonchus* spp. were the most common, but we also found resistance in *Ostertagia ostertagi*. On 1 of the 12 farms, *Cooperia* spp., *Haemonchus* spp., and *Ostertagia* were all resistant to AM drugs. We also have other recent data (K.L. Paras, personal communication, 2018) that indicates that AM drugs have lost the ability to kill inhibited Ostertagia L4 in calves in the southern United States. Overall in the southern United States, it seems that resistance to AM drugs is highly prevalent in *Cooperia* spp. and *Haemonchus* spp., and is in the emerging stages for *Ostertagia*. There are few published data on resistance in cattle nematodes in other parts of the United States, but based on unpublished data that this author is aware of, there is no reason to believe that there are major differences in other regions of the United States. This area is that needs further study. Increasing resistance in *Ostertagia* will pose a serious threat to cattle health and productivity in the United States, and this can be expected to occur in the near future, especially if the recommendations being made in this book are not instituted broadly and rapidly.

Outside the United States, there is a large amount of published data indicating that resistance is becoming a very serious problem; a study in New Zealand performed more than 10 years ago reported that ivermectin resistance was evident on 92% of cattle farms and resistance to both ivermectin and albendazole was evident on 74% of farms, with most of the resistance found in *Cooperia* spp.[20] More recently, resistance in *O ostertagi* has been found on numerous New Zealand beef farms.[21] Very high prevalences of resistance have also been reported in studies performed in Brazil, Argentina, and Australia.[22–24] *Cooperia* is consistently the species with the most resistance, but resistance in *Haemonchus* is also common. Resistance in *Oesophagostomum* and *Ostertagia* are reported less commonly, but recent evidence suggests increases in these species as well.

Historically, *Cooperia* was not considered a very important pathogen. However, over the past few decades, as a consequence of heavy use of AM drugs, the relative intensity of *Cooperia* compared with other species has risen substantially. Although *Cooperia* does not impact animal health and productivity to the degree that *Ostertagia* does, *Cooperia* infections do have a significant negative effect on growing cattle.[25] So, although clinical disease in cattle owing to *Cooperia* may be uncommon, there is little doubt that significant production losses can result from high levels of infection. Consequently, there is little evidence to support the opinion of some that AM resistance in *Cooperia* is not a major concern. Furthermore, the increasing levels of resistance in *Ostertagia* are especially concerning; *Ostertagia* is a serious pathogen that not only causes significant production loss, but also can produce clinical disease that can be severe.

Given this situation, the problem of anthelmintic resistance in parasites of cattle should not be ignored. Clearly, there is a great need for new research to address this issue, but waiting for this research before acting is not advisable. It is recommended that anthelmintic resistance in parasites of cattle be considered a major threat to cattle productivity and that steps be taken to mitigate the problem. Because almost no research has been done in this area, one cannot be certain which are the best approaches for decreasing the rate with which anthelmintic resistance evolves in cattle. However, there is a large amount of sound research in sheep, and it would seem logical to follow those recommendations for sheep that can be reasonably applied to cattle production systems. To do nothing seems irrational and short sighted. Modeling studies should help to address this issue so that different strategies can be compared with determine which are likely to be the most successful (see Hannah Rose Vineer's article, "What Modeling Parasites, Transmission, and Resistance can Teach Us," in this issue on modeling).

STRATEGIES FOR DELAYING AND MITIGATING THE PROBLEM OF ANTHELMINTIC RESISTANCE ON CATTLE FARMS

There are several approaches that have proven effective in reducing the rate with which resistance develops in sheep nematodes: (1) not treating the ewes and only treating the lambs, (2) leaving a percentage of the flock untreated (eg, the heaviest 10%), (3) treating selectively based on some measure of parasitism or growth rate, and (4) using drug combinations (≥ 2 active compounds from different drug classes administered at the same time).[26–28] The first three of these are covered in detail elsewhere in this issue (see Andrew W. Greer and colleagues' article, "Refugia-Based Strategies for Parasite Control in Livestock," in this issue); thus, they will only be addressed briefly here. However, some issues are discussed here, particularly with regard to implementing some of these strategies in cattle operations. Cattle are not sheep; thus, some practices are more difficult to implement on cattle farms, and some may be less effective in cattle. Nevertheless, some of these strategies are adapted easily for cattle and are likely to be effective. For instance, leaving cows untreated can be very beneficial as a source of refugia for *Ostertagia*. Cows are predominantly infected with *Ostertagia*; thus, not treating cows is likely to be quite beneficial for slowing the development of resistance in *Ostertagia* and is an easily implemented strategy. In contrast, this strategy would not be effective for *Cooperia*, because cows develop good immunity to this genus, and shed relatively few eggs of *Cooperia*. This is no longer very relevant, however, because the high levels of AM resistance that already exist in *Cooperia* make it too late to implement a refugia-based strategy.

Another easily implemented strategy for cattle that will provide refugia and slow down the development of anthelmintic resistance is leaving a portion of the herd (eg, 10%–20%) untreated. This is sometimes referred to as selective nontreatment; it differs from targeted selective treatments where the decision of which animals to treat is based on a measure of infection or productivity. In selective nontreatment, the farmer simply leaves some of the herd untreated when applying anthelmintics to the herd. The nontreated animals can be selected randomly, or preferably, the best-looking and/or heaviest (in growing animals) are left untreated. Because the best-looking animals are already performing well compared with the rest of the herd, they arguably will not gain as much benefit from anthelmintic treatment as the other animals. Thus, little production is lost by not treating these animals, while refugia is maintained and resistance is slowed.

I have often heard people say that cattlemen will not leave some animals untreated because this strategy goes against what they have been told for years, and goes against their common sense of what is best for maximizing productivity. This argument may sound reasonable at first, but how many of these same cattlemen are currently using anthelmintics that are poorly effective without knowing it? Based on this author's experience in testing cattle farms for resistance, this may be the majority of farms. So – yes, they are treating all animals with the full associated costs, but they are not getting a highly effective result, and in some cases getting almost no benefit. Some farms we have tested had 0% reduction in fecal egg count (FEC), and the cattleman had not suspected resistance at all before the test. Studies in sheep have clearly demonstrated that the production cost of subclinical parasitism as a result of using an anthelmintic product that is less than fully effective owing to resistance can greatly exceed the cost of routine testing of anthelmintic efficacy.[29] Cattle farmers would thus be much better off in the present, and have greater sustainability for the long term, if they used highly effective anthelmintic treatments and left some animals untreated. Highly effective is the key here; for refugia-based strategies to be successful in slowing the development of resistance, it is critical that treatments are highly effective. Testing the efficacy of drugs with a FEC reduction test (FECRT) is the best way for a farmer to make sure he or she is using effective drugs (**Boxes 1** and **2**). The reluctance of most cattlemen to test for anthelmintic resistance is not rational from an economic perspective.

Given the high levels of resistance that exist to some anthelmintics, to get the high efficacy desired, it is necessary to use multiple drugs from different anthelmintic classes simultaneously. This is referred to as combination treatment, and recent research has demonstrated quite clearly that the use of anthelmintics in combination is a beneficial practice. There are 3 major benefits to using drugs in combination. (1) There is an additive effect with each drug used, and thus the efficacy of the treatment increases with each additional drug given (**Table 1**). (2) There is a return to broad-spectrum efficacy; resistance is species and drug specific, and thus a second (or third) drug may kill any species resistant to the first (or second) drug. This will then return the broad-spectrum efficacy that one aims to achieve (and that is specified on the product label). (3) By achieving a higher efficacy, there are fewer resistant survivors, thus there is a greater dilution of resistant worms by the susceptible portion of the population (**Table 2**). For example, if 2 drugs each with 90% efficacy are used in rotation, then each time cattle are treated 10% of the worms (resistant) survive. In contrast if the 2 drugs are used in combination then the efficacy would be 99%; this yields 10 times fewer resistant survivors (the first drug kills 90%, he second drug kills 90% of the remaining 10%). Furthermore, as seen in **Table 2**, the sooner a combination treatment strategy is implemented the greater the benefits, because the greatest difference in the percent of resistant survivors is seen when efficacy of anthelmintics is high.

There are a few issues and precautions to be aware of before instituting the use of anthelmintic combinations. In New Zealand and Australia, products are sold that contain a combination of anthelmintics, so only 1 product needs to be administered. In contrast, in the United States, no anthelmintics are yet sold in this formulation, so

---

Box 1
Recommended procedures for performing a FECRT in cattle, sheep and goats

Note: Currently there are no standardized guidelines for performing a FECRT. However, a World Association for the Advancement of Veterinary Parasitology (WAAVP) subcommittee is in the process of developing such a guideline, with expected publication in 2020. Contents of the WAAVP will supersede any information found here. However, most of the recommendations provided here are likely to be consistent with those new guidelines.

- Fifteen animals per treatment group.
  - A minimum of 10 cattle should be used, but 20 is preferred when EPG are low.
  - The same cattle should be sampled for FEC both before and after treatment.

- If it is not logistically possible to test the same animals before and after treatment, then it is recommended to take 30 random grab samples. The higher number of samples is needed to decrease the impact of variability.

- Animals selected should be relatively uniform in age, breed, grazing history, anthelmintic exposure, other management considerations, and so on.

- For cattle, weaned animals less than 16 months of age, and for sheep, lambs 3 to 6 months of age are preferable. For goats. animals of all ages usually have sufficient EPG.
  - FEC of adult cows are generally too low to perform a FECRT (see note below).

- Weigh each animal so proper dose is given.
  - If each animal is not weighed and dosed individually, then all animals should be dosed to the heaviest in the same age group; never dose to the average weight, because this method results in one-half of the animals being underdosed.

- Use label recommendations for dosage and application.

- Ensure dosing equipment is calibrated and operating properly.

- Fecal samples should be collected per rectum at time of Tx and 14 to 21 days after treatment, depending on the drugs tested.
  - Non-AM drugs (eg, BZ or levamisole): 10 to 14 days
  - Ivermectin and other avermectin drugs: 14 to 17 days
  - Moxidectin: 17 to 21 days
  - If non-AM and AM tested at same time then use 14 days

- Use a FEC technique with sensitivity of 5 EPG or less for cattle; for sheep/goats a 25 or 50 EPG McMaster is adequate.
  - Mini-Flotac (and Fill Flotac) is the preferred method for cattle.
    - This is a new method that resembles McMaster, but provides a higher level of detection sensitivity and better precision.[32]
    - Modified Wisconsin can also be used, but this method is both more time consuming and less accurate than the mini-Flotac.[32]
  - Note: The detection sensitivity of the FEC method that is required will depend on the mean EPG of the group being tested.
    - For the most accurate result it is recommended that at least 200 eggs be counted before treatment (this means actual number of eggs counted under the microscope before applying a correction factor). However, so long as at least 100 eggs are counted, results will be accurate more often than not, and even 50 eggs counted may be enough.
    - Thus, if using a method with 5 EPG detection, then the mean EPG will need to be 100 if 10 cattle are tested and 65 is 15 cattle are tested. If mean FEC is less than 50 EPG, then there are 3 options:
      a. Use a procedure with a more sensitive detection level.
      b. Repeat the FEC or read an additional chamber for each animal.
      c. Test more animals.
    - If mean FEC are greater than 500 EPG (group size treated = 10) or greater than 250 EPG (group size treated = 20), then the McMaster method can used.
    - Adult cattle: adult cattle tend to have very low EPG, often averaging less than 2 EPG. Thus, it is extremely difficult to perform a FECRT in adult cattle with accuracy unless many cows are tested and a very sensitive FEC method (1 EPG or less) are used.

- The best (most accurate) method is to perform FEC on each individual fecal sample. However, research indicates that accurate results can often be obtained when feces are pooled and composite FEC performed.[33] This can reduce the number of FEC required by up to 80%. Thus, the composite FECRT has a lot benefits in terms of cost. (see **Box 2** for a recommended procedure for performing a composite FECRT).
- Data can be analyzed one of several ways
  - Measure the FEC of each sample and calculate the mean value. Then compare the mean pretreatment FEC and mean post-treatment FEC for the entire group.
    - [(Mean pretreatment FEC – Mean post-treatment FEC)/Mean pretreatment FEC] × 100.
    - This method is easiest but does not provide any statistical analysis, which is needed for proper interpretation.
    - Note: Do not interpret the results for any individual animal; only interpret the data for the group as a whole.
  - Analyze the data using an on-line analysis program.
    a. eggCounts[34]: http://shiny.math.uzh.ch/user/furrer/shinyas/shiny-eggCounts/
    b. Beta negative binomial method analysis tool for FECRT data by Matthew Denwood: https://mdenwood.shinyapps.io/fecrt_bnb/
    c. Note that these are great tools that provide detailed analysis, but one must enter the data correctly for them to work, which is a little tricky at first. Also, these cannot be used when performing the FECRT using a composite FEC approach.
  - Use a composite FEC protocol (see **Box 2**).
- Interpretation of egg count reduction
  - Note: Owing to many sources of variability the accuracy of results of FECRT are highly dependent on the number of animals tested and the number of eggs counted in the pretreatment FEC. If fewer animals are used then recommended, and/or too few eggs are counted, there is a possibility of the observed results being substantially different from the true efficacy.
  - To properly interpret results of a FECRT, it is necessary to calculate 95% CIs or perform a statistical analysis (see on-line programs above and WAAVP guidelines for detailed information on how to interpret the results using 95% CIs).
  - If 95% CIs are not calculated, a conservative interpretation is advised; the following values can be used to interpret the results:
    - Greater than 95% = effective, no evidence of resistance
    - 90% to 95% = reduced efficacy, suspected resistance
    - 80% to 90% = reduced efficacy, resistance is likely
    - Less than 80% = ineffective, resistance is highly likely
  - Of course, efficacy data can only be interpreted correctly if the following are true: (1) animals were treated with the proper dose, (2) animals were treated using proper administration technique, (3) drug used was within the expiration date and was stored properly, (4) fecal samples were labeled and stored correctly, (5) proper laboratory technique was used when performing FEC.
  - Note that when FEC reduction is greater than 98% and less than 80%, statistics are rarely needed to make a correct interpretation on whether the drug worked or not. Rather, when results are between these values in the gray or equivocal zone, variability can lead to errors in interpretation.

Abbreviations: CI, confidence interval; EPG, eggs per gram.

the anthelmintics need to be bought and administered separately. Additionally, the different groups of anthelmintics are not chemically compatible; thus, they cannot be mixed together in the same container or syringe. Rather, they need to be administered separately, but can be given concurrently, one immediately after the other. All anthelmintics used in a combination should be administered at the full recommended dose, and meat and milk withdrawal times will be equal to the anthelmintic used with the longest withdrawal time period. An extremely important consideration is that the presence of refugia is essential to realize the full benefits from combinations. If refugia

---

Box 2
Recommendations for performing a composite FECRT

- All recommendations provided in **Box 1** until the FEC step apply here as well.

- Sample preparation
  - Mix each sample to homogenize for about 10 to 15 seconds.
  - Weigh 1.0 g of feces from each individual sample and combine.
  - Mix for 1 minute to thoroughly homogenize the composite sample.
  - Repeat composite sample preparation for each treatment group tested.

- FEC
  - Follow parameters for selecting a FEC method as described in **Box 1**.
  - Using the composite fecal sample, perform 3 separate FEC. If less than 50 eggs are counted (actual number of eggs counted under the microscope) on these 3 FEC, then prepare and count as many additional slides/chambers as needed to count at least 50 eggs. If the 50-egg threshold is reached in the middle of counting a slide, finish counting that slide. Three slides must be examined no matter how many eggs are counted.
  - Record the FEC and the number of slides needed to reach the 50 eggs. Calculate the eggs per gram (EPG) for each slide, then calculate the average EPG for all of the slides counted
  - When performing the post-treatment FEC, prepare the composite samples from the same animals used for the pretreatment FEC and count the same number of slides needed to reach 50 eggs (or 3) as in the pretreatment samples.
  - Note: Fifty eggs counted are the fewest that will provide accurate data; however, counting more eggs will improve the accuracy of the results. Two hundred eggs are optimal for obtaining the most accurate results. However, the loss in accuracy with 50 eggs counted is small relative to the large decrease in work often required to reach 200.

- Efficacy calculations
  - Calculate the mean EPG for both the pretreatment and post-treatment FEC.
  - Calculate the percent reduction in FEC using the following formula:
    - %FECR = ([pretreatment EPG – post-treatment EPG]/pretreatment EPG) × 100

- Interpretation of results:
  - Use the parameters provided in **Box 1**.

- Example

A 25-EPG Modified McMaster slide was prepared and 14 eggs were counted on slide 1. This is less than 50 eggs, so another slide was counted that had 18 eggs. The total number of eggs is still less than 50 eggs (14 + 18 = 32). Additional slides were prepared and counted:

Slide Number	No. of Eggs Counted	FEC (EPG)
1	14	350
2	18	450
3	12	300
4	13	325
Total	57	1425
Mean EPG	1425/4 = 356.25	

  - Post-treatment samples were collected from the same calves and 4 composite sample 25-EPG Modified McMaster slides were prepared and counted.

Slide Number	No. of Eggs Counted	FEC (EPG)
1	3	75
2	4	100
3	4	100
4	5	125
Total	16	400
Mean EPG	400/4 = 100	

  - %FECR = ([pretreatment – post-treatment]/pretreatment) × 100
    - %FECR = ([356.25 – 100]/356.25) × 100

- %FECR = 71.9%
- In this example, the parasite population is interpreted as being resistant to the treatment because the decrease was less than 80%.

Abbreviations: EPG, eggs per gram.

are not maintained, the necessary dilution of the resistant survivors will not be achieved, and this will then lead to having multiple-resistant worms that can no longer be controlled with the combination treatment. Therefore, using anthelmintic combinations without managing refugia is not recommended. From a purely clinical perspective, if the efficacy of an anthelmintic (used singly) is greater than 80%, it is very possible that the farmer will not notice any difference in the clinical response of treatments when applied singly versus in combination. However, the impact on the further development of resistance could be quite substantial (see **Table 2**).

Thus, cattleman should perform a FECRT to determine which drugs are effective, and then knowing this, they should optimally use 2 (or 3) drugs in combination. The expected efficacy of the combination is easily calculated based on the efficacy of the individual drugs. Additionally, 10% to 20% of the herd should be left untreated (selected from best looking animals; upper quartile) to provide untreated refugia. Using this new approach, cattlemen will be getting a highly effective treatment in most of the herd, which will provide excellent herd-level parasite control, and will greatly diminish egg shedding thus reducing subsequent pasture contamination and reinfection. Additionally, by leaving some animals untreated they will be maintaining a drug-susceptible refugia, which will dilute out the small number of resistant worms that survive the treatment. This strategy will result in a worm population that remains predominantly drug susceptible, greatly slowing the development of resistance. The production loss in the 10% to 20% that are untreated will likely be small because these were in the upper quartile of animals before the treatment, and so their growth or productivity was apparently not being heavily impaired by parasites. Studies in sheep comparing productivity of groups where both traditional and targeted selective

Table 1
Impact of using anthelmintics in combination on the efficacy of treatments

Drug 1 (%)	Drug 2 (%)	Drug 3 (%)	Combination (%)
80	80	–	96
80	80	80	99.2
90	90	–	99
90	90	90	99.9
60	95	–	98
60	60	95	99.2
99	99	–	99.99
60	60	60	93.6
50	50	50	87.5

The increases in efficacy are due to a simple additive effect as per the equation below: where D1 = efficacy of drug 1, D2 = efficacy of drug 2, D3 = efficacy of drug 3, C2 = efficacy of D1+D2, and C3 = efficacy of D1 + D2 + D3.

$$C2\% = D1\% + (100 - D1\%) \times D2\%.$$
$$C3\% = C2\% + (100 - C2\%) \times D3\%.$$

Table 2
Impact of using anthelmintic combinations on the percent of resistant worms that survive

Efficacy of Anthelmintic	Single Anthelmintic	Two Anthelmintics in Combination	Fold Difference
99			
% Killed	99	99.99	1.01×
% Surviving	1	0.01	100×
98			
% Killed	98	99.96	1.02×
% Surviving	2	0.04	50×
95			
% Killed	95	99.75	1.05×
% Surviving	5	0.25	20×
90			
% Killed	90	99	1.1×
% Surviving	10	1	10×
80			
% Killed	80	96	1.2×
% Surviving	20	4	5×

Table shows the percent of worms killed by a single anthelmintic versus a combination treatment with 2 anthelmintics, both with the same efficacy, ranging from 80% to 99%. The last column shows the magnitude of the difference between the percent of worms killed and the percent surviving when 1 or 2 anthelmintics in combination are used. Note that the higher the efficacy of the drugs, the smaller the difference in efficacy when used in combination, but the greater the difference in the percent of resistant survivors.

treatment programs were used demonstrated no significant differences in growth of lambs.[30,31] By using effective drugs (and preferably combinations of drugs) and managing refugia by leaving some animals untreated is highly likely to improve overall herd productivity, and the susceptibility of the worms to the drugs will be sustained much longer into the future.

Summary of Recommended Practices to Reduce the Development of Resistance

- Know the resistance status of the worms infecting the herd by performing a FECRT every few years.
- Keep resistant worms off the farm by quarantining all new additions to the herd in a dry lot (without any grass) and treating them with a triple anthelmintic combination. An FEC should be performed at the time of treatment and again after 14 days, and the animal should only be allowed to enter the herd if the FEC is negative.
- Administer the proper dose to animals. Optimally, animals should be weighed before treatment, because several studies have demonstrated that livestock producers often underestimate the weight of their animals. Underdosing exposes worms to sublethal doses of drug, increasing the selection for resistance.
- Use a refugia-based strategy; leaving 10% to 20% of the herd untreated or leaving cows untreated when treating calves provides refugia and slows the development of resistance without causing significant levels of production loss.
- Use a combination of anthelmintics, rather than rotating between anthelmintics. Rotation is not recommended; it does virtually nothing to slow the development of resistance and gives farmers (and veterinarians) a false sense that they are

actually doing something worthwhile in terms of resistance prevention. Additionally, given the high prevalence of resistance, it is likely that rotation will frequently lead to switching from an effective to an ineffective drug. Instead, it is recommended to use multiple anthelmintics in combination. Anthelmintic combinations maximize treatment efficacy, thereby minimizing the number of resistant worms that survive the treatment. The fewer resistant worms that survive, the greater is the dilution from the existing refugia.

- Use nondrug approaches (see David S. Lindsay and J. P. Dubey's article, "Neosporosis, Toxoplasmosis, and Sarcocystosis in Ruminants," in this issue for more details).

SUMMARY

Anthelmintic resistance is a natural evolutionary process that is impossible to prevent if anthelmintics are used on a farm. However, the rate with which resistance develops can be greatly reduced by following recommendations provided here and in several other articles in this issue. The prevalence of multiple-drug resistance in gastrointestinal nematodes of small ruminants is very high, and many goat farms now are in a situation where there is resistance to all available anthelmintics. This situation creates serious problems for parasite control and demands that novel nonchemical approaches be integrated into parasite control programs. The problems with drug resistance in cattle are less severe, but are worsening. The lower levels of resistance in gastrointestinal nematodes of cattle provide an opportunity to use what has been learned from sheep to modify how anthelmintics are used to improve sustainability of chemical-based control. Given the large amount of data showing the magnitude of the resistance problem, livestock farm managers should no longer assume high efficacy of their treatments, and need test for drug resistance using the FECRT. Doing so will allow farms to make future treatment decisions based on the knowledge of which drugs are effective and which are not. Additionally, all livestock farms should move immediately to the use of anthelmintic combinations.

DISCLOSURE

The Kaplan laboratory at University of Georgia serves as the North American distributor of Mini-FLOTAC and Fill FLOTAC devices.

REFERENCES

1. Kaplan RM. Drug resistance in nematodes of veterinary importance: a status report. Trends Parasitol 2004;20:477–81.
2. Kaplan RM, Vidyashankar AN. An inconvenient truth: global worming and anthelmintic resistance. Vet Parasitol 2012;186:70–8.
3. Shoop WL, Haines HW, Michael BF, et al. Mutual resistance to avermectins and milbemycins: oral activity of ivermectin and moxidectin against ivermectin-resistant and susceptible nematodes. Vet Rec 1993;133:445–7.
4. Prichard R, Hall C, Kelly J, et al. The problem of anthelmintic resistance in nematodes. Aust Vet J 1980;56:239–51.
5. Wolstenholme AJ, Fairweather I, Prichard R, et al. Drug resistance in veterinary helminths. Trends Parasitol 2004;20:469–76.
6. Anderson TJC, Blouin MS, Beech RN. Population biology of parasitic nematodes: applications of genetic markers Adv Parasitol. San Diego: Academic Press Inc 1998;41:219–83.

7. Prichard RK. Is anthelmintic resistance a concern for heartworm control? What can we learn from the human filariasis control programs? Vet Parasitol 2005; 133:243–53.
8. Borgsteede F, Duyn S. Lack of reversion of a benzimidazole resistant strain of Haemonchus contortus after six years of levamisole usage. Res Vet Sci 1989; 47:270–2.
9. Hall CA, Ritchie L, Kelly JD. Effect of removing anthelmintic selection pressure on the benzimidazole resistance status of Haemonchus contortus and Trichostrongylus colubriformis in sheep. Res Vet Sci 1982;33:54–7.
10. Zajac AM, Gipson TA. Multiple anthelmintic resistance in a goat herd. Vet Parasitol 2000;87:163–72.
11. Howell SB, Burke JM, Miller JE, et al. Prevalence of anthelmintic resistance on sheep and goat farms in the southeastern United States. J Am Vet Med Assoc 2008;233:1913–9.
12. Crook EK, O'Brien DJ, Howell SB, et al. Prevalence of anthelmintic resistance on sheep and goat farms in the mid-Atlantic region and comparison of in vivo and in vitro detection methods. Small Rumin Res 2016;143:89–96.
13. Ploeger HW, Everts RR. Alarming levels of anthelmintic resistance against gastrointestinal nematodes in sheep in the Netherlands. Vet Parasitol 2018;262:11–5.
14. Lamb J, Elliott T, Chambers M, et al. Broad spectrum anthelmintic resistance of Haemonchus contortus in Northern NSW of Australia. Vet Parasitol 2017;241: 48–51.
15. Playford MC, Smith AN, Love S, et al. Prevalence and severity of anthelmintic resistance in ovine gastrointestinal nematodes in Australia (2009-2012). Aust Vet J 2014;92:464–71.
16. Falzon LC, Menzies PI, Shakya KP, et al. Anthelmintic resistance in sheep flocks in Ontario, Canada. Vet Parasitol 2013;193:150–62.
17. Verissimo CJ, Niciura SCM, Alberti ALL, et al. Multidrug and multispecies resistance in sheep flocks from Sao Paulo state, Brazil. Vet Parasitol 2012;187:209–16.
18. Edmonds MD, Johnson EG, Edmonds JD. Anthelmintic resistance of Ostertagia ostertagi and Cooperia oncophora to macrocyclic lactones in cattle from the western United States. Vet Parasitol 2010;170:224–9.
19. Gasbarre LC, Smith LL, Hoberg E, et al. Further characterization of a cattle nematode population with demonstrated resistance to current anthelmintics. Vet Parasitol 2009;166:275–80.
20. Waghorn TS, Leathwick DM, Rhodes AP, et al. Prevalence of anthelmintic resistance on 62 beef cattle farms in the North Island of New Zealand. N Z Vet J 2006;54:278–82.
21. Waghorn TS, Miller CM, Leathwick DM. Confirmation of ivermectin resistance in Ostertagia ostertagi in cattle in New Zealand. Vet Parasitol 2016;229:139–43.
22. Suarez VH, Cristel SL. Anthelmintic resistance in cattle nematode in the western Pampeana Region of Argentina. Vet Parasitol 2007;144:111–7.
23. Soutello RGV, Seno MCZ, Amarante AFT. Anthelmintic resistance in cattle nematodes in northwestern Sao Paulo state, Brazil. Vet Parasitol 2007;148:360–4.
24. Rendell DK. Anthelmintic resistance in cattle nematodes on 13 south-west Victorian properties. Aust Vet J 2010;88:504–9.
25. Stromberg BE, Gasbarre LC, Waite A, et al. Cooperia punctata: effect on cattle productivity? Vet Parasitol 2012;183:284–91.
26. Leathwick DM, Waghorn TS, Miller CM, et al. Managing anthelmintic resistance – use of a combination anthelmintic and leaving some lambs untreated to slow the development of resistance to ivermectin. Vet Parasitol 2012;187:285–94.

27. Bartram DJ, Leathwick DM, Taylor MA, et al. The role of combination anthelmintic formulations in the sustainable control of sheep nematodes. Vet Parasitol 2012; 186:151–8.

28. Leathwick DM, Miller CM, Atkinson DS, et al. Managing anthelmintic resistance: untreated adult ewes as a source of unselected parasites, and their role in reducing parasite populations. N Z Vet J 2008;56:184–95.

29. Miller CM, Waghorn TS, Leathwick DM, et al. The production cost of anthelmintic resistance in lambs. Vet Parasitol 2012;186:376–81.

30. Kenyon F, McBean D, Greer AW, et al. A comparative study of the effects of four treatment regimes on ivermectin efficacy, body weight and pasture contamination in lambs naturally infected with gastrointestinal nematodes in Scotland. Int J Parasitol Drugs Drug Resist 2013;3:77–84.

31. Busin V, Kenyon F, Laing N, et al. Addressing sustainable sheep farming: application of a targeted selective treatment approach for anthelmintic use on a commercial farm. Small Rumin Res 2013;110:100–3.

32. Paras KL, George MM, Vidyashankar AN, et al. Comparison of fecal egg counting methods in four livestock species. Vet Parasitol 2018;257:21–7.

33. George MM, Paras KL, Howell SB, et al. Utilization of composite fecal samples for detection of anthelmintic resistance in gastrointestinal nematodes of cattle. Vet Parasitol 2017;240:24–9.

34. Wang C, Torgerson PR, Kaplan RM, et al. Modelling anthelmintic resistance by extending eggCounts package to allow individual efficacy. Int J Parasitol Drugs Drug Resist 2018;8:386–93.

Refugia-Based Strategies for Parasite Control in Livestock

Andrew W. Greer, PhD[a],*, Jan A. Van Wyk, PhD[b], Joseph C. Hamie, PhD[a,c], Charles Byaruhanga, PhD[b], Fiona Kenyon, PhD[d]

KEYWORDS

- Targeted selective treatment • Targeted treatment • Parasitism
- Anthelmintic resistance

KEY POINTS

- Refugia-based strategies are intended to help slow the development of anthelmintic resistance by leaving a population unexposed to a treatment.
- Refugia can be supplied in several forms and through a variety of means that vary immensely in their complexity, and not all will fit with every livestock farming system.
- Three main forms of refugia-based strategies are whole flock-targeted treatment, part flock-targeted selective treatments, and selectively leaving a portion of the flock untreated.
- Incorporating refugia-based strategies into production systems typically requires a change in farm management and greater inputs, which may hinder farmer uptake.

THE CONCEPT OF REFUGIA

With the emphasis on anthelmintics for worm management, "refugia" are defined primarily by the proportions of a given parasite population on pasture (mainly worm eggs and larvae) or in untreated hosts that not only escape exposure to deleterious substances,[1,2] but also contribute to the next generation thereof.[3] The concept of refugia was first described by ecologists with regard to the Last Glacial Maximum for categorizing habitats with spatial and/or temporal dimensions with potential for maintaining the viability of biota.[4] However, it was not until the need for application of the principles of refugia to the use of chemicals for management of mosquito vectors of various infective diseases was pointed out[5] that it was considered in the fields of parasitology and pests.

[a] Faculty of Agriculture and Life Sciences, Lincoln University, PO Box 85084, Christchurch, Canterbury 7647, New Zealand; [b] Department of Veterinary Tropical Diseases, Faculty of Veterinary Science, University of Pretoria, P/Bag X04, Onderstepoort 0110, South Africa; [c] Department of Agricultural Research Services, Lunyangwa Agricultural Research Station, PO Box 59, Choma Road, Mzuzu, Malawi; [d] Disease Control, Moredun Research Institute, Pentlands Science Park, Bush Loan, Penicuik, Midlothian EH26 0PZ, Scotland
* Corresponding author.
E-mail address: Andy.Greer@lincoln.ac.nz

Vet Clin Food Anim 36 (2020) 31–43
https://doi.org/10.1016/j.cvfa.2019.11.003
0749-0720/20/© 2019 Elsevier Inc. All rights reserved.

vetfood.theclinics.com

the respondents (95.1%) agreed that sIPM training made a difference in their ability to control and monitor parasitism in their herd or flock, and 96.3% used sIPM practices to control GIN. In addition, the vast majority of the respondents reported fewer problems with GIN (71.9%) and were still using FAMACHA to help them make deworming decisions (87.3%) at the time the follow-up survey was conducted. These data emphasize that the optimal benefits of a refugia-based system, such as FAMACHA, are best achieved with personalized training that teaches farmers why this approach is recommended, and how to integrate methods to achieve improved and sustainable parasite control on their farm.

Several performance-based indicators have also been evaluated as part of a TST regime. In dairy goats/ewes, milk yield has proved to be an appropriate indicator, with multiparous nannies/ewes and those with lower milk yield able to remain untreated without any negative effects on the overall fecal egg counts compared with a midseason treatment of all animals.[39] The use of live weight as a marker of treatment need in lambs has had variable results. Although live weight was selected as the most suitable criterion in modeling studies,[20] this has not always been supported in empirical studies[40] where lambs were identified as either heaviest or lightest and either given anthelmintic or not. The untreated animals had lower production scores and higher fecal egg counts than treated animals, with no evidence that heavier animals were more resilient than lighter animals, presumably reflecting that live weight is a measure of the animals historical status rather than simply its current status. This was also observed where treatment was withheld from the heaviest 10% of lambs at each monthly treatment.[32] On three of the five treatment occasions, those that were in the 10% heaviest that remained untreated had significantly lower ADG in the following month than their treated contemporaries, which were lighter. Importantly, however, although individual untreated animals had reduced ADG, the overall mean herd performance was not affected. Thus, refugia were maintained, and presumably anthelmintic resistance was delayed with only minimal herd-level production loss.

In contrast to the studies cited above, other studies have demonstrated that ADG is a useful criterion, but it is influenced by many environmental and genetic factors. By taking into account some of the major nonparasitological factors that influence lamb growth, such as pasture availability, pasture quality, and the relative maturity of the animal, the use of ADG was refined through inclusion of the so-called Happy Factor,[41] that is, the calculation of a production efficiency value whereby the decision to treat animals, or not, is based on their ability to perform at a predetermined efficiency. This approach has been successfully used in research[33] and on commercial farms in a range of lowland and upland environments and in both the United Kingdom and in New Zealand, with a consistent halving of anthelmintic use with no or relatively little associated losses in lamb productivity.[14,42,43]

From a practical implementation standpoint, various treatment indicators do not have to be used in isolation. In fact, there are many studies where a combination of criteria, for example, high FEC, low body condition score (BCS), low diarrhea score, and/or low weight gain have been used to optimize anthelmintic use. In a recent study fecal samples were only collected from ewes if they had low BCS and/or high FAMACHA scores and then only treated if their FEC was over a threshold of 750 eggs per gram of feces.[44] This approach allowed the focusing of the effort required for FEC to those animals that were most likely to be in need of anthelmintic. The results suggested that using BCS can accurately identify animals with FEC over the threshold, and using this approach resulted in treatment of only 36.5% of ewes. In addition, in a Canadian study ewes at lambing were treated only if they exhibited any 1 of 4 criteria, namely ewe age (if the last season grazing was their first season grazing), poor BCS (equal or <2), FAMACHA score of equal to or less than 3, or if they were nursing 3 or more lambs.[28] Because grazing animals are likely to be exposed to an array of parasite species, using multiple criteria seems worthy of consideration to safeguard both anthelmintic efficacy and animal welfare. This approach has been used in the 5-point check system, which has been promoted as an extension of the FAMACHA system.[45] Furthermore, TST do not necessarily need to be within the same stock class. For example, a field study suggested that untreated ewes, when grazed in conjunction with lambs, could provide a source of refugia to most, but not all, nematode parasite species.[46] Also relevant to this study is that the field study was performed to test the results of a computer model, and both the in silico and in situ experiments yielded consistent results.

Targeted Treatment in Cattle

Overall, most of the support for TT in cattle originates from European studies in dairy cattle, which typically have shown the value of either plasma pepsinogen or bulk milk tank enzyme-linked immunosorbent assay (ELISA) optical density ratio (ODR) measurement of O ostertagi antibodies for an assessment of whether to treat the whole herd. In lactating adult cattle, the relative ease of collecting bulk milk tank ELISA ODR measurements has been demonstrated as an effective tool for determining the levels of exposure to parasite challenge and the likely response to treatment,[47] even though this may also be influenced by animal age, level of animal confinement,[48] and season.[49] Individual milk ELISA ODR have been shown to correlate well ($r = 0.72$) with mean individual milk ELISA results;[50] although from this study 3 major conclusions were drawn that: (1) O ostertagi ELISA results from individual milk samples could provide more information on the parasitic status of a given herd than a single bulk-tank milk result; (2) a need to include lactation numbers when interpreting ELISA results from individual milk samples, which might have reflected higher acquired immunity after repeated exposure to GIN infections; and (3) that the value of O ostertagi antibody level in individual cow milk samples remains ambiguous as a means to predict individual production responses after anthelmintic treatment. In a meta-analysis,[51] it was reported that anthelmintic treatment based on the bulk milk ODR to O ostertagi antibodies could be expected to yield an overall combined estimate of increase in milk of 0.35 kg per cow per day.[49] Thus, the approach of bulk milk antibody ODR cannot only provide an indicator for the need for treatment of cows infected with O ostertagi, but also of quantification of the expected benefit. All of these strategies will help to maintain refugia, while simultaneously providing both good parasite control and levels of productivity.

Targeted Selective Treatment in Cattle

By comparison with the number of studies carried out in small ruminants there have been relatively few that have investigated TST regimes in cattle. As mentioned above, investigations in lactating cattle have included milk ODR to parasite antibodies, which can be taken on an individual basis, although the preference is now to use a bulk milk ODR test as part of a whole herd-targeted regime. Conversely, the individual cow milk production response to treatment over time was relative to the time of effective contact (TEC) with parasites on pasture before first calving.[52] Although a TEC of 8 months was identified as the optimal indicator for a TT treatment, the high level of individual cow variability associated with number of parity, days in milk, and ODR suggested that taking these parameters into account may provide a useful TST indicator. For growing cattle, ADG has gained favor as a performance indicator of choice. This presumably reflects the relative ease with which this can be recorded and its relevance for cattle to reach target weights. More specifically, Swedish studies have suggested that measurements of midseason ADG (6–8 weeks after turnout) can provide a simple and practical means of identifying whether animals should be given an anthelmintic or not; they reported that ADG at this time provided the best predictor of final season live weight, with an optimal cutoff target weight of 0.75 kg per day at midseason.[53] This value is in general agreement with both the required growth rates needed to achieve anticipated mating weights and also the New Zealand studies,[54,55] which used breed-specific predetermined live weight targets to set ADG targets, ranging from 0.30 to 0.68 kg per day in winter and summer, respectively. Overall, these New Zealand-based studies showed a 47% and 72% reduction in anthelmintic use, with an associated 2% and 5% reduction in ADG compared with a monthly whole herd treatment. Greater reductions in both anthelmintic use and animal performance have also been reported in Swedish studies[56] where an anthelmintic was administered only to those TST calves with the ADG of approximately one-quarter of the continuously treated animals; this resulted in a reduction of both anthelmintic use by 92% and growth from 0.39 to 0.61 kg per day to 0.36 to 0.50 kg per day. Overall, although the number of TST studies in cattle are limited, using ADG as a decision criterion does seem to provide a useful means of reducing anthelmintic use while safeguarding animal productivity.

As with small ruminants, setting TST indicators based on animals reaching predetermined performance targets is problematic because attributes, such as growth, are greatly influenced by nonparasite factors. These can be alleviated somewhat, however, through the use of one of a range of growth calculators that are freely available on the Internet but these still do not fully account for individual animal variability. Alternatively, recent interest in changes in animal behavior associated with parasitism may provide a more sensitive method of individualizing treatment. For example, differences in daily and diurnal activity patterns, such as an increase in the number of lying-bouts in parasitized cattle compared with nonparasitized cattle[57] and increased total grazing time after anthelmintic treatment.[58] The potential to monitor individual animal behavior as an indicator of welfare and parasitologic status has recently been made possible through the use of accelerometers, GPS, fixed cameras and drones, combined with sophisticated analysis algorithms. Though still in its early stages of refinement, this is an exciting prospect for the future refinement of TST indicators in cattle.

All of the approaches discussed above for TST rely on the measurement of specific production and or pathologic parameters. However, in many cattle operations, particularly small holders, this type of data collection is often impractical given the farm management structure, and thus will rarely be done by the farmer. Because true TST is not possible without collection of animal-specific data, an alternative approach to maintain refugia is to perform selective nontreatment. Here, the farmer treats most the herd, but leaves 10% to 20% of the cattle untreated. These untreated animals can be selected randomly or based on visual characteristics (eg, leave the best looking animals untreated). This strategy will provide a source of refugia, and based on available data, the loss of productivity will be rather small. Furthermore, when using this strategy it is recommended to use a combination of anthelmintics to maximize the level of efficacy from the treatment. Given the high levels of anthelmintic resistance in many areas, using both selective nontreatment of 10% to 20% of the herd combined with a combination anthelmintic treatment, will likely yield better overall parasite control and production compared to using a drug with suboptimal efficacy in the entire herd (see Ray M. Kaplan's article, "Biology, Epidemiology, Diagnosis, and Management of Anthelmintic Resistance in Gastrointestinal Nematodes of Livestock," in this issue for more information on anthelmintic resistance and optimal strategies for using anthelmintics).

FUTURE PROSPECTS AND CHALLENGES WITH REFUGIA-BASED APPROACHES

Incorporating refugia into anthelmintic treatment regimes generally requires a change in farming practice and farmer mindset. However, in many instances current parasite control practices are no longer effective and are unsustainable. Thus, continuing to use traditional herd-wide treatments often is no longer a reasonable option. This is reflected in the current recommendations of several national parasite advisory schemes, such as Wormwise in New Zealand, Wormboss in Australia, SCOPS in the United Kingdom, and the ACSRPC in the United States. Including refugia invariably requires greater inputs of some degree, whether that be time, labor, or investment in technology. In part this is balanced in the short term by the generally lesser need to treat animals, thus saving in anthelmintic costs, and, in the long term, maintenance of anthelmintic efficacy. The economic impacts of refugia-based strategies are yet to be comprehensively analyzed, but limited data are available. Studies using FEC to target treatment and reduce anthelmintic use in the United Kingdom showed savings of £660 ($1000) per annum.[59] However, farmers will also consider the whole system rather than just savings in costs of anthelmintics. Using a combination of precision livestock farming approaches (TST in lambs and optimized ewe feeding over winter) on an upland/hill flock showed that labor can be reduced and costs saved. Labor was reduced by 36%, and anthelmintic use by 40%, compared with a more conventional approach whereby the animals were dealt with in batches. This equated to savings of £3 ($4.50)/ewe.

There is no single way for optimally providing refugia. Rather, there are a range of options depending on the complexity and diversity of both the parasite epidemiology and farming systems.[27] Each of these has its own advantages and disadvantages, but it is worthwhile considering that the incorporation of refugia does not have to be an all-or-nothing approach. For example, it may be incorporated into part of the system, such as a TT or TST directed to replacement female lambs, which has the potential to provide sufficient refugia to allow for more suppressive parasite control in animals destined for slaughter and for which production loss is unacceptable to the farmer. It is generally agreed that any attempt to provide refugia, even if on a small scale, will be expected to provide some benefit in slowing resistance compared with the alternative.

Although it must be left to the individual farmer/advisor to identify what fits best with a given production system, regardless of what option is selected, a major shift in mentality is required to make these approaches common practice in parasite control.[11] This is particularly the case because reduced development of anthelmintic resistance will not be readily apparent to farmers.[12] Although the provision of refugia can be achieved through relatively simple means (ie, leaving some animals untreated at each time) the relative complexity and compatibility of TT or TST strategies need to be taken into consideration by the farming industry[60] and their application may be hindered by farm-specific factors. Among others, a lack of detailed socioecological analysis and understanding of farmers' preconceptions, attitude, behavior, and beliefs regarding the implementation of TT/TST approaches are among current barriers to their uptake.[11] Moreover, it may be that the delay in anthelmintic resistance alone may not be enough of an incentive. For example, TST in combination with electronic animal identification provides an opportunity to not only identify and select animals that were less reliant on anthelmintics as replacements,[61] but also provide a signal to the markets that the saleable product has been produced sustainably with responsible use of chemicals in food-producing animals. Therefore, benefits of refugia-based strategies for parasite control can extend beyond the provision of refugia, and these benefits are likely to increase in the future.

DISCLOSURE

The authors have nothing to disclose.

REFERENCES

1. Martin PJ, Le Jambre LF, Claxton JH. The impact of refugia on the development of thiabendazole resistance in *Haemonchus contortus*. Int J Parasitol 1981;11: 35–41.
2. Michel JF. Strategies for the use of anthelmintics in livestock and their implications for the development of drug resistance. Parasitology 1985;90:621–8.
3. Martin PJ. Selection for thiabendazole resistance in *Ostertagia* spp. by low efficiency anthelmintic treatment. Int J Parasitology 1989;19:317–25.
4. Dahl E. On different types of unglaciated areas during ice ages and their significance to phytogeography. New Phytol 1946;45:225–42.
5. Axtel RC. Principles of integrated pest management (IPM) in relation to mosquito control. Mosq News 1979;39:709–18.
6. Van Wyk JA. Refugia overlooked as perhaps the most potent factor concerning the development of anthelmintic resistance. Onderstepoort J Vet Res 2001;68: 55–67.
7. Van Wyk JA, Hoste H, Kaplan RM, et al. Targeted selective treatment for worm management—how do we sell rational programs to farmers? Vet Parasitol 2006;139:336–46.
8. Jackson F, Waller P. Managing refugia. Trop Biomed 2008;25:34–40.
9. Leathwick DM, Hosking B. Managing anthelmintic resistance: modelling strategic use of a new anthelmintic class to slow the development of resistance to existing classes. N Z Vet J 2009;57:181–92.
10. Fleming SA, Craig T, Kaplan RM, et al. Anthelmintic resistance of gastrointestinal parasites in small ruminants. J Vet Intern Med 2006;20:435–44.
11. Charlier J, Morgan ER, Rinaldi L, et al. Practices to optimise gastrointestinal nematode control on sheep, goat and cattle farms in Europe using targeted (selective) treatments. Vet Rec 2014;175:250–5.
12. Berk Z, Laurenson YSCM, Forbes AB, et al. Modelling the consequences of targeted selective treatment strategies on performance and emergence of anthelmintic resistance amongst grazing calves. Int J Parasitol Drugs Drug Resist 2016;6:258–71.
13. Kenyon F, Greer AW, Coles GC, et al. Refugia-based approaches to the control of gastrointestinal nematodes of small ruminants. Vet Parasitol 2009;164:3–11.
14. Greer AW, McAnulty RW, Logan CL, et al. Suitability of the happy factor decision support model as part of a targeted selective anthelmintic regime in Coopworth sheep. Proceedings of the New Zealand Society of Animal Production. Palmerston North (New Zealand): New Zealand Society of Animal Production, Inc; 2010. p. 213–6.
15. Cabaret J. Pro and cons of targeted selective treatment against digestive-tract strongyles of ruminants. Parasite 2008;15:506–9.
16. Charlier J, Levecke B, Devleesschauwer B, et al. The economic effects of whole-herd versus selective anthelmintic treatment strategies in dairy cows. J Dairy Sci 2012;95:2977–87.
17. Hodgkinson JE, Kaplan RM, Kenyon F, et al. Refugia and anthelmintic resistance: concepts and challenges. Int J Parasitol Drugs Drug Resist 2019;10:51–7.

18. Gaba S, Cabaret J, Sauve C, et al. Experimental and modelling approaches to evaluate different aspects of the efficacy of targeted selective treatments against sheep parasite nematodes. Vet Parasitol 2010;171:254–62.

19. Learmount J, Taylor MA, Bartram DJ. A computer simulation study to evaluate resistance development with a derquantel-abamectin combination in UK sheep farms. Vet Parasitol 2012;187:244–53.

20. Laurenson YCSM, Kahn LP, Bishop SC, et al. Which is the best phenotypic trait for use in a targeted selective treatment strategy for growing lambs in temperate climates? Vet Parasitol 2016;226:174–88.

21. Cornelius MP, Jacobson C, Dobson R, et al. Computer modelling of anthelmintic resistance and worm control outcomes for refugia-based nematode control strategies in Merino ewes in Western Australia. Vet Parasitol 2016;220:59–66.

22. Berk Z, Laurenson YCSM, Forbes AB, et al. Modelling the impacts of pasture contamination and stocking rate for the development of targeted selective treatment strategies for *Ostertagia ostertagi* infection in calves. Vet Parasitol 2017; 238:82–6.

23. Ravinet N, Lehebel A, Bareille A, et al. Design and evaluation of multi-indicator profiles for targeted-selective treatment against gastrointestinal nematodes at housing in adult dairy cows. Vet Parasitol 2017;237:17–29.

24. Merlin A, Chauvin A, Lehebel A, et al. End-season daily weight gains as rationale for targeted selective treatment against gastrointestinal nematodes in highly exposed first-grazing season cattle. Prev Vet Med 2017;138:104–12.

25. Leathwick DM, Vlassoff A, Barlow ND. A model for nematodiasis in New Zealand lambs: the effect of drenching regime and grazing management on the development of anthelmintic resistance. Int J Parasitol 1995;25:1479–90.

26. Leathwick DM. Modelling the benefits of a new class of anthelmintic in combination. Vet Parasitol 2012;186:93–100.

27. Van Wyk JA, Reynecke DP. Blueprint for an automated specific decision support system for countering anthelmintic resistance in *Haemonchus* spp. at farm level. Vet Parasitol 2011;177:212–23.

28. Westers T, Jone-Bitton A, Menzies P, et al. Identification of effective treatment criteria for use in targeted selective treatment programs to control haemonchosis in periparturient ewes in Ontario, Canada. Prev Vet Med 2016;134:49–57.

29. Van Wyk JA, Bath GF. The FAMACHA© system for managing haemonchosis in sheep and goats by clinically identifying individual animals for treatment. Vet Res 2002;33:509–29.

30. Suter RJ, Besier RB, Perkins NR, et al. Sheep-farm risk factors for ivermectin resistance in *Ostertagia circumcincta* in Western Australia. Prev Vet Med 2004; 63:257–69.

31. Waghorn TS, Leathwick DM, Miller CM, et al. Brave or gullible: testing the concept that leaving susceptible parasites in refugia will slow the development of anthelmintic resistance. N Z Vet J 2008;56:158–63.

32. Leathwick DM, Waghorn TS, Miller CM, et al. Selective and on-demand drenching of lambs: impact on parasite populations and performance of lambs. N Z Vet J 2006;54:305–12.

33. Kenyon F, McBean D, Greer AW, et al. A comparative study of the effects of anthelmintic treatment regime on ivermectin efficacy and performance in lambs naturally infected with gastrointestinal nematodes in Scotland. Int J Parasitol Drugs Drug Resist 2013;3:77–84.

34. Malan FS, Van Wyk JA. The packed cell volume and colour of the conjunctivae as aids for monitoring *Haemonchus contortus* infestations in sheep. Proc SA Vet Assoc Bie Nat Vet Cong. 1992. p. 139.
35. Bath GF, Malan FS, Van Wyk JA. The "FAMACHA" Ovine Anaemia Guide to assist with the control of haemonchosis. Proc 7th Annual Congress Livestock Health Production Group SA Vet Assoc. 1996. p. 5.
36. Kaplan RM, Burke JM, Terrill TH, et al. Validation of the FAMACHA eye color chart for detecting clinical anemia in sheep and goats on farms in the southern United States. Vet Parasitol 2004;123:105–20.
37. Burke JM, Kaplan RM, Miller JE, et al. Accuracy of the FAMACHA system for on-farm use by sheep and goat producers in the southeastern United States. Vet Parasitol 2007;147:89–95.
38. Whitley NC, Oh SH, Lee SJ, et al. Impact of integrated gastrointestinal nematode management training for U.S. goat and sheep producers. Vet Parasitol 2014;200: 271–5.
39. Cringoli G, Veneziano V, Jackson F, et al. Effects of strategic anthelmintic treatments on the milk production of dairy sheep naturally infected by gastrointestinal strongyles. Vet Parasitol 2008;156:340–5.
40. Keegan JD, Good B, Hanrahan JP, et al. Live weight as a basis for targeted selective treatment of lambs post-weaning. Vet Parasitol 2018;258:8–13.
41. Greer AW, Kenyon F, Bartley DJ, et al. Development and field evaluation of a decision support model for anthelmintic treatments as part of a targeted selective treatment (TST) regime in lambs. Vet Parasitol 2009;164:12–20.
42. Busin V, Kenyon F, Parkin T, et al. Production impact of a targeted selective treatment system based on liveweight gain in a commercial flock. Vet J 2014;200: 248–52.
43. McBean D, Nath M, Lambe N, et al. Viability of the happy factor™ targeted selective treatment approach on several sheep farms in Scotland. Vet Parasitol 2016; 218:22–30.
44. Soto-Barrientos N, Chan-Pérez JI, España-España E, et al. Comparing body condition score and FAMACHA© to identify hair-sheep ewes with high faecal egg counts of gastrointestinal nematodes in farms under hot tropical conditions. Small Rum Res 2018;167:92–9.
45. Bath GF. The "BIG FIVE"—a South African perspective on sustainable holistic internal parasite management in sheep and goats. Small Rumin Res 2014;118: 48–55.
46. Leathwick DM, Miller C, Atkinson D, et al. Managing anthelmintic resistance: untreated adult ewes as a source of unselected parasites, and their role in reducing parasite populations. N Z Vet J 2008;56:184–95.
47. Charlier J, Demeler J, Höglund J, et al. *Ostertagia ostertagi* in first-season grazing cattle in Belgium, Germany and Sweden: general levels of infection and related management practices. Vet Parasitol 2010;171:91–8.
48. Vanderstichel R, Dohoo I, Sanchez J, et al. Predicting the effect of anthelmintic treatment on milk production of dairy cattle in Canada using an *Ostertagia ostertagi* ELISA from individual milk samples. Prev Vet Med 2013;111:63–75.
49. Sanchez J, Dohoo I, Leslie K, et al. The use of an indirect *Ostertagia ostertagi* ELISA to predict milk production response after anthelmintic treatment in confined and semi-confined dairy herds. Vet Parasitol 2005;130:115–24.
50. Charlier J, Vercruysse J, Smith J, et al. Evaluation of anti-*Ostertagia ostertagi* antibodies in individual milk samples as decision parameter for selective anthelmintic treatment in dairy cows. Prev Vet Med 2010;93:147–52.

51. Sanchez J, Dohoo I, Carrier J, et al. A meta-analysis of the milk-production response after anthelmintic treatment in naturally infected adult dairy cows. Vet Parasitol 2004;63:237–56.
52. Ravinet N, Bareille N, Lehebelc A, et al. Change in milk production after treatment against gastrointestinal nematodes according to grazing history, parasitological and production-based indicators in adult dairy cows. Vet Parasitol 2014;201:95–109.
53. Höglund J, Morrison DA, Charlier J, et al. Assessing the feasibility of targeted selective treatments for gastrointestinal nematodes in first-season grazing cattle based on mid-season daily weight gains. Vet Parasitol 2009;164:80–8.
54. Greer AW, McAnulty RW, Gibbs JSJ. Performance-based targeted selective anthelmintic treatment regime for grazing dairy calves. Proc 4th Austral Dairy Sci Symp. 2010. p. 385–9.
55. McAnulty RW, Gibbs SJ, Greer AW. Liveweight gain of grazing dairy calves in their first season subjected to a targeted selective anthelmintic treatment (TST) regime. Proceedings of the New Zealand Society of Animal Production. Palmerston North (New Zealand): New Zealand Society of Animal Production, Inc; 2011. p. 301–3.
56. Höglund J, Dahlström F, Sollenberg S, et al. Weight gain-based targeted selective treatments (TST) of gastrointestinal nematodes in first-season grazing cattle. Vet Parasitol 2013;196:358–65.
57. Högberg N, Lidfors L, Hessle A, et al. Effects of nematode parasitism on activity patterns in first-season grazing cattle. Vet Parasitol X 2019;1:100011.
58. Forbes AB, Huckle CA, Gibb MJ. Impact of eprinomectin on grazing behaviour and performance in dairy cattle with sub-clinical gastrointestinal nematode infections under continuous stocking management. Vet Parasitol 2004;125:353–64.
59. Kenyon F, Jackson F. Targeted flock/herd and individual ruminant treatment approaches. Vet Parasitol 2012;186:10–7.
60. Woodgate RG, Love S. WormKill to WormBoss-Can we sell sustainable sheep worm control? Vet Parasitol 2012;186:51–7.
61. Greer AW, Pettigrew CA, Logan CM. Evaluation of lambs subjected to a targeted selective treatment anthelmintic regime. Proceedings of the New Zealand Society of Animal Production. Palmerston North (New Zealand): New Zealand Society of Animal Production, Inc; 2013. p. 175–9.

Epidemiology and Control of Gastrointestinal Nematodes of Cattle in Southern Climates

Christine B. Navarre, DVM, MS

KEYWORDS

- Cattle • Gastrointestinal • Parasites • GIN

KEY POINTS

- The biology of gastrointestinal nematodes (GIN) is influenced by the warm climate and variable rainfall patterns in the southern United States, and this affects recommendations for parasite control measures in this region.
- The GIN of cattle that have the highest prevalence and veterinary importance in the southern United States are *Cooperia spp (Cooperia oncophora, Cooperia punctata*, and *Cooperia pectinata), Hemonchus placei* and *Hemonchus contortus,* and *Ostertagia ostertagi.* Of these *O ostertagi* is the most pathogenic.
- With increasing levels of anthelmintic resistance, current deworming practices are not sustainable and may no longer make economic sense. Control programs need to be tailored for individual ranches to maximize the benefits of deworming while minimizing development of resistance.
- Refugia-based control programs for GIN offer the best balance of short-term economic benefits and long-term sustainability of anthelmintic efficacy.
- Control programs should integrate grazing management and management of the immune system (proper nutrition, preventive herd health program, etc.) with the use of anthelmintics so cattle can resist infection and anthelmintic use can be minimized.

INTRODUCTION

Control of gastrointestinal nematodes (GIN) has positive economic and health benefits for cattle operations in the southern United States. In the past several decades, GIN control has been based almost exclusively on the use of anthelmintics. Now with the increase in anthelmintic resistance (AR), new strategies must be developed and implemented.

Cattle production and management as well as GIN biology and control in the southern United States are influenced by climate and weather. Warm climate predominates but weather can be highly variable. The gulf coast states typically have higher rainfall than the southcentral region, whereas the southwestern region is more arid. Climate

School of Animal Sciences, Louisiana State University Agricultural Center, Louisiana State University, 111 Dalrymple Building, 110 LSU Union Square, Baton Rouge, LA 70803-0106, USA
E-mail address: cnavarre@agcenter.lsu.edu

Vet Clin Food Anim 36 (2020) 45–57
https://doi.org/10.1016/j.cvfa.2019.11.006
0749-0720/20/© 2019 Elsevier Inc. All rights reserved.

and weather conditions affect grazing management and stocking density, both of which can affect GIN transmission. The generally low stocking density[1] and low rainfall in the southwestern United States greatly lessen GIN transmission compared with the gulf coast states.[2] This article focuses on the epidemiology and control of GIN in the gulf coast states and southcentral states where GIN transmission and disease have a greater impact. For specific situations in the southwest, such as more intensive grazing of irrigated pastures, the principals of control outlined here are still applicable. This article also focuses on the beef cow-calf and stocker industries, as these sectors of the cattle industry predominate and transmission of GIN in concentrated feeding operations is negligible. Dairy production is concentrated in more northern climates[3] and is not addressed here. However, control of GIN in grazing dairies and in dairy heifer raising operations are virtually the same as for grazing beef cattle.

MAJOR GASTROINTESTINAL NEMATODES OF CONCERN IN SOUTHERN CLIMATES

The GIN of cattle that have significant prevalence and veterinary importance in the southern United States are *Cooperia* spp. (*Cooperia oncophora*, *Cooperia punctata*, and *Cooperia pectinata*), *Hemonchus placei and Hemonchus contortus*, and *Ostertagia ostertagi*.[4,5] Porter reported in 1942 an overall prevalence of 91% for *C punctata*, 83% for *Hemonchus* spp., and 74% for *O ostertagi* in cattle from the gulf coast states (Alabama, Florida, Georgia, Louisiana, and Mississippi). National Animal Health Monitoring System data from 2007 to 2008 showed that this prevalence has changed little over time.[2,6]

O ostertagi is the most important GIN of cattle because of its high pathogenicity and its impact on a wider age range of cattle.[7] *H placei* and *H contortus* are also very pathogenic but usually only affect weanlings and yearlings. *Cooperia spp.* are less pathogenic than either *Hemonchus* or *Ostertagia* but in warm wet conditions may be present in very large numbers and become economically and clinically significant.

AR is covered in more depth in Ray M. Kaplan's article, "Biology, Epidemiology, Diagnosis, and Management of Anthelmintic Resistance in Gastrointestinal Nematodes of Livestock," in this issue but warrants mention here. Research into AR in the southern United States is mostly from the gulf coast states, Arkansas and Missouri. Results are highly variable, but there is no question that AR is reported for all of the major GIN. Of particular concern is the emergence of AR to *Ostertagia*.[8,9] Deaths in adult beef cattle from *Ostertagia* recently have been reported in Louisiana in herds previously dewormed with macrocyclic lactones, which highly suggests that AR may be present in this species (C. Navarre, personal communication, 2019).

GOALS OF CONTROL PROGRAMS

There are 2 goals in controlling GIN: controlling economic losses and controlling clinical disease. The level of infection determines both health and economic impacts of GIN. At low levels, there may be minimal economic impact and development of immunity can be protective to health. At moderate levels, production losses occur without evident clinical disease. The most studied impact from GIN is on weight gains in young growing animals, but impact on reproductive efficiency and milk production in adult cows is also reported.[5,7,10] A study published in 2013 looking at efficacy and production benefits following use of extended-release injectable eprinomectin showed significant differences in weight gain of 30.4 kg, 19.1 kg, and 8.6 kg in calves from Louisiana, Arkansas, and Missouri, respectively.[11] In this study efficacy was high, with fecal egg count reductions (FECR) greater than 95% at all sites; this level of FECR and these levels of weight gains likely would not be obtained today in the face of increasing levels of AR, which is increasingly common. Clinical disease from high GIN burdens can occur, even in adults, especially when other stressors occur, particularly nutritional stress.

There is no question that there are economic and sometimes health benefits from controlling GIN in cattle, but predicting the outcomes of deworming on an individual ranch or in individual animals is difficult. Extrapolating research findings to individual farms and expecting similar gains in growing cattle is risky. Levels of AR as well as management factors (weather, nutrition, other diseases, etc.) all affect growth in young cattle. Deworming benefits in older cattle are even less predictable. It is important to remember that AR is not static and that extrapolating gains from studies from even a few years ago can be misleading. On ranch monitoring of anthelmintic efficacy and production levels are the best ways to optimally adapt recommendations to individual ranches.

BACKGROUND INFORMATION NEEDED TO DEVELOP CONTROL PROGRAMS

Parasite control programs should integrate grazing management and management of the immune system (proper nutrition, preventive herd health program, etc.) with use of anthelmintics so cattle can resist infection and anthelmintic use can be minimized. The first step is to understand what is happening on an individual ranch. This takes knowledge of GIN biology and epidemiology in the region based on climate and weather and specific information from the individual ranch, such as quantitative fecal egg counts, estimates of AR through FECRT, ages of the cattle, and pasture management. **Box 1** lists the factors that can affect the prevalence and degree of cattle GIN on a ranch. The reader is encouraged to see other articles in this issue to gain more in-depth knowledge in these areas. This article focuses on how to put this information into practice to develop integrated GIN control programs.

Climate and Weather

A basic understanding of how climate and weather affect GIN biology is advantageous when developing pasture management plans. In the southern United States the climate is too hot most of the summer for the free-living stages of O ostertagi and C oncophora to survive. The greatest infection risk for *Ostertagia* is from fall through spring.[10] *Ostertagia* does not survive at any time in southern most parts of Florida and Texas,[12] although this may be changing (T. Craig, personal communication). C punctata and Hemonchus spp. are more heat tolerant than *Ostertagia* and can be problematic during wet summers. Areas with higher rainfall tend toward higher GIN problems. It should be noted that rainfall may be increasing across the United States above what is typical,[13] which may change GIN epidemiology from what has been seen in the past.

Climate also affects seasonal arrestment of development of GIN, the most important of which is the late spring and early summer arrestment of *Ostertagia* in the south.[14] Resumed development in the fall can lead to type II ostertagiasis, which is not common but is severe when it occurs. It most commonly occurs in older steers, replacement heifers, and bulls.[10]

Weather plays an important role in GIN transmission by affecting the rate of development and success of survival of the free-living larval stages on pasture. This varies somewhat depending on the species, but under conditions of moderate temperatures (7–25°C) and moisture (at least 1 inch of precipitation per month), the period from egg hatching to the infective larval stage is 7 to 14 days.[15,16] Colder weather can lengthen this period as well as decrease the percent hatch of eggs.[7] Larvae must have moisture

> **Box 1**
> **Determinants of the prevalence and degree of cattle nematodosis**
>
> Nature of challenge
>   Overriding determinants
>   Climate
>   Weather
>   Season
>   Region
>   Pasture and management determinants
>   Pasture quality and productivity
>   Pasture type
>   Pasture topography and drainage
>   Grazing management: age group separation, alternate species, stocking rates, rotation, supplemental feeding
>   Production type: dairy (confined vs pastured), beef (stocker vs cow/calf vs feedlot, etc)
>   Animal-based determinants
>   Immunologic status
>   Physiologic status
>   Health
> Nature of parasiticidal effort
>   Effectiveness of parasiticide usage
>   Effectiveness of product: spectrum of activity, larvicidal versus adulticidal, degree of resistance
>   Persistence of product
>   Diminished efficacy: formulation considerations (topicals vs injectables, etc), dietary considerations (gut flow, ingredients, closures, etc), generics
>   Coordination of epidemiology with treatment
>   Time and extent of posttreatment challenge
>
> *From* Yazwinski TA., Tucker CA. A sampling of factors relative to the epidemiology of gastrointestinal nematode parasites of cattle in the united states. *Vet Clin North Am Food Anim Pract.2006;* 22(3):501-527; with permission.

to migrate from the fecal pat, so drought can delay pasture contamination.[17] Thus, there can be a buildup of infective larvae within the fecal pats, which are then released over a short period of time once rains resume. This can lead to an overwhelming infection, precipitating more severe economic losses and even clinical disease.

Weather also affects the longevity of the infective stages of larvae, which can range from days to several months.[15,18] Infective larvae have limited energy stores. In hot weather, their metabolism is faster and these energy stores are used up quickly. Leaving pastures unoccupied for a few months in the summer can greatly reduce the levels of larval contamination on pastures. The opposite is true in cooler weather; during cooler periods of the year L3 can survive on pasture for many months.

Pasture and Grazing Management

Pasture management is an important component of GIN control and delaying and/or reversing AR. Although pasture type, quality, topography, and drainage can all influence prevalence of GIN on pasture, these are usually factors that are difficult to change. Grazing management offers the most practical solution.

Pastures with reduced GIN contamination ("safe" or "clean" pastures) can be especially helpful in controlling GIN in stocker cattle.[5] There are several ways of decreasing larval contamination of pastures:

- Pasture rest in summer

    o Must have rain at the beginning of the rest period
- Alternating land use as pasture and crop/hay production
- Annual or biannual pasture renovation
- Cograzing with alternate, less suitable hosts
    o Alternate calves with adult dry cows
    o Horses
    o Sheep and goats can also be beneficial but are not as suitable because *H. contortus* can also infect cattle, particularly young cattle

Avoidance of overstocking is a common recommendation to avoid buildup of GIN on pasture but "over stocking" should be defined. It usually refers to too many animals grazing continuously on limited land. Some high-intensity "mob" grazing systems have very high stocking rates but for very short periods of time with extended periods of rest. This type of grazing could be detrimental in the short term if pastures are contaminated because cattle will graze close to the ground. But it may have benefits in the long term by decreasing GIN levels from long rest periods. The cost-benefit and rest time necessary to affect GIN transmission varies considerably depending on climate, weather, and forage type. More research is needed to elucidate specific benefits and risks, but due to the farm-related and climate variabilities, each farm will need to make judgments to determine optimal approaches.

The combination of safe pastures and suppressive anthelmintic use can hasten the development of AR. Treating an entire group of cattle and turning onto safe pasture will produce high selection pressures for AR. This can be minimized if the pasture is made "safe" again by rest or alternate use for crops between groups of cattle. However, if that pasture is used continuously, AR will increase.

Pasture rotation at a set length of time is frequently cited as a way to control GIN. This might be true if the life cycle was predictable. But, many factors (temperature, moisture, etc.) determine if larvae develop into infective stages,[15,19] so predicting when the GIN will lie in wait to try to thwart them with grazing management is difficult and impractical. What can be predicted is that infective larvae usually remain in the lower 8 to 10 cm of the grass.[5] Therefore, maintaining forage height of at least 8 cm in combination with following best management practices for a particular forage should maximize forage sustainability while minimizing the impact of GIN. Tracking FECs over time can also help determine when parasites are a problem in different grazing systems.

Management that Affects the Immune System

Understanding how GIN burdens affect the immune system of cattle is beyond the scope of this article, but readers are encouraged to consider the impact of GIN on vaccine response and disease resistance when developing comprehensive herd health plans.[7,20] Conversely, understanding how the immune system of cattle affects GIN burdens is also an important component of developing GIN control programs. Age, sex, breed, genetics, and overall health all influence susceptibility to GIN.

Young grazing cattle, especially stocker calves and replacement heifers, are most susceptible to GIN.[10] Although uncommon, older cattle can also have severe parasitic disease including mortality, when high GIN burdens are combined with other stressors. This is most evident in brood cows in winter that are either nursing a calf or heavily pregnant depending on the calving season. Poor nutrition as a consequence of poor-quality pastures in combination with high GIN contamination of the pastures, along with severe weather and/or other parasites (liver flukes in particular), can lead to serious disease.

Males are more susceptible to GIN than females, thus bulls should not be overlooked when designing GIN control programs.[21] There is some evidence that differences in GIN susceptibility exist between *Bos taurus* and *Bos indicus* breeds,[22] and it has been suggested that *B indicus* breeds may be particularly susceptible to *Ostertagia* (Thomas Craig, personal communication). The hypothesis is that *B indicus* cattle were developed in parts of the world that were too hot for *Ostertagia* to survive, so there was no evolutionary pressure to develop an immune response to *Ostertagia*. Research is needed to clarify whether there are true breed and species differences in susceptibility of cattle to GIN, including the role of hybrid vigor.

Some individual cattle within each herd are genetically more susceptible to GIN than others. It is estimated that 20% of cattle harbor 80% of the GIN in a herd and with a moderate heritability index of 0.3, thus genetic selection for GIN resistance should be possible over time.[13,23–25] FECs could theoretically be used as one selection tool in cattle but only in young animals and only with *Cooperia* and *Hemonchus*, not *Ostertagia*. Unfortunately, putting this into practice is more complicated, as several other factors may influence FECs. Time of year affects both the FECs and the heritability index; therefore, it affects the power of genetic selection based on FECs.[24] Also, the milking ability of the dam may be inversely correlated with GIN burdens in nursing calves[26] and may influence FECs and selection. Selecting for GIN resistance may have positive or negative impacts on other production traits, and there is currently no efficient and accurate means to achieve this goal. More research is needed to reveal gene alleles that may confer GIN resistance and how selection of these alleles may affect other traits of importance.

Diagnostics

Given all of the variables discussed so far, it is easy to see why collecting data on individual ranches is necessary to develop optimal parasite control programs. Diagnostic methods are covered in detail in Guilherme G. Verocai and colleagues' article, "Diagnostic Methods for Detecting Internal Parasites of Livestock," in this issue. Regardless of the specific techniques chosen and the challenges of interpreting FECs and FECRT data, this information is still critical to developing control programs on individual ranches. FECs are most useful for monitoring patterns for grazing management and for determining treatment thresholds rather than assessing infection levels of individual animals.[27] Magnitude of change in weight gains between treated and untreated groups of calves are generally correlated with FECs. Kunkle and colleagues[11] (2013) showed that the greatest change in gains was in Louisiana where egg counts were higher (140–271 eggs per gram; EPG) than in Arkansas and Missouri (60–68 and 51–77 EPG, respectively). However, nematode species differ in their fecundity, thus in mixed-species infections, which is the normal situation, the FEC does not necessarily correlate with the number of worms, particularly the number of *Ostertagia*, which are the most pathogenic and also the least fecund. Consequently, a true universal FEC treatment threshold recommendation is illusive and is best determined with on-ranch trials. In herds where management and nutrition are optimal and FECs remain low, deworming may not be necessary or at least may be needed less frequently.

Surveillance of FECs over time in different groups of cattle at different times of year and under different management schemes and stressors give insight into the magnitude and timing of GIN burdens. When FEC data over years are combined with production, weather, and grazing data, more accurate targeted treatment decisions can be made. Surveillance of young cattle, particularly at the later part of the nursing period and 6 to 8 weeks after turnout of stocker cattle is a top priority. Monitoring adult cattle under nutritional stress may also be helpful. Changes in management or weather, particularly rain events, should be taken into consideration when comparing FECs from year to year. FEC data are a must for guiding refugia-based treatment and management recommendations (see Andrew W. Greer and colleagues' article, "Refugia-Based Strategies for Parasite Control in Livestock," in this issue for more information). The cost of performing FECs should be offset by more targeted use and timing of anthelmintic treatments leading to cost savings and better animal performance. Appropriate pooling of fecal samples can also decrease cost of FECs significantly (see Ray M. Kaplan's article, "Biology, Epidemiology, Diagnosis, and Management of Anthelmintic Resistance in Gastrointestinal Nematodes of Livestock," in this issue).

PRINCIPLES OF CONTROL

Refugia-based control strategies for GIN offer the best balance of short-term economic benefits from deworming and long-term sustainability of anthelmintic efficacy. These strategies are discussed in detail in Andrew W. Greer and colleagues' article, "Refugia-Based Strategies for Parasite Control in Livestock," in this issue but are mostly focused on sheep. **Box 2** lists some of the principles of control of GIN in cattle in the southern United States. The following recommendations are meant to be a starting place for developing control programs. These recommendations are made somewhat in a "vacuum" and must be integrated with other herd health and production management decisions.

Refugia can come from 2 sources; free-living stages on pasture and in animals not treated with anthelmintic, and both need to be considered. Deworming all animals in a group and moving them shortly to a "clean" pasture should be avoided. Also avoid deworming all cattle at times when the climate and/or weather is not conducive to survival of larvae in the environment. For example, "strategic" deworming of all cattle in

---

Box 2
Principles of control of gastrointestinal nematodes in cattle in the Southern United States

- Increase overall herd immunity
  - Proper nutrition
  - Decrease stressors
  - Decrease other disease pressures

- Graze cows after calves

- Maintain biosecurity practices to prevent introduction of resistant GIN with herd additions

- Incorporate resistance to GIN in genetic selection programs

- Keep refugia
  - Avoid deworming all animals before turnout onto clean pastures
    - Especially critical with macrocyclic lactones and other long-acting products
  - In cow/calf operations consider only deworming cattle younger than 5 years and allow older cows to serve as refugia
    - Be aware of special circumstances that may alter this recommendation such as nutritional stress, treatment of liver flukes

- Use and store products properly
  - Always use at least 2 classes of anthelmintics at the same time
  - Dose based on actual weights if possible
  - Do not store products at the processing area unless it is climate controlled
    - Follow label directions for storage

continually with no rest is not sustainable given the current levels of AR that calves are expected to have on arrival. The 2 most practical options are to leave at least 10% of the calves untreated or to have enough pasture to allow for rest. Only grazing stockers in the fall/spring allow pastures to rest in the summer, which is the best time to decrease contamination in the south. Resting pastures in the winter may not affect contamination very much. More research is needed on high-intensity ("mob") grazing techniques, as this might offer some solutions.

SAMPLE CONTROL PROGRAMS FOR COW-CALF HERDS

The following are *templates* for developing GIN control programs based on calving season. As discussed earlier, results of FECs and FECRT monitoring as well as knowledge of grazing management, nutrition, health, etc. should be used to fine tune these recommendations for individual ranches. *These recommendations assume use of multiple classes of anthelmintics and refugia-based grazing management as discussed earlier and are not meant as stand-alone recommendations.*

For FEC monitoring, 15 to 20 samples per grazing group should suffice. These samples can be pooled as directed in Ray M. Kaplan's article, "Biology, Epidemiology, Diagnosis, and Management of Anthelmintic Resistance in Gastrointestinal Nematodes of Livestock," in this issue for cost savings. On-farm trials may be necessary to determine the economic benefits of deworming young cattle at given FEC thresholds. FECs in adult females on good nutrition are usually quite low and should generally be less than 50. FECs that are increasing in the face of other stressors may indicate the need for treatment. After a few years of FEC surveillance, the frequency and timing of FECs can be adjusted as needed.

Spring Calving Herds

- Summer
  - Monitor FECs in calves midsummer, especially in warm, wet weather
  - Preweaning
    - Deworm calves at least 1 month before weaning
      - Earlier if heavy burdens
- Fall
  - Monitor FECs in cows, including flukes if necessary
  - Deworm young cows and replacement heifers
  - Deworm adult cows if deemed necessary for liver fluke control
  - Deworm calves depending if and when calves were dewormed preweaning
- Winter
  - Monitor FECs in adult cows and replacement heifers, especially if under nutritional and weather stress
  - Consider deworming bulls at time of breeding soundness examinations
- Spring
  - Monitor FECs in cows as an indicator of potential pasture contamination for calves

Fall Calving Herds

- Winter
  - Monitor FECs in calves midwinter
  - Preweaning
    - Deworm calves at least 1 month before weaning
      - Earlier if heavy burdens

- Monitor FECs in adult cows, replacement heifers, and bulls, especially if under nutritional and weather stress
  - Fall calving cows have the additional stress of lactation during this time
- Spring
  - Deworm calves depending if and when calves were dewormed preweaning
- Fall
  - Monitor FECs in cows, including flukes if necessary
  - Deworm young cows and replacement heifers
  - Deworm adult cows if deemed necessary for liver fluke control
  - Monitor FECs in bulls and consider deworming at time of breeding soundness examinations

SUMMARY

There is a large body of knowledge regarding GIN and their control in cattle, but there are still many gaps in that knowledge. Much of the recent research has focused on the economic benefits of treating with anthelmintics, but much of that research is no longer valid as a consequence of drug resistance. In addition, most epidemiologic data are decades old, and there is evidence of changes due to both climate change and decades of anthelmintic use. More recent epidemiologic data as well as documentation of the effectiveness of refugia-based control programs and nonanthelmintic alternatives are needed.

Waiting for all of these knowledge gaps to be filled is not an option. GIN control in cattle can no longer be just about which anthelmintic product to use and when. Changing practices from simple (scheduled deworming of entire groups) to complex (refugia-based strategies) is not easy but is necessary if we are to sustain some anthelmintics for future use. Designing control programs for a given farm needs to take into account what we know about GIN epidemiology and combine that knowledge with specific information from diagnostic testing and ranch management. Gathering FEC and FECRT data is necessary and costly in the short term but in the long term can better equip ranches to make sound management and cattle selection decisions that result in more productive and sustainable ranches.

DISCLOSURE

Author has nothing to disclose.

REFERENCES

1. Asem-Hiablie S, Rotz CA, Stout R, et al. Management characteristics of beef cattle production in the western United States. Prof Anim Sci 2017;33(4):461–71.
2. Stromberg BE, Gasbarre LC, Ballweber LR, et al. Prevalence of internal parasites in beef cows in the United States: results of the National Animal Health Monitoring System's (NAHMS) beef study, 2007-2008. Can J Vet Res 2015;79(4):290–5. Available at: http://www.ncbi.nlm.nih.gov/pubmed/26424909. Accessed June 26, 2019.
3. USDA ERS - Dairy data. 2019. Available at: https://www.ers.usda.gov/data-products/dairy-data/dairy-data/. Accessed June 26, 2019.
4. Stuedemann JA, Kaplan RM, Miller JE, et al. Ecology/physiology workgroup importance of nematode parasites in cattle grazing research. Available at: https://agrilife.org/spfcic/files/2013/02/stuedemann.pdf.

5. Yazwinski TA, Tucker CA. A sampling of factors relative to the epidemiology of gastrointestinal nematode parasites of cattle in the United States. Vet Clin North Am Food Anim Pract 2006;22(3):501–27.

6. Porter D. Incidence of gastrointestinal nematodes of cattle in the Southeastern United States. Am J Vet Res 1942;3:304–8.

7. Stromberg BE, Gasbarre LC. Gastrointestinal nematode control programs with an emphasis on cattle. Vet Clin North Am Food Anim Pract 2006;22(3):543–65.

8. Hunter JS, Yoon S, Yazwinski TA, et al. The efficacy of eprinomectin extended-release injection against naturally acquired nematode parasites of cattle, with special regard to inhibited fourth-stage Ostertagia larvae. Vet Parasitol 2013; 192(4):346–52.

9. Yazwinski TA, Tucker CA, Wray E, et al. Control trial and fecal egg count reduction test determinations of nematocidal efficacies of moxidectin and generic ivermectin in recently weaned, naturally infected calves. Vet Parasitol 2013; 195(1–2):95–101.

10. Williams JC, Loyacano AF. Internal parasites of cattle in Louisiana and other Southern States. 2001. Available at: https://www.lsuagcenter.com/~/media/system/3/d/3/1/3d31b74693c6eccd47125d34100c80e1/ris104cattleparasites.pdf. Accessed June 26, 2019.

11. Kunkle BN, Williams JC, Johnson EG, et al. Persistent efficacy and production benefits following use of extended-release injectable eprinomectin in grazing beef cattle under field conditions. Vet Parasitol 2013;192(4):332–7.

12. Courtney CH. Strategic parasite control - practices that pay. Available at: https://animal.ifas.ufl.edu/beef_extension/bcsc/1995/docs/courtney.pdf. Accessed June 27, 2019.

13. USGCRP. Climate science special report 2017. p. 1–470. Available at: https://science2017.globalchange.gov/chapter/front-matter-about/. Accessed June 26, 2019.

14. Williams JC, Knox JW, Baumann BA, et al. Seasonal changes of gastrointestinal nematode populations in yearling beef cattle in Louisiana with emphasis on prevalence of inhibition in Ostertagia ostertagi. Int J Parasitol 1983;13(2):133–43.

15. Williams JC, Bilkovich FR. Distribution of Ostertagia ostertagi infective larvae on pasture herbage. Am J Vet Res 1973;34(10):1337–44. Available at: http://www.ncbi.nlm.nih.gov/pubmed/4748245. Accessed June 26, 2019.

16. Levine ND. Weather, climate, and the bionomics of ruminant nematode larvae. Adv Vet Sci 1963;8:215–61. Available at: https://www.cabdirect.org/cabdirect/abstract/19650802833. Accessed June 28, 2019.

17. Barger IA, Lewis RJ, Brown GF. Survival of infective larvae of nematode parasites of cattle during drought. Vet Parasitol 1984;14(2):143–52.

18. Williams JC, Bilkovich FR. Develpoment and survival of infective larvae of the cattle nematode, Ostertagia ostertagi. J Parasitol 1971;57(2):327–38. Available at: http://www.ncbi.nlm.nih.gov/pubmed/5102817. Accessed June 26, 2019.

19. Stromberg BE. Environmental factors influencing transmission. Vet Parasitol 1997;72(3–4):247–64.

20. Gasbarre LC. Effect of gastrointestinal nematode infection on the ruminant immune system. Vet Parasitol 1997;72:327–43.

21. Barger IA. Influence of sex and reproductive status on susceptibility of ruminants to nematode parasitism. Int J Parasitol 1993;23(4):463–9.

22. Suarez VH, Busetti MR, Lorenzo RM. Comparative effects of nematode infection on Bos taurus and Bos indicus crossbred calves grazing on Argentina's Western Pampas. Vet Parasitol 1995;58(3):263–71.

23. Leighton EA, Murrell KD, Gasbarre LC. Evidence for genetic control of nematode egg-shedding rates in calves. J Parasitol 1989;75:498–504. Available at: https://about.jstor.org/terms. Accessed June 28, 2019.
24. Gasbarre LC, Leighton EA, Davies CJ. Genetic control of immunity to gastrointestinal nematodes of cattle. Vet Parasitol 1990;37(3–4):257–72.
25. Mackinnon M, Meyer K, Hetzel DJ. Genetic variation and covariation for growth, parasite resistance and heat tolerance in tropical cattle. Livest Prod Sci 1991;27(2–3):105–22.
26. Snyder DE. Epidemiology of ostertagia ostertagi in cow-calf herds in the Southeastern USA. Vet Parasitol 1993;46:277–88.
27. Eysker M, Ploger HW. Value of present diagnostic methods for gastrointestinal nematode infections in ruminants. Parasitology 2000;120(7):109–19.

Epidemiology and Control of Gastrointestinal Nematodes of Cattle in Northern Climates

Michael B. Hildreth, PhD*, John B. McKenzie, BS

KEYWORDS

- Cattle gastrointestinal nematodes • Northern climates • Ostertagia • Cooperia
- Haemonchus • Economic losses • Winter survival • Anthelmintic resistance

KEY POINTS

- A shorter grazing season and extended freezing winter conditions help keep gastrointestinal nematode intensities in Canada and the northern United States at levels lower than in southern states with warmer climates.
- *Ostertagia ostertagi* and *Cooperia oncophora* are still the most prevalent gastrointestinal nematodes (GIN) in Canada but their relative prevalence seems to be diminishing throughout the United States because other trichostrongyles, such as *Haemonchus* spp, have expanded their distribution into northern states.
- Studies suggest that GINs in stocker cattle and preweaned calves from northern North America typically diminish weight gains by roughly 0.05 to 0.15 kg/d during the grazing season.
- Spring deworming programs designed to attack the GIN life-cycle during its weakest time-period using persistent anthelmintics with persistent efficacies has been a popular strategy among cattle producers throughout the northern region as a way to maximize the economic benefits of anthelmintic use. These anthelmintics should persist long enough for a significant portion of the postwinter larvae on pastures to die off during the spring. Postwinter larvae can only survive a few weeks after coming out of hypobiosis before they die from starvation. However, this strategy likely is not sustainable given the increasing levels of anthelmintic resistance.
- The absence of pasture refugia for trichostrongyle species with L3s that die during freezing winter conditions may accelerate the development of anthelmintic resistance within northern North America, and therefore, it is absolutely necessary for cattle producers to incorporate refugia into any deworming program in this region.

UNIQUE FEATURES OF CATTLE PRODUCTION IN NORTHERN CLIMATES

Cattle management systems are heavily influenced by environmental factors (discussed in Johannes Charlier and colleagues' article, "Biology and Epidemiology of Gastrointestinal

Department of Biology and Microbiology, South Dakota State University, SNP 252, Brookings, SD 57007, USA
* Corresponding author.
E-mail address: michael.hildreth@sdstate.edu

Vet Clin Food Anim 36 (2020) 59–71
https://doi.org/10.1016/j.cvfa.2019.11.008
0749-0720/20/© 2019 Elsevier Inc. All rights reserved.

vetfood.theclinics.com

Nematodes in Cattle," in this issue), and predominant weather conditions are primary. Climatic parameters specific to the colder winter conditions of northern North America significantly influence the clinical effects that parasites can have on their hosts and the strategic approaches used to control these negative effects. This is particularly true for gastrointestinal nematodes (GIN) because their free-living transmittal stages are significantly affected by the harsh climates specific to this region. This article focuses on the epidemiology and control of GIN in the northern regions of North America, where transmittal stages are exposed to prolonged freezing temperatures during the winter season. These climatic factors have their primary influence on transmission of these parasites while cattle are grazing on pastures, and therefore, this article focuses primarily on GIN issues in grazing cattle in the region.

The distribution and management of beef and dairy cattle herds within the various US climatic zones has been reviewed.[1] Significant changes in the dairy production industry have resulted in less than 5% of lactating cows within the United States grazing on pastures.[2,3] The only segments of the dairy industry using pastures are producers of dairy replacement heifers, and stock-growers involved in dairy beef production. Pasture management systems used in these instances are the same as those used for beef cattle. Beef cattle production throughout North America is commonly compartmentalized into four segments consisting of (1) seedstock breeders, (2) commercial cow-calf producers, (3) yearling-stocker operators, and (4) feedlot/confinement feeding operations. Only the feedlot beef segment does not use pastures. The needs for profitability affect the locations for each segment, causing a clustering of the industries. Of the roughly 90 million beef breeding cows in the United States, more than 70% are located in the 15 central US states of Montana, North Dakota, South Dakota, Minnesota, Colorado, Wyoming, Nebraska, Iowa, Kansas, Oklahoma, Missouri, New Mexico, Arkansas, Louisianan, and Texas. About half of these breeding cows are located in the northern eight of these states.[4] Approximately 90% of the roughly 4 million beef breeding cows in Canada are located in the three providences of Manitoba, Saskatchewan, and Alberta, which are located directly north of the high calf producing areas from the northern United States.[5]

The Köppen Climate Classification System is the most widely used system for classifying climatic zones, and is based on annual and monthly average temperatures and precipitation.[6] In this system, the major cattle-rearing areas in the southeastern half of Canada and northeastern half of United States are classified as hot (Dfa) or warm (Dfb) summer humid continental climates with their coldest month averaging less than $-0°C$ and at least 4 months averaging above 10°C. The southern edge of Dfa includes Nebraska and Iowa, and the northern halves of Illinois, Indiana, Ohio, and Pennsylvania. Climates in the major cattle-rearing areas west of Dfa/Dfb are heavily influenced by the Rocky Mountains. Areas east of the mountains are part of the dry rain-shadow zone occupied by the western parts of the Dakotas and Nebraska, plus the eastern parts of Wyoming and Montana. They contain the cold semiarid climate zone (Bsk) where temperatures are similar to Dfa, but where precipitation is much lower. Climates within the mountainous areas of western Montana and Wyoming and eastern Idaho vary depending on altitude and precipitation, but include significant areas of Dfa to Bsk. Within Washington and Oregon, the climate is more Mediterranean-like where precipitation is plentiful, and temperatures are somewhat warmer.

Within these areas, cow-calf production generally involves grazing the pairs in pastures until calves are weaned and either put into feedlots or into additional grazing systems. Depending on climate, cows are either placed back onto pastures and/or maintained under feedlot conditions to build up body-condition-scores for the next calving season. Although cold winters generally force livestock producers to use harvested forage and grains to sustain their animals through long winters, these times away from grazing interrupts the GIN lifecycle helping to keep their populations at levels significantly lower than those in warmer, more southern, climates. A lack of moisture in the drier areas the northern North America can limit GIN intensities in cattle to some of the lowest levels in North America.

DISTRIBUTION AND PREVALENCE OF GASTROINTESTINAL PARASITES IN CATTLE FROM NORTH AMERICAN REGIONS WITH FREEZING WINTER SOIL TEMPERATURES

With few exceptions, the various parasite species that infect cattle throughout Canada and the Northern United States are generally the same as those found throughout North America, although generally in lower numbers. A large September 1993 survey involving 98 cattle herds grazing in major portions of the Dakotas and western Minnesota illustrates the relative prevalence of gastrointestinal (GI) parasites present in cattle from the northern portion of the high-calf-producing region of North America.[7] The most common type of GI parasites reported among these cow-calf herds was the complex of GIN nematodes producing trichostrongyle-type eggs. Most genera in the superfamily Trichostrongyloidea produce this oval egg with a thin eggshell filled with multiple blastomeres. Species in the genus *Oesophagostomum* (superfamily Strongyloidea) infecting ruminants also produce a similar-type egg. Throughout North America, four genera of trichostrongyles have been most frequently identified in cattle" (1) *Haemonchus*, (2) *Ostertagia*, (3) *Trichostrongylus*, and (4) *Cooperia*.[8] Even in colder climates, trichostrongyle-type nematodes infect virtually all grazing cattle. For example, 94% of the calves from the Dakota/Minnesota study showed the presence of at least one trichostrongyle egg in 3-g fecal samples.[7] Of the 1772 calf samples analyzed in a recent national survey 86% contained at least one trichostrongyle egg, with a mean fecal egg count (FEC) of 32.5 eggs per gram of feces (EPG).[9] Mean egg counts were highest for calves from the southeastern region (58.1 EPG) and lowest in the western region (11.3 EPG). Mean FECs for the Dakota/Minnesota study (33.8 EPG) was similar to the grazing season mean FECs for the central region (30.3 EPG) of the national study. Similar trichostrongyle FEC results have been found among various other calf studies from northern North America.[10–16] Trichostrongyle FECs were significantly lower among the cows in all of these studies.

Nematodirus sp, *Moniezia* sp, and *Trichuris* sp eggs were also found within calves from the Dakota/Minnesota study, but only present in 35%, 20%, and 10% of the samples, respectively. It is not uncommon to find species of *Nematodirus* temporarily present in high numbers among young calves from northern regions. Although *Nematodirus* is a member of the superfamily Trichostrongyloidea, its egg morphology is distinctive from the other trichostrongyles, and so are often reported separately. Evidence suggest Nematodirinae nematodes originated in a holarctic environment, and they seem to be particularly well suited to surviving extreme cold and dry conditions.[17] Surveys also suggest that *Nematodirus* might be more important in cooler climates.[9,18] The lifecycle of *Nematodirus* spp is similar to other trichostrongyles, but its infectious larvae are particularly resistant to environmental conditions and can remain infectious through two winters and one summer, at least in milder northern climates.[19] *Nematodirus helvetianus* is the most common species in cattle from the northern regions, and most calves quickly develop an effective immunity against this species, eliminating or reduce it to low levels.

Because it is not possible to reliably differentiate trichostrongyle genera (apart from *Nematodirus*) based on egg morphology, surveys have historically relied on identifying adults in necropsy samples. *Ostertagia ostertagi* (98% prevalence), *Cooperia* oncophora (60.6%), Ostertagia bisonis (41.8%), Cooperia bisonis (33.6%), and Trichostrongylus axei (27.9%) were the predominant trichostrongyles identified in a necropsy survey involving 208 cattle from Wyoming.[11] O ostertagi and C oncophora were also predominant in tracer calves from Minnesota and Oregon epizootiology studies.[14,20] Advances in molecular biology have made it possible to use egg samples in surveys to conveniently determine the genera and/or species of trichostrongyles from different regions. Recently, a method for simultaneously identifying all possible trichostrongyle species in cattle fecal samples has been developed using deep amplicon next-generation sequencing (nemabiome metabarcoding) of the internal transcribed spacer 2 rDNA locus.[21] This approach was used to evaluate the trichostrongyle species composition of 20 calf fecal samples that had been collected from 50 cattle herds located in the major cattle-producing Canadian provinces, and 38 calf fecal samples each entering into different feedlots from Oklahoma, Arkansas, and Nebraska.[18] The Canadian data indicate that 59.1% of the DNA came from O ostertagi and 37.6% came from C oncophora. Most of the remaining 3.3% DNA came from C punctata, but notable amounts of Haemonchus placei and Oesophagostomum radiatum were found in more than one herd. With 96.7% of the DNA coming from only two species, diversity was low among Canadian samples, but slightly higher in Ontario where all but one of the C punctata–infected herds were located. Similar results were also found among dairy replacement heifers collected from 47 dairy farms across Canada.[22] Species diversity was much higher among the US herds, where C punctata was the predominant species in 12 of the 13 herds sold to Nebraska feedlots. Surprisingly, the second most common species in 6 of the 13 herds from the Nebraska study was H placei, and this was the predominant species in one of these herds. Prevalence was lower and at similar levels for O radiatum, O ostertagi, and C oncophora among these herds. These results were different from older necropsy studies where O ostertagi and C oncophora were the most prevalent, and where C punctata and H placei were only rarely found.[11,20,23] Although the origins of the Nebraska calves were not known, at least some were from cow-calf herds in northern states. A genus level polymerase chain reaction survey of 239 fall calves from 13 eastern South Dakota herds provides even stronger evidence that Haemonchus spp have become established into the northern Great Plains.[24] In this survey, Cooperia spp was found in 64% of the samples, Ostertagia spp in 59%, and Haemonchus spp in 26%. Haemonchus spp eggs were present in at least one calf for 69% of these herds. These results are consistent with genus-level polymerase chain reaction results from the recent national study where the total US prevalence was highest for Cooperia spp (91%) followed by Ostertagia spp (79%); however, almost half of the samples contained Haemonchus spp DNA (53%).[9]

Collectively, these various results show that the historical prevalence of H placei and Haemonchus contortus among northern cattle has been low,[8] and Canada still does not contain significant amounts of Haemonchus spp in cattle.[18] However, recent studies from the United States suggest that H placei and C punctata has expanded their distribution into the northern states. Potential explanations for the expansion of these two southern species northward are likely related to changes in their overwintering strategies (discussed later), and warming of the climate.

ECONOMIC COSTS OF TRICHOSTRONGYLE PARASITES IN NORTHERN NORTH AMERICA

Even among northern cattle, trichostrongyles adversely affect numerous performance parameters including: weight gain, feed efficiency, forage utilization, carcass quality, reproductive efficiency, milk production, and immune responses to other pathogens.[25–27] Most data used in quantifying the economic effects of trichostrongyles have come from anthelmintic efficacy studies using a separate-but-equal "twin" pasture experimental approach that necessitates separating a single contaminated pasture into multiple paddocks where each paddock is the unit of observation. The objective of these studies has not been to measure production losses from parasitism, but rather measuring treatment effects for specific products. Yet, results from these studies are helpful in providing estimates for the costs of parasitism when highly efficacious anthelmintics virtually eliminate all nematodes from the treated groups for extended periods so that differences in performance parameters between the treated and untreated cattle represent the economic effects of the worms. Average daily gain (ADG) has been the most frequently measured production parameter used in beef cattle studies, and most weight-gain studies have involved stockers.[27]

Unfortunately, twin-pasture studies are expensive and logistically difficult to set up, limiting the number and geographic distribution of these type studies. This has limited the understanding of the real-world economic impacts that cattle trichostrongyles have, especially in the northern portions of North America. A single pasture approach to estimating nematode impacts has been developed based on using an effective and long-acting anthelmintic to protect a small portion (ie, 10%) of "wormless" cattle within a larger population of untreated cattle (ie, 90%) containing normal parasite loads.[28] Using this approach, economic losses were measured for nine commercial stocker herds primarily in northeastern South Dakota.[29] Combined results from these trials indicated that wormless cattle gained an additional 0.05 kg/head/d compared with the wormy control animals. This resulted in an additional gain of 7.2 kg (14.5 lb) over the average 143-day grazing season. There was considerable variation in the weight-gain advantage among the different herds, but collectively this increase was highly significant, and individually significant within two of the trials. Mean FEC at the end of the season for the untreated stockers was only 14.4 EPG and for the treated stockers 1.2 EPG. The Ivomec SR (sustained release) boluses (Merial Animal Health, Rahway, NJ) used in this study were designed to deliver ivermectin at a rate of 12 mg/d over a 135-day period. More recently, an extended-release injectable formulation of eprinomectin has been developed that can provide nematode control in cattle for up to 150 days.[30]

In twin-pasture studies involving the extended-release injectable formulation, daily weight gain advantages among three northern states (Idaho, Minnesota, and Wisconsin) averaged about one-half (0.07, 0.05, and 0.18 kg/d, respectively) the weight gain advantage seen in similar trials in Louisiana and Arkansas.[31] A meta-analysis study of 23 stocker-trials from seven northern US states (Wisconsin, Illinois, Missouri, Minnesota, South Dakota, Nebraska, and Kansas) showed an ADG advantage of 0.05 kg/d among the anthelmintic-treated animals in these states.[32] These pasture studies suggest that if left untreated, trichostrongyles in northern North America stockers are diminishing weight gains by roughly 0.05 to 0.15 kg/d. Cost-benefit analyses of nematode control in stockers from this region should consider these ADG advantages as the upper limits for potential gains in an average-type herd. In more recent years, anthelmintic resistance (AR) among many trichostrongyle populations in most areas has reduced anthelmintic efficacies and thereby the expected economic benefits of nematode control strategies that rely on treatments with one class of anthelmintic.[33]

Measuring production effects from trichostrongyle infections in cow-calf herds is more complicated than in stockers, and there have been only a few cow-calf treatment studies from the northern region using a twin-pasture format. In most of these treatment studies, ADG did not increase among treated cows but cow treatment did increase ADG for their calves. In a 2-year Minnesota study involving two treatments with fenbendazole, mean ADGs increased by 0.14 and 0.11 kg/d during Year 1 and Year 2, respectively.[15] Pregnancy rates were also 11.8% and 12.4% higher during Year 1 and Year 2, respectively. A 2-year North Dakota study used ivermectin injectable on cows at spring turn-out to compare weight gains in cows and their calves.[34] Grazing days were not reported in this study, but assuming 170 days separated beginning and ending weights, then calves from the treated herd outgained control animals by 0.04 kg/d over the 2-year study. During this time, pregnancy rates were 3.4% higher. A single pour-on treatment of cows from an Idaho herd with doramectin pour-on yielded a 0.07 kg/d advantage in their calves after 140 days.[35] Collectively, these few studies suggest that trichostrongyle nematodes from US northern states diminish weight gains in calves at levels similar to those reported for stockers in the region. Although these effects on production parameters are generally lower that those measured in cattle from the more southern states, they are significant enough to justify treatment and control strategies designed to limit their effects as long as AR has not significantly reduced the dewormer's efficacy.

PARTICULAR CHALLENGES FOR SURVIVAL OF TRICHOSTRONGYLE POPULATIONS CREATED BY COLD-WINTER CLIMATES

Trichostrongyle nematodes use a direct lifecycle consisting of four free-living stages (egg, first-, second-, and third-larval stages) dwelling on pastures and two parasitic stages (fourth-larval stage and adult stage) living in the host's GI tract. Eggs are released from adult females, excreted into the fecal pat, and there develop quickly to the third larval stage (L3). L3s then migrate onto vegetation where they are accidently ingested by a proper ruminant host. Depending on environmental conditions, L3 can survive for extended periods on pastures. Once ingested, L3s penetrate into the wall of the GI tract and develop to the fourth-larval stage (L4) before re-emerging back into the lumen to develop into the adult stage. For most economically important cattle trichostrongyles, L4s are able to arrest their development within the host and remain there in a hypobiotic state for extended periods.[36]

Trichostrongyle populations in the northern portions of North America have at least two challenges not experienced by the more southern populations. The first challenge is the short grazing season, which limits the number of generations possible for each nematode species each year. This time limitation helps keep populations low and parasite problems subclinical. Even during years with adequate precipitation, grazing seasons throughout Canada and northern United States typically range from 140 to 180 days. The second challenge is needing to survive the 185 to 225 days between each grazing season. Trichostrongyle adults are thought to have a life expectancy of roughly 50 to 80 days,[37,38] and so without the ability of L4 stages to arrest development during the fall and winter months, it would not be possible for trichostrongyles to consistently survive through the winter inside its host. The percentage of L4s entering into hypobiosis generally increases before adverse climatic events (eg, the onset of winter) and L4 maturation resumes at or before the ending of that event.[39] In cold winter climates, initiation of hypobiosis is highest during the late summer and fall, and resumption of development and maturation is highest during late winter and spring.[11] Several authors have reported a significant periparturient increase in trichostrongyle egg shedding in sheep, which is associated with a relaxation of immunity particularly in response to lactation.[40,41] This rise is less pronounced in sheep breeds that are more resistant to trichostrongyles and is much less notable in cattle.[42,43]

In addition to overwintering as hypobiotic L4s within their hosts, some trichostron-gyle species can also overwinter as L3s within the soil of pastures. In southwest Ontario, *O ostertagi*, *C oncophora*, *Cooperia mcmasteri*, and *N helvetianus* L3s were found to survive winters; however, *C punctata* and *Bunostomum phlebotomum* did not.[44] Additional tracer-calf studies have confirmed these results for *O ostertagi* and *C oncophora* in New Brunswick, Maine, Minnesota, and South Dakota.[14,19,45–50] In Maine, Gibbs[46] found that overwinter survival of *Ostertagia* sp and *Cooperia* sp L3s on pasture was more important than L4s within the hosts; however, their relative importance likely varies with species, regional climate, and yearly variations in weather. The inability of *H contortus* L3s to survive South Dakota and Ontario winters has been documented in tracer-lamb studies,[45,51–53] but there have been no such studies for *H placei*. Given its close relationship with *H contortus* and its historical dis-tribution, it is unlikely that *H placei* L3s can survive winters in northern North America.

Historically, benzimidazole and macrocyclic lactone (ML) anthelmintics killed most arrested L4s among nonresistant populations, and so winter survival of trichostron-gyles in fall- or spring-treated cattle largely depended on the survivability of L3s on pasture.[46] In fall seasons as soil temperatures cool, remaining L3s on pastures migrate into the soil during winter, reemerging back onto vegetation as temperatures warm during spring. For this population to survive, at least some of these postwinter L3s (PW-L3s) must remain infective long enough during spring to be ingested by suscep-tible grazing cattle. Survival times for these larvae are influenced by environmental conditions on the pasture, particularly temperature.[54] This is because a remnant L2 cuticle completely encloses L3s preventing them from ingesting food after their molt to the L3. Although this larval sheath aids in winter survivability, it later causes starva-tion as increasing spring temperatures increase the L3's metabolic rate. In regions with cold winters, this postwinter phase is the most vulnerable period of the trichos-trongyle lifecycle, and therefore, forms the basis for strategic deworming programs in this region.

POTENTIAL FOR CATTLE TRICHOSTRONGYLES TO DEVELOP ANTHELMINTIC RESISTANCE IN NORTHERN CLIMATES

AR to the MLs has been recently documented within most cattle-producing regions of the world, including the United States.[55,56] Although AR is described in detail else-where in this issue, there are a few AR issues that are specific to ruminants raised in a cold-winter climate. Because AR to all three anthelmintic classes has been a prob-lem within small ruminant production systems for many years, the epidemiologic fac-tors contributing to AR are better understood in relation to sheep trichostrongyles. Even though AR is a more significant problem for sheep production in warm climates, including the southern United States, recent studies have described AR within sheep herds living in cold-winter climates across the globe.[53,57–60] It is likely that some of these AR cases have resulted from the translocation of infected southern sheep into cold-climate herds; however, the development of AR in a population of *H contortus* within a closed sheep herd from South Dakota, United States demonstrates that it can originate within herds from cold-winter climates.[53] It may even be possible that selective pressures driving *H contortus* toward AR are higher in cold climates because freezing soil conditions eliminates L3 pasture refugia that would normally exist throughout the winter months in warm climates.

L3s from the two most common cattle trichostrongyles in cold-winter regions, *O ostertagi* and *C oncophora*, can easily survive subfreezing soil temperatures and so provide a refugia population for these two species even for herds receiving fall and/or spring anthelmintics treatments. For these overwintering species, the shorter grazing season and the lower parasite loads may help slow the development of AR within Canada and the US northern states. Ironically, the two documented cases of AR were described in northern US states: a stocker herd in Wisconsin[61,62] and feedlot cattle in Idaho.[63] In both cases, however, the cattle originated from milder climates. Stockers in the Wisconsin study came from auction barns throughout the southeastern United States before their inclusion to an intensive grazing program in Wisconsin. Resistance to avermectins, milbemycins, and benzimidazoles was documented for H contortus and C punctata, whereas H placei was resistant to both classes of MLs. Pasture survival of Haemonchus spp and C punctata L3s through a Wisconsin winter is unlikely and suggests that imported calves brought these AR species with them each year. The feedlot cattle from the Idaho study originated from northern California, where soil temperatures rarely fall lower than freezing. In this study, Cooperia spp adults were significantly resistant to avermectins and mildly resistant to milbemycins. Although avermectin was effective against O ostertagia adults, it did not reduce developing and arrested L4s by 90%. Although both the Wisconsin and Idaho studies demonstrate the existence of AR in the United States, they do not provide any evidence for a more rapid development of AR in cattle trichostrongyle populations from climates with freezing soil temperatures.

The growing prevalence of H placei, H contortus, and C punctata in anthelmintic-treated cattle from regions with yearly freezing soil temperatures highlights a need to measure AR among these species in northern cattle.[24] The only way that populations of Haemonchus can survive through winter in dewormed cattle herds is if the L4s have become AR. Certainly, these results indicate that AR studies are needed within Canada and the northern US states. Lastly, it should be kept in mind that the results of studies performed in previous decades demonstrating significant production and economic benefits of various anthelmintic treatment strategies may no longer be representative of what can be expected from similar treatment regimens given the rising levels of AR.

CONTROL STRATEGIES FOR CATTLE PARASITES IN NORTHERN NORTH AMERICAN CLIMATES

General strategies for controlling cattle GI parasites are described in Johannes Charlier and colleagues' article, "Biology and Epidemiology of Gastrointestinal Nematodes in Cattle," in this issue and in previous reviews.[64-67] Some of these strategies also apply to cattle segments in the northern regions of North America. For example, general treatment approaches for cattle entering feedlots in southern states have been used effectively in northern states and Canada. Additionally, these approaches are appropriate for treating cows entering their winter quarters. Anthelmintic-based control programs for GIN in this region originally focused primarily on fall deworming of retained heifers and first year cows with a benzimidazole drench product.[68] For a variety of reasons including convenience and lice control, many producers then switched to avermectin/milbemycin (ML) pour-on products when they became available. Control of lice is still a major motivator for northern producers to continue using MLs in the fall. Eventually, most of these producers added an additional springtime treatment, taking advantage of the persistent anthelmintic activity of MLs, to minimize losses from trichostrongyles while cattle are on pastures. The primary objectives for springtime deworming programs in this region are to kill adults and arrested L4s in cows and stockers, and then also kill any PW-L3s (and other newly shed L3s) consumed once cattle are released onto summer pastures. Both persistent activity against incoming

L3 and high efficacy against the arrested L4 stages are necessary features of the drug used to achieve these objectives.

The PW-L3s need to live off of their depleted energy reserves, and thus have a limited lifespan once the temperatures begin to warm. Thus, anthelmintics with persistent activity can prevent new infections from establishing while PW-L3 populations are collapsing from starvation. Consequently, knowing how long PW-L3s survive on pastures can help cattle producers optimize the efficacy of their control efforts. In northern North America, survival times for PW-L3s have been measured in only two regions. Tracer-calf studies along the east coast in New Brunswick and Maine found that infectivity of O ostertagi and C oncophora L3s decreased significantly during early summer, dropping by at least 90% by the second week in July.[19,46,49,50] A more recent 2-year study from eastern South Dakota showed that most PW-L3 infectivity decreased before the second week in June, and virtually no L3s were infectious by the second half of July.[48] This study also involved O ostertagi and C oncophora but started measuring PW-L3 populations earlier and in 2-week intervals instead of the month intervals for the previous studies. For every 14-day period, pasture survival dropped by an average of 44.1%, and therefore, pasture infectivity decreased by about 90% in 8 weeks. An average survival half-life of 15 days was calculated for the South Dakota region. The rate of decline depends on the general temperature and moisture levels of the region, and on the available microhabitats present in pastures, and thus survival times vary somewhat from year to year.

The depressed metabolic rate of arrested L4s makes them less susceptible to anthelmintics.[39] Thus, reduced efficacy of anthelmintics caused by resistance is first seen against this stage, even while the drugs remain effective against adult worms. Originally, all ML anthelmintics provided high efficacy against arrested L4s, and persistent activity against new incoming L3 that ranged from about 14 to 35 days.[69,70] Newer long-acting ML formulations extended this persistent activity for up to 120 days.[31] These features of MLs made them ideal drugs to use for these spring treatments. However, as resistance to MLs develops, the first detectable changes in efficacy are the loss of persistency, and the loss of efficacy against the arrested L4s. Although most data demonstrating these effects are in small ruminants[71] and horses,[72] there is growing anecdotal evidence that the increasing levels of ML resistance in GIN of cattle are decreasing or even eliminating the persistent effect and efficacy against arrested L4. Thus, increasing levels and spectrum of AR has important implications for parasite control in this region.

In summary, strategic spring-time deworming programs are designed to attack the GIN life-cycle during its weakest time-period, using anthelmintics with persistent efficacies that are long enough to permit significant natural die-off of PW-L3. Using this strategy has been popular among cattle producers throughout the northern region as a way to maximize the economic benefits of anthelmintic use. However, these highly effective programs also create high selective pressures that are responsible for hastening the development of AR, particularly among GIN species whose larvae cannot survive winter while on pastures. Given the impact that AR will have on the success of this strategy and evidence suggesting that AR is increasing throughout North America, it is absolutely essential that northern producers test for resistance, and incorporate strategies to reduce these pressures by modifying parasite control practices to incorporate and manage refugia (discussed in Ray M. Kaplan's article, "Biology, Epidemiology, Diagnosis, and Management of Anthelmintic Resistance in Gastrointestinal Nematodes of Livestock," in this issue and Andrew W. Greer and colleagues' article, "Refugia-Based Strategies for Parasite Control in Livestock," in this issue).

DISCLOSURE

This review was supported by South Dakota State University Agricultural Experiment Station.

REFERENCES

1. Bull LS. Distribution and management of cattle in relation to climatic zones within North America. Vet Clin North Am Food Anim Pract 1986;2:205–10.
2. Barkema HW, von Keyserlingk MA, Kastelic JP, et al. Invited review: changes in the dairy industry affecting dairy cattle health and welfare. J Dairy Sci 2015;98: 7426–45.
3. USDA. Dairy 2007, part I: reference of dairy cattle health and management practices in the United States, 2007. Fort Collins (CO): USDA-APHIS-VS, CEAH; 2007.
4. Field TG. An overview of the U.S. Beef industry. In: Beef production and management decisions. University of Nebraska; 2018. p. 1–15. Available at: https://www.amazon.com/Production-Management-Decisions-Trades-Technology/dp/013460 2692.
5. Statistics-Canada. Table 32-10-0424-01 cattle and calves on census day. 2016. Available at: https://www150.statcan.gc.ca/t1/tbl1/en/tv.action?pid=3210042401. Accessed June 8, 2019.
6. Kottek M, Grieser J, Beck C, et al. World map of the Köppen-Geiger climate classification updated. Meteorol Z 2006;15:259–63.
7. Hildreth MB, Epperson WB, Mertz KJ. Effect of longitude and latitude on fecal egg and oocyst counts in cow-calf beef herds from the United States Northern Great Plains. Vet Parasitol 2007;149:207–12.
8. Gibbs HC, Herd RP. Nematodiasis in cattle: importance, species involved, immunity, and resistance. In: Gibbs HC, Herd RP, Murrell KD, editors. Veterinary Clinics of North America: food animal practice. Food animal practice. Philadelphia: W.B. Saunders Company; 1986. p. 211–24.
9. Stromberg BE, Gasbarre LC, Ballweber LR, et al. Prevalence of internal parasites in beef cows in the United States: results of the National Animal Health Monitoring System's (NAHMS) beef study, 2007-2008. Can J Vet Res 2015;79:290–5.
10. Jelinski M, Gilleard J, Rocheleau L, et al. Epidemiology of gastrointestinal nematode infections in grazing yearling beef cattle in Saskatchewan. Can Vet J 2017; 58:1044–50.
11. Malczewski A, Jolley WR, Woodard LF. Prevalence and epidemiology of trichostrongylids in Wyoming cattle with consideration of the inhibited development of *Ostertagia ostertagi*. Vet Parasitol 1996;64:285–97.
12. Polley L, Bickis MG. Gastrointestinal nematode parasites in Saskatchewan cattle: egg count distribution in beef animals. Can J Vet Res 1987;51:465–9.
13. Slocombe JOD, Curtis RA. Aspects of the epidemiology of nematode infections in a cow-calf herd in Ontario. Can J Vet Res 1989;53:336–9.
14. Stromberg BE, Schlotthauer JC, Haggard DL, et al. Epizootiology of helminth parasitism in a beef cow/calf herd in Minnesota. Am J Vet Res 1991;52:1712–6.
15. Stromberg BE, Vatthauer RJ, Schlotthauer JC, et al. Production responses following strategic parasite control in a beef cow/calf herd. Vet Parasitol 1997; 315-322:315–22.
16. Werner BA, Bergstrom RC. Numbers of gastrointestinal helminth eggs of Wyoming cattle in two surveys: 1957 to 1961 and 1973 to 1977. Am J Vet Res 1983;44: 301–3.

17. Hoberg EP, Lichtenfels JR, Rickard LG. Phylogeny for genera of Nematodirinae (Nematoda: Trichostrongylina). J Parasitol 2005;91:382–9.
18. Avramenko RW, Redman EM, Lewis R, et al. The use of nemabiome metabarcoding to explore gastro-intestinal nematode species diversity and anthelmintic treatment effectiveness in beef calves. Int J Parasitol 2017;47:893–902.
19. Gibbs HC. Persistence on pasture of the infective larvae of nematodes parasitizing Maine dairy cattle. Am J Vet Res 1980;41:1694–5.
20. Rickard LG, Zimmerman GL. The epizootiology of gastrointestinal nematodes of cattle in selected areas of Oregon. Vet Parasitol 1992;43:271–91.
21. Avramenko RW, Redman EM, Lewis R, et al. Exploring the gastrointestinal "Nemabiome": deep amplicon sequencing to quantify the species composition of parasitic nematode communities. PLoS One 2015;10:e0143559.
22. Scott H, Gilleard JS, Jelinski M, et al. Prevalence, fecal egg counts, and species identification of gastrointestinal nematodes in replacement dairy heifers in Canada. J Dairy Sci 2019;102:8251–63.
23. Stromberg BE, Corwin RM. Epizootiology of Ostertagia ostertagi in cow-calf production systems in the American midwest. Vet Parasitol 1993;46:297–302.
24. Harmon AF, Lucas BC, Hildreth MB. PCR comparison of trichostrongyle genera present in South Dakota cattle with and without springtime deworming. Proc Natl Acad Sci U S A 2009;88:147–54.
25. Corwin RM. Economics of gastrointestinal parasitism of cattle. Vet Parasitol 1997; 72:451–60.
26. Gibbs HC. The effects of subclinical disease on bovine gastrointestinal nematodiasis. Compend Contin Educ Pract Vet 1992;14:669–77.
27. Hawkins JA. Economic benefits of parasite control in cattle. Vet Parasitol 1993;46: 159–73.
28. Epperson WB, Kenzy BD, Mertz KJ, et al. A single pasture limited treatment approach to estimate productive loss from internal nematodes in grazing stocker cattle. Vet Parasitol 2001;97:269–76.
29. Mertz KJ, Hildreth MB, Epperson WB. Assessment of the effect of gastrointestinal nematode infestation on weight gain in grazing beef cattle. J Am Vet Med Assoc 2005;226:779–83.
30. Soll MD, Kunkle BN, Royer GC, et al. An eprinomectin extended-release injection formulation providing nematode control in cattle for up to 150 days. Vet Parasitol 2013;192:313–20.
31. Kunkle BN, Williams JC, Johnson EG, et al. Persistent efficacy and production benefits following use of extended-release injectable eprinomectin in grazing beef cattle under field conditions. Vet Parasitol 2013;192:332–7.
32. Baltzell P, Engelken T, O'Connor AM. A critical review and meta-analysis of the magnitude of the effect of anthelmintic use on stocker calf production parameters in Northern US States. Vet Parasitol 2015;214:2–11.
33. Edmonds MD, Vattab AF, Marchiondob AA, et al. Concurrent treatment with a macrocyclic lactone and benzimidizole provides season long performance advantages in grazing cattle harboring macrocyclic lactone resistant nematodes. Vet Parasitol 2018;252:157–62.
34. Wohlgemuth K, Melancon JJ. Relationship between weaning weights of North Dakota beef calves and treatment of their dams with ivermectin. Agri-Pract 1988;9:23–6.
35. Ballweber LR, Evans RR, Siefker C, et al. The effectiveness of doramectin pour-on in the control of gastrointestinal nematode infections in cow-calf herds. Vet Parasitol 2000;90:93–102.

36. Armour J, Duncan M. Arrested larval development in cattle nematodes. Parasitol Today 1987;3:171–6.

37. Saccareau M, Salle G, Robert-Granie C, et al. Meta-analysis of the parasitic phase traits of *Haemonchus contortus* infection in sheep. Parasit Vectors 2017; 10:201.

38. Verschave SH, Rose H, Morgan ER, et al. Modelling *Cooperia oncophora*: quantification of key parameters in the parasitic phase. Vet Parasitol 2016;223:111–4.

39. Ikpeze OO. Arrested development in nematodes of grazing ruminants: a review. Int J Zool 2009;1:25–31.

40. Falzon LC, Menzies PI, Shakya KP, et al. A longitudinal study on the effect of lambing season on the periparturient egg rise in Ontario sheep flocks. Prev Vet Med 2013;110:467–80.

41. Fleming MW. Selection for a strain of *Haemonchus contortus* that exhibits periparturient egg rise in sheep. J Parasitol 1993;79:399–402.

42. Hammerberg B, Lamm WD. Changes in periparturient fecal egg counts in beef cows calving in the spring. Am J Vet Res 1980;41(10):1686–9.

43. Romero-Escobedo E, Torres-Hernández G, Miguel BecerrilPérez C, et al. A comparison of Criollo and Suffolk ewes for resistance to *Haemonchus contortus* during the periparturient period. J Appl Anim Res 2016;46:17–23.

44. Slocombe JOD. Overwintering of bovine gastrointestinal nematodes in southwestern Ontario. Can J Comp Med 1974;38:90–3.

45. Ayalew L, Gibbs HC. Seasonal fluctuations of nematode populations in breeding ewes and lambs. Can J Comp Med 1973;37:79–89.

46. Gibbs HC. Relative importance of winter survival of larval nematodes in pasture and infected carrier calves in a study of parasitic gastroenteritis in calves. Am J Vet Res 1979;40:227–31.

47. Gibbs HC. The epidemiology of bovine ostertagiasis in the north temperate regions of North America. Vet Parasitol 1988;27:39–47.

48. Mertz KJ, Epperson WB, Hildreth MB. Survival-time for post-winter thirdstage juvenile trichostrongyles of cattle in the U.S.A. Northern Great Plains. Proc SD. Acad Sci 2019;98:41–52.

49. Smith HJ. On the persistence of infective *Ostertagia ostertagi*, *Cooperia oncophora* and *Nematodirus helvetianus* on pastures. Can J Comp Med 1972;36: 333–8.

50. Smith HJ, Archibald RM. On the survival of overwintering bovine gastrointestinal nematode larvae during the subsequent grazing season. Can J Comp Med 1969; 33:44–7.

51. Campbell DJ, Needham EN. An attempt to eliminate *Haemonchus contortus* from a sheep flock in Ontario. Can Vet J 1964;5:61–4.

52. Falzon LC, Menzies PI, VanLeeuwen J, et al. Pilot project to investigate overwintering of free-living gastrointestinal nematode larvae of sheep in Ontario, Canada. Can Vet J 2014;55:749–56.

53. Grosz DD, Eljaki AA, Holler LD, et al. Overwintering strategies of a population of anthelmintic-resistant *Haemonchus contortus* within a sheep flock from the United States Northern Great Plains. Vet Parasitol 2013;196(1–2):143–52.

54. Stromberg BE. Environmental factors influencing transmission. Vet Parasitol 1997;72:247–64.

55. Gasbarre LC. Anthelmintic resistance in cattle nematodes in the US. Vet Parasitol 2014;204:3–11.

56. Kaplan RM, Vidyashankar AN. An inconvenient truth: global worming and anthelmintic resistance. Vet Parasitol 2012;186:70–8.

57. Falzon LC, Menzies PI, Shakya KP, et al. Anthelmintic resistance in sheep flocks in Ontario, Canada. Vet Parasitol 2013;193:150–62.
58. Hoglund J, Gustafsson K, Ljungstrom BL, et al. Anthelmintic resistance in Swedish sheep flocks based on a comparison of the results from the faecal egg count reduction test and resistant allele frequencies of the beta-tubulin gene. Vet Parasitol 2009;161:60–8.
59. Papadopoulos E, Gallidis E, Ptochos S. Anthelmintic resistance in sheep in Europe: a selected review. Vet Parasitol 2012;189:85–8.
60. Ploeger HW, Everts RR. Alarming levels of anthelmintic resistance against gastrointestinal nematodes in sheep in the Netherlands. Vet Parasitol 2018;262:11–5.
61. Gasbarre LC, Smith LL, Hoberg E, et al. Further characterization of a cattle nematode population with demonstrated resistance to current anthelmintics. Vet Parasitol 2009;166:275–80.
62. Gasbarre LC, Smith LL, Lichtenfels JR, et al. The identification of cattle nematode parasites resistant to multiple classes of anthelmintics in a commercial cattle population in the US. Vet Parasitol 2009;166:281–5.
63. Edmonds MD, Johnson EG, Edmonds JD. Anthelmintic resistance of *Ostertagia ostertagi* and *Cooperia oncophora* to macrocyclic lactones in cattle from the western United States. Vet Parasitol 2010;170:224–9.
64. Rew R, Vercruysse J. Use of macrocyclic lactones to control cattle parasites in the USA and Canada. In: Vercruysse J, Rew R, editors. Macrocyclic lactones in antiparasitic therapy. Wallingford (England): CABI Publishing; 2002. p. 248–61.
65. Stromberg BE, Averbeck GA. The role of parasite epidemiology in the management of grazing cattle. Int J Parasitol 1999;29:33–9.
66. Stromberg BE, Gasbarre LC. Gastrointestinal nematode control programs with an emphasis on cattle. Vet Clin North Am Food Anim Pract 2006;22:543–65.
67. Williams JC. Anthelminthic treatment strategies: current status and future. Vet Parasitol 1997;72:461–77.
68. Corwin RM, Stromberg BE. Internal parasitism and deworming of beef cattle: status in the 1990s. Vet Med 1995;90:486–92.
69. Craig TM. The anthelmintic dilemma. Compend Contin Educ Pract Vet 1999;21: S125–43.
70. Vercruysse J, Rew R. General efficacy of the macrocyclic lactones to control parasites of cattle. In: Vercruysse RSRAJ, editor. Macrocyclic lactones in antiparasitic therapy. Wallingford (England): CABI Publishing, CAB International; 2002. p. 185–222.
71. Sutherland IA, Brown AE, Leathwick DM, et al. Resistance to prophylactic treatment with macrocyclic lactone anthelmintics in *Teladorsagia circumcincta*. Vet Parasitol 2003;115:301–9.
72. Molento MB, Nielsen MK, Kaplan RM. Resistance to avermectin/milbemycin anthelmintics in equine cyathostomins: current situation. Vet Parasitol 2012;185: 16–24.

Biology, Epidemiology, and Control of Gastrointestinal Nematodes of Small Ruminants

Anne M. Zajac, DVM, PhD[a],*, Javier Garza, PhD[b]

KEYWORDS

- Nematodes • *Haemonchus contortus* • Trichostrongyles • Anthelmintics
- Combination treatments

KEY POINTS

- Gastrointestinal nematodes of small ruminants, especially *Haemonchus contortus*, are a principal cause of morbidity and mortality in the United States.
- The geographic distribution and success of important trichostrongyle parasites depend on the development and survival of their larvae in the environment.
- Current recommendations for anthelmintic use include combination treatments and targeted treatment.

In the United States, internal parasites are a leading cause of known, nonpredator goat and kid losses reported to the National Animal Health Monitoring System.[1] The internal parasites responsible for most of these deaths are gastrointestinal nematodes (GINs) belonging to the order Strongylida, superfamily Trichostrongyloidea. Grazing sheep and goats throughout North America are infected with a community of these strongylid nematodes, whose combined clinical effect is the condition known as parasitic gastroenteritis (PGE).[2] Basic knowledge of the biology of these organisms is important for the design of effective management programs.

Nematodes belonging to other taxonomic orders also commonly parasitize the intestines of small ruminants in the United States and Canada. These nematodes include *Aoncotheca* (formerly *Capillaria*) and *Strongyloides* (small intestine), and *Skrjabinema* and *Trichuris* (large intestine).[2–4] These parasites are not important pathogens and cause disease only in unusual circumstances. The presence of their eggs in fecal examinations is usually considered incidental and most are controlled by anthelmintics used for treatment of the more important species.

---

[a] Department of Biomedical Sciences and Pathobiology, Virginia/Maryland College of Veterinary Medicine, Virginia Tech, Blacksburg, VA 24061-0442, USA; [b] Leica Biosystems, 1700 Leider Lane, Buffalo Grove, IL 60089, USA
* Corresponding author.
E-mail address: azajac@vt.edu

Vet Clin Food Anim 36 (2020) 73–87
https://doi.org/10.1016/j.cvfa.2019.12.005
0749-0720/20/© 2020 Elsevier Inc. All rights reserved.

IMPORTANT STRONGYLID SPECIES

Although all grazing sheep and goats are infected with GINs, low worm burdens usually have little impact on animal health. As worm numbers increase, subclinical effects, including reduced weight gain and decreased appetite, occur. With heavier worm burdens, clinical signs may develop, including weight loss, anemia, submandibular edema, and diarrhea.[2–5]

The most important of the strongylid nematodes in North America and many other regions is *Haemonchus contortus*, the barber pole worm (also referred to as barber's pole or wireworm). *H contortus* adults parasitize the small ruminant abomasum. Female *H contortus* reach about 3 cm in length, making this species one of the largest strongylid nematodes of ruminants. During necropsy, *H contortus* and its distinctive barber pole appearance are readily seen in the abomasal contents,[2,3] whereas other species are much smaller and easily overlooked unless the contents are examined under a microscope.

Haemonchus is a highly fecund nematode. A female worm may produce 10,000 eggs daily, and larvae on pastures can accumulate rapidly during the grazing season.[2–5,6] The prepatent period (length of time elapsing between host infection and parasite maturity to the egg-laying stage) is usually 17 to 21 days. Adult worms are short lived, typically surviving in the host for only a few months,[7] although the length of time can be much longer in some animals and circumstances.

The pathogenic potential of *H contortus* is the result of the blood-feeding behavior of the parasites in the abomasum. Heavy infections can cause fatal anemia. Unlike many other parasites of the gastrointestinal tract, *H contortus* is not a primary cause of diarrhea.[2,6] Consequently, the course of infection is often insidious because routine observation of animals may not detect disease until deaths occur. Haemonchosis and PGE in general occur most often in young, nonimmune animals (those less than about 1 year of age), adult animals whose immunity is compromised, or in sheep or goats exposed to very high levels of infection.[2–4,6] Although other trichostrongylid nematodes can add to the burden of parasitism in small ruminants, *H contortus* is the primary cause of parasite-related disease in most of the United States[8,9] Because of the overriding importance of *H contortus*, it is the most frequently studied GIN and is the focus of this article.

OTHER STRONGYLID SPECIES

Species of the genus *Trichostrongylus* are also common GINs that are usually secondary contributors to PGE in North America. Several species of *Trichostrongylus* infect small ruminants, including *Trichostrongylus axei* in the abomasum, and *T colubriformis* and *T vitrinus* in the small intestine. These small, thin worms (<1 cm) are not readily visible in gastrointestinal contents, and detection usually requires removal and close examination of gut contents under a microscope.[5] Adult *Trichostrongylus* are longer lived than *H contortus* adults and can survive over winter as adults in the host.[3] Heavy burdens of *Trichostrongylus* can cause severe diarrhea, weight loss, and death,[3,5] and *T colubriformis* is often the second most common species infecting small ruminants in the United States. Although GINs are generally not considered to be zoonotic, 2 cases of human infection with *Trichostrongylus* sp were reported from Australia. Infected individuals used fresh goat manure as fertilizer for vegetables that were consumed raw.[10]

Another trichostrongylid nematode that contributes to PGE in the United States and Canada is *Teladorsagia (Ostertagia) circumcincta*. Like *H contortus*, *T circumcincta* is an abomasal parasite. Following infection, *T circumcincta* larvae spend a variable period of time developing in abomasal gastric glands. These larvae cause changes in the glands that lead to formation of visible nodules on the mucosal surface of the abomasum. In heavy infections the most common clinical signs are diarrhea, anemia, and hypoproteinemia, and in severe cases death can occur. More commonly, moderate levels of infection with *T circumcincta* contribute to PGE, with signs including diarrhea and poor weight gain or weight loss.[2,3] *T circumcincta* is a smaller parasite than *H contortus* (females are ~1 cm long).[5] On necropsy of infected animals, the abomasal nodules produced by larvae are readily seen, but the worms are very difficult to see and are often missed unless contents are removed and examined more closely. The prepatent period of this parasite is approximately 3 weeks.[2,3,5] Although *T circumcincta* is found throughout the United States and Canada, this genus is most important in more northern areas because of the environmental preference of its larvae for cooler climatic conditions.[11]

Cooperia curticei, *Nematodirus spathiger*, and *Nematodirus filicollis* are common small intestinal parasites of sheep and goats, as is *Oesophagostomum venulosum* in the large bowel. *Bunostomum trigonocephalum* and *Chabertia ovina* are less common parasites of the small intestine and large intestine, respectively.[3–5] These species are rarely pathogenic alone because of low numbers typically being present, but may contribute to PGE.[2] *Nematodirus battus*, which causes severe diarrhea in lambs in some European countries, was identified in the United States in sheep and llamas for the first time in the 1980s.[12] The discovery of the parasite aroused concern that it could become an important pathogen in North America. However, disease problems associated with this parasite have not developed to date.

HOST SPECIFICITY

Grazing of small ruminants with cattle or horses or alternating grazing of small ruminant pastures with cattle or horses is often recommended as a component of small ruminant integrated parasite management programs.[13–16] However, producers are often concerned that mixing livestock species will result in cross-infection. Although cattle are infected by the same genera of parasites as small ruminants, most of the species are different, and cross-infection leading to PGE is rarely reported. In general, strongylid species that parasitize small ruminants do not establish well when ingested by other species. One exception to this is *H contortus*, which is capable of infecting cattle, and clinical haemonchosis has been reported in calves less than a year of age.[17–19] Investigators in New Zealand have recently suggested that preweaned cattle could be a significant source of *H contortus* on sheep pastures.[20] Also, *T axei* can successfully infect cattle, horses, and pigs,[2,3] but *T axei* infections in the United States are usually minor and the parasite has not been reported as a clinical problem for mixed or alternate grazing systems in Canada or the United States.[8]

Producers are often interested to know whether small ruminant nematodes can infect white-tailed deer, which frequently invade pastures. Natural infections with several small ruminant trichostrongyles have been described, and clinical haemonchosis has been reported in fawns,[21] but there is no clear evidence from the United States or Canada suggesting that deer are important in *H contortus* transmission. However, researchers in Europe have suggested that various deer species may be important reservoirs of small ruminant parasites,[22] and the role of white-tailed deer should be examined more closely in the United States and Canada.

LIFE CYCLE

The same life cycle generally applies to all the economically important strongylid parasites of small ruminants in the United States and Canada. In this simple cycle, adult female parasites in the abomasum or intestines produce eggs that are passed in the manure. Development occurs within the fecal mass, which provides some protection from environmental conditions. A first-stage larva (L1) forms and hatches out of the egg. After hatching, larvae feed on bacteria, molt to the second larval stage (L2), and then undergo another molt to reach the infective third larval stage (L3). Third-stage larvae move out of the fecal material and onto the forage, where they are ingested by sheep and goats while grazing.[2,3,5] Nematodirus spp are an exception to the life cycle described earlier. The L3 develops inside the egg before hatching occurs. Eggs are generally cold tolerant, and, in some species, hatching is stimulated by a period of low temperature followed by higher temperature.[23]

STRONGYLID LARVA BIOLOGY

The fortunes of strongylid larvae in the microenvironment of the fecal pellets and on herbage ultimately determine whether or not a producer will battle parasitic disease. Appreciating the biology of the immature parasite stages is critical for predicting parasite distribution and for formulating integrated parasite management programs.

In general, development of trichostrongylid larvae in the manure from egg to L3 occurs in a temperature range of approximately 10°C to 36°C (50°F–96°F).[5,11] However, within this range individual species have specific preferences. H contortus is the most important GIN of small ruminants in the United States, not only because of its pathogenic potential but because this prolific parasite finds the climate in a large part of the country highly favorable for development and survival of its infective larvae.[5] H contortus is often described as a parasite of the tropics and develops to L3 most successfully in temperatures of about 25°C to 38°C.[11] Southeast and parts of southcentral United States, in particular, with hot, humid summers and a long grazing season, are ideal for H contortus.[24–27] In the remainder of the United States and southern Canada, H contortus is still a common, and typically dominant, component of the GIN population, capable of causing significant losses. In the northern limits of the parasite's distribution the shorter transmission season may not regularly allow accumulation of parasites to clinically important levels.[28–31] For example, based on 1960s temperature and rainfall data, Levine predicted that optimum conditions for transmission of H contortus occurred from May through September in Urbana, Illinois, but were present from mid-March to mid-October in Columbus, Georgia.[32] Even within broader environmental preferences for each species, there is evidence of some local adaptation. Eggs of H contortus from the United Kingdom, where summer temperatures are cooler, hatched at lower temperatures than H contortus strains from Kentucky and New York.[33,34] Despite some strain variation, environmental stages of H contortus are cold intolerant and do not survive freezing winter weather.[11]

Teladorsagia circumcinta and Trichostrongylus spp are also found throughout the United States. Teladorsagia is the most cold tolerant of the 3 genera, with egg to L3 development occurring best at temperatures between 16°C and 30°C[11]. After eggs of Haemonchus and Teladorsagia isolated in the state of Washington were exposed to a 15-hour period of 18°C, greater than 87% of T circumcincta eggs but less than 4% of H contortus eggs were able to hatch.[35] Similarly, when L3 of the 2 species were exposed to −18 C for 5 hours, the viability of H contortus L3 declined to less than 5%; T circumcincta L3 viability was 85%.[36] Trichostrongylus is between Haemonchus and Teladorsagia in terms of temperature preference, but is the most drought tolerant of these genera.[11] In the United States and Canada the contribution of these genera to the total GIN population may increase where shorter transmissions seasons and/or dry summers reduce the success of H contortus.[28,31,37,38]

Equally important for successful development of eggs to L3 is moisture. Moisture level in feces during the larval developmental period is affected by moisture level at the time of feces deposition, soil moisture levels, and precipitation. These factors interact in complex ways to affect whether successful parasite development occurs.[6,11,32,39–41] In general, it is reasonable to assume that drought disadvantages parasite development and moist conditions are favorable. For this reason, the arid summers in some regions of the western United States have historically reduced transmission rates of most GINs.[37,38] However, *H contortus* can become an important parasite in dry regions where irrigation occurs. In a study conducted in the 1970s in Utah, conditions were suitable for transmission of *H contortus* on irrigated pasture during 5 of the 6 months of the experiment. In contrast, conditions were never suitable for transmission on the nonirrigated pasture during the study.[42] Recent growth in smaller flocks that may use irrigated land is likely to be accompanied by an increase in the importance of *H contortus*, and changes in parasite epidemiology in this region should be closely monitored.[43]

The length of time required for development to the L3 stage varies most directly with temperature. The minimum length of time required for the development of *H contortus* L3 is about 3 to 4 days,[5,11] which can rapidly lead to massive pasture contamination in hot, humid weather. In contrast, eggs deposited in cool spring weather develop more slowly and may require weeks to become L3. As a result, spring pastures in more northern states may not carry a substantial burden of infective larvae until late in spring or early summer.[6,11,28]

Once larvae reach the infective stage they must leave fecal pellets and migrate onto forage. Rain is important in releasing larvae from the manure. During dry weather, larvae are retained in the pellets and can accumulate. A subsequent rain event results in larval release. Producers may see an outbreak of parasitic disease a few weeks after the end of a period of drought when animals are exposed to large numbers of newly available L3.[6,11,41–45] If small ruminant producers are made aware of this epidemiologic issue, then proactive monitoring of animals a few weeks after the end of a drought period, together with application of targeted treatments, can yield important benefits for animal health and productivity.

L3 can migrate both laterally and vertically, but this migration is affected by air temperature, soil moisture, and relative humidity. The random movement of larvae is highly dependent on the availability of moisture. Some *H contortus* larvae can migrate up to 90 cm away from fecal pellets, but most remain within about 10 cm of the feces.[41,46] In addition, most GIN larvae cannot migrate vertically more than 5 cm from the ground.[41,47] This limitation has important implications for how the pasture forage is managed; animals forced to graze on short forage ingest many more larvae than when grazing tall forage. In hot, dry weather, when no moisture is on the grass and humidity is low, larvae are unable to migrate on the herbage.[46] Forage type also seems to influence migration of larvae on pastures, possibly because of differences in temperature and humidity in stands of different forages or the ease with which the moisture film required by L3 develops on leaves.[48,49]

The length of time that L3 can survive on pasture is also important for pasture management programs. Nematodes are covered by a tough semipermeable outer layer called the cuticle. The cuticle is replaced with each molt, but the L3 retains the L2 cuticle, yielding a double cuticle that is protective to the worm.[3,6] Although the double cuticle layer provides L3 greater resistance to environmental conditions, it also prevents feeding. Once L3 deplete their stored energy reserves, they die. Consequently, the best conditions for survival of L3 are cool, dry weather, because dry weather reduces movement of larvae and use of their stored reserves. Cool, moist weather also supports survival of L3 for many months. L3 survive for much shorter periods in hot weather because of the higher metabolic rate, which rapidly depletes energy reserves. In temperate portions of the United States, a pasture that has been grazed by sheep or goats should be rested for 6 months during cool weather to be considered safe (limited number of larvae remaining). In hot weather, most larvae are cleared from pasture in 3 months,[8] although even periods as short as 4 to 6 weeks greatly reduce pasture larvae numbers during hot, wet, tropical-like weather.[11,50] Other factors affecting larval survival include parasite species, larval location on pasture, and forage height, making precise predictions of survival at a specific location very difficult.

HYPOBIOSIS

The epidemiology of important GINs is also strongly influenced by aspects of host/parasite biology after infection occurs. Larvae of important GINs are able to undergo a period of arrested development (hypobiosis) in the host. Following infection, larvae may become metabolically inactive for a period up to several months and then resume development.[51] Immunity seems to be 1 factor associated with larval arrest, because immune animals have a higher proportion of hypobiotic larvae than nonimmune animals. The highest rates of hypobiosis typically occur at times of the year when conditions in the environment are least favorable for development and survival of eggs and larvae.[51–53] In areas of the United States with cold winters, Haemonchus survives the winter months primarily as arrested larvae, because most environmental stages are unlikely to survive the winter. In lambs in Ohio, Maine, Virginia, Pennsylvania and South Dakota, most, H contortus and some other GINs in animals were present as arrested larvae in winter.[29,54,55] Even without anthelmintic treatment in states with cold winters, problems with Haemonchus usually resolve at the end of the grazing season because most newly ingested larvae become arrested in the host. Consequently, as existing adult worms die they are not immediately replaced. Also, eggs shed at the end of the grazing season are unlikely to develop or develop very slowly, preventing further L3 buildup on pasture. Where winters are very mild, hypobiosis seems to be less important in the epidemiology of parasite transmission. In Louisiana, levels of hypobiotic larvae were never substantial in tracer lambs followed throughout the year, although the highest proportion of hypobiotic larvae tended to be in the fall.[26]

In areas where winter arrest of parasite larvae occurs, emergence and development of adult worms in late winter and spring are followed by an increase in fecal egg counts. The increase in egg counts is magnified in periparturient animals by a relaxation of immunity that increases survival and egg production in existing parasites and also increases susceptibility to further infection. The periparturient egg "rise" (PPR) can make an important contribution to L3 populations on pastures as young, susceptible animals begin grazing.[51] The PPR and its epidemiologic importance is well documented in sheep, but less so in goats.[56,57]

IMPACT OF CLIMATE CHANGE

Increased temperatures and extended growing seasons occurring as a result of changes in the climate caused by global warming are expected to increase the risk of PGE generally, and haemonchosis in particular. However, the complexity of management and environmental factors that influence the transmission of GINs complicate the ability to measure the changes caused by climate change.[58,59] Computer modeling has predicted that infection pressure from H contortus will increase in northern temperate areas and that even small temperature changes could increase the infection intensity of parasites at the limit of their geographic range enough to cause increased clinical disease outbreaks.[60–62] Clinical haemonchosis in the United Kingdom, previously uncommon, has been increasingly reported in recent years, probably related, at least in part, to climate change. The range of *H contortus* and reports of clinical haemonchosis have also increased in Australia.[63,64] At present there are no similar reports clearly linking changes in distribution of GINs in the United States and Canada with climate change, although anecdotal reports strongly suggest that *H contortus* populations are increasing in more northern areas as average temperatures increase.

ANTHELMINTICS

Highly effective broad-spectrum anthelmintics with wide safety margins first became available in the 1960s and producers have relied on these products for control of GINs ever since. In areas where *H contortus* causes substantial losses, frequent treatments throughout the grazing season were recommended, which most likely contributed to current widespread resistance seen in GIN populations, especially in *H contortus*.[8,27,65–67] For most producers, parasite control continues to include some level of anthelmintic use, but veterinarians working with sheep and goats should stress the importance of alternative methods of parasite control; for example, genetic selection and pasture management (see Joan M. Burke and James E. Miller's article, "Sustainable Approaches to Parasite Control in Ruminant Livestock," in this issue) used in combination with anthelmintics. A further incentive to look beyond anthelmintic-based control programs is the increased public demand for animal products raised more sustainably, and using organic production methods.

All of the approved available anthelmintics for sheep and/or goats in the United States belong to 1 of 3 major drug groups: the benzimidazoles, the cholinergic agonists, and the macrocyclic lactones. When a population of worms becomes resistant to 1 member of a drug group, it effectively becomes resistant to the other members of the group.[68] The drugs discussed next are currently approved for use in sheep or goats in the United States.

Benzimidazoles

Albendazole (ABZ) and fenbendazole (FBZ) are the benzimidazole (BZ) drugs marketed in the United States for small ruminants. At this time, ABZ is only approved for use in sheep for GINs, and FBZ is only approved for goats. However, ABZ is approved for both sheep and goats for treatment of the liver fluke, *Fasciola hepatica*. The primary mode of action of benzimidazoles is inhibition of microtubule formation.[68,69] Resistance to BZ drugs is extremely common in GINs in the United States, and evidence suggests that resistance is present on most farms.[70] Thus, farms using BZ drugs should check the efficacy before relying on them. ABZ is contraindicated for use in the first 30 days of gestation because of embryotoxic effects in early pregnancy.[68]

Macrocyclic Lactones

The macrocyclic lactones (MLs) include 2 products approved for oral use in sheep: ivermectin and moxidectin. Other MLs approved only for use in cattle in the United States are eprinomectin and doramectin, but there is rarely a justification for using these drugs in place of ivermectin or moxidectin for control of GINs in small ruminants. The ML group has activity against both nematodes and arthropods and is widely used in livestock and horses. Drugs in this group interfere with chloride channel neurotransmission.[69,71] MLs have been extensively used by small ruminant producers and, like

BZ, widespread resistance to the group is seen in *H contortus* and other trichostrongyles.[65–67,70] Thus, similar to BZ drugs, farms using ML drugs, especially ivermectin, should check the efficacy before relying on them.

Nicotinic Agonist Anthelmintics

This designation covers 2 groups (imidazothiazoles and tetrahydropyrimidines) with very similar modes of action that target the parasite nervous system; these act as nicotinic agonists and cause nematode paralysis.[68,69] Drugs in this group approved for use in small ruminants include levamisole and morantel; pyrantel, a very similar drug, is not approved for use in any ruminant. Although levamisole is chemically different from pyrantel and morantel, there is evidence that parasites that develop resistance to 1 compound will be resistant to all.[68] However, this is not known to occur in every case and the different drugs should be tested separately to confirm efficacy. In the United States, morantel is approved for use in medicated feed for goats, and in dairy goats can be used with no milk withdrawal required.

Other Anthelmintics

Two additional anthelmintic products have recently become available in Canada as prescription-only products, but they are not marketed in the United States: closantel and a combination of abamectin plus derquantel. Closantel is a salicylanilide compound that inhibits energy metabolism by uncoupling oxidative phosphorylation in blood-feeding parasites such as *H contortus* and *F hepatica*. However, it has limited efficacy against other GINs. The drug has a long half-life and continues to have activity against *H contortus* for several weeks after administration.[3,16] Derquantel is a nicotinic cholinergic antagonist in the spiroindole group. Because it is not uniformly effective against GINs, it is only marketed in combination with abamectin, with which it has a synergistic interaction.[72] Also, because both closantel and derquantel/abamectin contain compounds in drug groups that are distinct from those already discussed, they have efficacy against populations of GINs resistant to the common anthelmintic products sold in the United States and Canada. However, reduced efficacy of the derquantel/abamectin combination has been observed in other countries with high levels of macrocyclic lactone resistance.[73]

USE OF ANTHELMINTICS IN PARASITE MANAGEMENT PROGRAMS

Anthelmintics remain an important component in the arsenal for controlling GINs. Current recommendations for the use of available anthelmintics are designed to maximize efficacy and reduce further selection for resistant parasites. Multiple factors act in combination to influence the rate at which anthelmintic resistance develops. One important selection pressure contributing to drug resistance in small ruminants has been widespread use of frequent treatments in suppressive treatment programs. Sustainable anthelmintic use should minimize the number of anthelmintic treatments while maintaining a population of drug-susceptible parasites in refugia. The concept and use of refugia are important for recommendations for anthelmintic use[74] and are the subject of another Andrew W. Greer and colleagues' article, "Refugia-Based Strategies for Parasite Control in Livestock," in this issue.

ANTHELMINTIC CHOICE AND DOSE

Sheep and goat owners often believe their anthelmintics are fully effective because their animals are alive and appear normal. However, drug resistance is so pervasive in the United States that it is likely that most producers are using products that are far less effective than they were when first introduced, and those products are continuing to lose efficacy. Anthelmintic efficacy can be tested with a fecal egg count reduction test, which calculates the percentage reduction in posttreatment egg counts compared with pretreatment counts (see Ray M. Kaplan's article, "Biology, Epidemiology, Diagnosis, and Management of Anthelmintic Resistance in Gastrointestinal Nematodes of Livestock," in this issue). The DrenchRite larval development assay is an in vitro test that simultaneously tests for resistance against all major anthelmintics used in small ruminants in the United States by evaluating development of GIN eggs to the infective stage in the presence of the anthelmintics. Despite recommendations to test anthelmintic efficacy, most owners fail to do this and so continue to use drugs with suboptimal to poor anthelmintic activity.

Anthelmintics with reduced efficacy can still be used in a combination treatment.[75–77] A combination treatment consists of 2 or 3 drugs from different drug groups (MLs, BZs, nicotinic agonists) administered sequentially at the same time. In some countries, commercial products are sold that contain mixtures of multiple anthelmintics, but currently in the United States there are no approved combination products. Instead, products from different groups can be given sequentially over a short period. Withdrawal times for all products used must be followed, thus when given in combination the withdrawal time of the drug with the longest withdrawal period must be adhered to. Anthelmintics given in combination typically work in an additive fashion, even if neither is fully effective; as an example, if one drug is 60% effective and the other is 75% effective, then the first can remove 60% of the worms and the second will remove 75% of the remaining worms, yielding an efficacy of 90%. Use of combination treatments has 2 important advantages. First, it is far more likely than use of a single product to provide an effective treatment. Second, because each drug removes parasites resistant to the other, the rate of growth of resistant worm populations is slowed for both drugs, particularly when adequate refugia containing susceptible worms are available to provide reinfection.[75,78] As a general rule, use of a combination treatment is now preferred to single-drug use. Although use of combination treatments extends the useful life of commercial anthelmintics, combinations must be used in conjunction with a strategy that preserves a refugium of anthelmintic-susceptible parasites. An example is use of the FAMACHA program of targeted selective treatment.[79] Combination treatments should not be used in all animals in a suppressive treatment program because they exert high selection pressure for multiple drug resistance.

Another type of combination treatment composed of a BZ and a copper oxide wire particle bolus was also found in 1 study to be more effective than either product alone when administered to BZ-resistant parasites in a sheep flock.[80] Copper oxide wire particle boluses are an alternative to commercial anthelmintics that have activity primarily against *H contortus*.[81,82]

In general, dose levels of commercial anthelmintics do not differ for sheep and cattle. However, goats metabolize anthelmintics faster than sheep and cattle and thus require higher doses.[76,83] Because so few products in the United States and Canada are approved for use in goats, owners often have used cattle and sheep label doses of anthelmintics, resulting in widespread underdosing. Subtherapeutic anthelmintic levels are an additional selection factor for resistance and the common use of cattle/sheep doses in goats has probably contributed to the rapid development of drug resistance in *H contortus* and other GINs.[84] For useful information on correct doses of common anthelmintic products for sheep and goats, see the Web site of the American Consortium for Small Ruminant Parasite Control (https://www.wormx.info/dewormers). As an additional resource, the US Food Animal Residue Avoidance

Databank has published information on suggested withdrawal times for meat and milk for fenbendazole, ivermectin, and moxidectin.[85]

ANTHELMINTIC FORMULATION

It is noteworthy that all products approved for small ruminants in the United States and Canada are sold only as oral formulations. Several studies have shown that levels of anthelmintic present in worms recovered from treated animals are highest when MLs are delivered orally.[72] Therefore, anthelmintic products used for treatment of GINs in small ruminants should be delivered only by the oral route.

USE OF ANTHELMINTICS IN PARASITE MANAGEMENT PROGRAMS

Regardless of which anthelmintics are used by sheep and goat owners, the rate of development of resistance can usually be reduced by using drugs selectively and in combination while also preserving parasite refugia. In the United States, the FAMA-CHA program of targeted selective treatment is highly recommended where *H contortus* is the predominant GIN. Animals can be assessed individually by matching the color of the conjunctival mucous membranes to a color on the FAMACHA card, which then directs whether treatment is needed. When used regularly this system is an efficient and effective way to administer treatment selectively and prevent severe anemia.[9] Training in the use of FAMACHA is required for producers and can be provided by extension programs, veterinarians, or by an on-line certification program provided by the University of Rhode Island (https://web.uri.edu/sheepngoat/famacha/) Use of the FAMACHA system not only reduces, often dramatically, the number of animals dewormed, thereby increasing the refugia, but it also alerts owners to developing anemia in their flocks or herds before severe disease or death losses occur. Even in large flocks and herds, the system can be used by scoring a group of sentinel animals, usually kids or lambs, that are the most susceptible animals and, therefore, most likely to be anemic. Based on the scores of these animals, the need for additional testing can be determined. Further information on the FAMACHA system and obtaining cards can be obtained at the Web site of the ACSRPC (https://www.wormx.info/famacha). Andrew W. Greer and colleagues' article, "Refugia-Based Strategies for Parasite Control in Livestock," in this issue provides detailed information on refugia-based strategies.

Two common practices used for parasite management in the United States and Canada may increase the rate of accumulation of resistant worms by administering anthelmintic to animals when the refugia are low. In the first case, owners deworm all sheep or goats in conjunction with a move to pasture contaminated with few or no GIN infective larvae. Because resistant worms remain in the treated animals, the new pasture becomes contaminated primarily with resistant parasites.[3] Better strategies are to assess animals individually (FAMACHA) and treat accordingly or treat only a portion of the animals before moving them to lightly infected or clean pastures. In this way, both drug-resistant and drug-susceptible GINs are introduced onto the new pasture.

The second case is the routine practice of treating periparturient animals, which is routinely recommended by veterinarians for all ewes and does to avoid clinical and/or subclinical disease in lactating females and their offspring. In the case of small ruminants lambing/kidding in the spring in the northern United States and Canada, this treatment often occurs at a time when the refugia are low following freezing winter weather. Thus, it is important that treatment of periparturient animals be done in a targeted selective manner.[86] In Canada, clinical haemonchosis is often seen in lambing ewes as a result of synchronous resumed development by hypobiotic larvae. Investigators in Ontario found that FAMACHA scores in periparturient ewes were significantly associated with *H contortus* egg counts and recommended deworming animals with a score greater than 3.[87] If desired, body condition score and litter size could also be considered in identifying animals for treatment.

The rapid increase in anthelmintic resistance in *H contortus* and other GINs combined with changing global climate conditions can be expected to increase the clinical significance of PGE. Appreciating the climatic requirements and behavior of environmental stages of the parasites will be important in formulating management programs to complement sustainable practices for anthelmintic use.

DISCLOSURE

Dr. Zajac receives research support from USDA-NIFA (Engineered Probiotics for Farm Animal and Human Nematodes MASW-2015-11323).

REFERENCES

1. National Animal Health Monitoring System, US Department of Agriculture. Goat and kid predator and nonpredator death loss in the United States, 2015. Available at: https://www.aphis.usda.gov/animal_health/nahms/general/downloads/goat_kid_deathloss_2015.pdf. Accessed June 15, 2019.
2. Bowman DD. Georgi's parasitology for veterinarians. 10th edition. St Louis (MO): Elsevier; 2014.
3. Sutherland I, Scott I. Gastrointestinal nematodes of sheep and goats. Chichester (England): Wiley-Blackwell; 2010.
4. Smith MC, Sherman DM. Goat medicine. 2nd edition. Ames (IA): Wiley-Blackwell; 2009.
5. Levine N. Nematode parasites of domestic animals and of man. Minneapolis (MN): Burgess Publishing Company; 1980.
6. Besier RB, Kahn LP, Sargison ND, et al. The pathophysiology, ecology and epidemiology of *Haemonchus contortus* infection in small ruminants. Adv Parasitol 2016;93:95–143.
7. Courtney CH, Parker CF, McClure KE, et al. Population dynamics of *Haemonchus contortus* and *Trichostrongylus* spp in sheep. Int J Parasitol 1983;13:557–60.
8. Fleming S, Craig T, Kaplan RM, et al. Anthelmintic resistance of gastrointestinal parasites in small ruminants. J Vet Intern Med 2006;20:435–44.
9. Whitley NC, Oh SH, Lee SJ, et al. Impact of integrated gastrointestinal nematode management training for U.S goat and sheep producers. Vet Parasitol 2014;200: 271–5.
10. Ralph A, O'Sullivan MVN, Sangster NC, et al. Abdominal pain and eosinophilia in suburban goat keepers. Med J Austral 2006;184:467–9.
11. O'Connor LJ, Waldken-Brown SW, Kahn LP. Ecology of the free-living stages of major trichostrongylid parasites of sheep. Vet Parasitol 2006;142:1–15.
12. Zimmerman GL, Hoberg EP, Rickard LG, et al. Broadened geographic range and periods of transmission for *Nematodirus battus* in the United States. Proc Annu Meet US Anim Health Assoc 1986;90:404–12.
13. Barger IA. The role of epidemiological knowledge and grazing management for helminth control in small ruminants. Int J Parasitol 1999;29:41–7.
14. Jordan HE, Phillips WA, Morrison RD, et al. A 3-year study of continuous mixed grazing of cattle and sheep: parasitism of offspring. Int J Parasitol 1988;18: 77–784.

15. Marshall R, Gebrelul S, Gray L, et al. Mixed species grazing of cattle and goats on gastrointestinal infections of *Haemonchus contortus*. Amer J Anim Vet Sci 2012;7:61–6.

16. Besier RB, Kahn LP, Sargison ND, et al. Diagnosis, treatment and management of *Haemonchus contortus* in small ruminants. Adv Parasitol 2016;93:183–238.

17. DeVaney JA, Craig TM, Rowe LD. Resistance to ivermectin in *Haemonchus contortus* in goats and calves. Int J Parasitol 1992;22:369–76.

18. Fávero FC, Buzzulini C, Cruz BC, et al. Experimental infections of calves with *Haemonchus placei* and *Haemonchus contortus:* assessment of parasitological parameters. Vet Parasitol 2016;217:25–8.

19. Hogg R, Whitaker K, Collins R, et al. Haemonchosis in large ruminants in the UK. Vet Rec 2010;166:373–4.

20. Waghorn TS, Bouchet CLG, Bekelaar K, et al. Nematode parasites in young cattle: what role for unexpected species? NZ Vet J 2019;67:40–5.

21. Hoberg EP, Kocan AA, Rickard LG. Gastrointestinal strongyles in wild ruminants. In: Samuel WM, Pybus MJ, Kocan AA, editors. Parasitic diseases of wild mammals. 2nd edition. Ames (IA): Iowa State University Press; 2001. p. 193–228.

22. Chintoan-Uta C, Morgan ER, Skuce PJ, et al. Wild deer as potential vectors of anthelmintic-resistant abomasal nematodes between cattle and sheep farms. Proc R Soc B 2014;281:20132985.

23. Rickard LG, Hoberg E, Zimmerman GL, et al. Late fall transmission of *Nematodirus battus* (Nematoda:Trichostrongyloidea) in Western Oregon. J Parasitol 1987; 73:244–7.

24. Craig TM. Epidemiology and control of gastrointestinal nematodes and cestodes in small ruminants: Southern United States. Vet Clin N Amer Food Anim Prac 1986;2:367–72.

25. Amarante AFT, Craig TM, Ramsey WS, et al. Comparison of naturally acquired parasite burdens among Florida Native, Rambouillet and crossbreed ewes. Vet Parasitol 1999;85:61–9.

26. Miller JE, Bahirathan M, Lemarie SL, et al. Epidemiology of gastrointestinal nematode parasitism in Suffolk and Gulf Coast Native sheep with special emphasis on relative susceptibility to *Haemonchus contortus* infection. Vet Parasitol 1998;74: 55–74.

27. Mortensen LL, Williamson LH, Terrill TT, et al. Evaluation of prevalence and clinical implications of anthelmintic resistance in gastrointestinal nematodes of goats. J Amer Vet Med Assoc 2003;223:495–500.

28. Herd RP. Epidemiology and control of gastrointestinal nematodes and cestodes in small ruminants: Northern United States. Vet Clin N Amer Food Anim Prac 1986;2:367–72.

29. Coyne MJ, Smith G, Johnstone C. Fecundity of gastrointestinal trichostrongylid nematodes of sheep in the field. Am J Vet Res 1991;52:1182–8.

30. Aaylew L, Gibbs HC. Seasonal fluctuations of nematode populations in breeding ewes and lambs. Can J Comp Med 1973;37:79–89.

31. Mederos A, Fernández S, VanLeeuwen J, et al. Prevalence and distribution of gastrointestinal nematodes on 32 organic and conventional commercial sheep farms in Ontario and Quebec, Canada (2006-2008). Vet Parasitol 2010;170: 244–52.

32. Levine ND. Weather, climate and the bionomics of ruminant nematode larvae. Adv Vet Sci 1963;8:215–61.

33. Crofton HD, Whitlock JH, Glazer RA. Ecology and biological plasticity of sheep nematodes. II. Genetic X environmental plasticity in *Haemonchus contortus* (Rud. 1803). Cornell Vet 1965;55:251–9.
34. LeJambre LF, Whitlock JH. Changes in the hatch rate of *Haemonchus contortus* eggs between geographic regions. Parasitol 1976;73:223–38.
35. Jasmer DP, Wescott RB, Crane JW. Influence of cold temperatures upon development and survival of eggs of Washington isolates of *Haemonchus contortus* and *Ostertagia circumcincta*. Proc Helminthol Soc Wash 1986;53:244–7.
36. Jasmer DP, Wescott RB, Crane JW. Survival of third-stage larvae of Washington isolates of *Haemonchus contortus* and *Ostertagia circumcincta*. Proc Helminthol Soc Wash 1987;54:48–52.
37. Wescott RB. Epidemiology and control of nematodes and cestodes in small ruminants: Western states. Vet Clin N Amer: Food Anim Prac 1986;2:363–6.
38. Craig TM, Miller D. Controlling internal parasites. Ranch Magazine 1989;14–20.
39. O'Connor LJ, Kahn LP, Walkden-Brown SW. Interaction between the effects of evaporation rate and amount of simulated rainfall on development of the free-living stages of *Haemonchus contortus*. Vet Parasitol 2008;155:223–34.
40. Leathwick DM. The influence of temperature on the development and survival of the pre-infective free-ling stages of nematode parasites of sheep. NZ Vet J 2013; 61:32–40.
41. Molento MB, Buzatti A, Sprenger LK. Pasture larval count as a supporting method for parasite epidemiology, population dynamic and control in ruminants. Livestock Sci 2016;192:48–54.
42. Bullick GR, Andersen FL. Effect of irrigation on survival of third-stage *Haemonchus contortus* larvae (Nematoda: Trichostrongylidae). Great Basin Nat 1978; 38:369–78.
43. National Research Council. Changes in the sheep industry in the United States: making the transition from tradition. Washington, DC: The National Academies Press; 2008. https://doi.org/10.17226/12245.
44. van Dijk J, Morgan ER. The influence of water on the migration of infective trichostrongyloid larvae onto grass. Parasitol 2011;138:780–8.
45. Wang T, Vineer HR, Morrison A, et al. Microclimate has a greater influence than macroclimate on the availability of infective *Haemonchus contortus* larvae on herbage in a warmed temperate environment. Agr Ecosyst Environ 2018; 265:31–6.
46. Skinner WD, Todd KS. Lateral migration of *Haemonchus contortus* larvae on pasture. Am J Vet Res 1980;41:395–8.
47. Krecek RC, Hartman R, Groeneveld HT, et al. Micoclimatic effect on vertical migration of *Haemonchus contortus* and *Haemonchus placei* third-stage larvae on irrigated Kikuyu pasture. Onderstepoort J Vet Res 1995;62:117–22.
48. Niezen JH, Charleston WAG, Hodgson J, et al. Effect of plant species on the larvae of gastrointestinal nematodes which parasitize sheep. Int J Parasitol 1998;28:791–803.
49. Amaradasa B, Lane R, Manage A. Vertical migration of *Haemonchus contortus* infective larvae on *Cynodon dactylon* and *Paspalum notatum* pastures in response to climatic conditions. Vet Parasitol 2010;170:78–87.
50. Gruner L, Berbigier P, Crotet J, et al. Effect of irrigation on appearance and survival of infective goat gastro-intestinal nematodes in Guadeloupe (French West Indies). Int J Parasitol 1989;19:409–15.
51. Gibbs HC. Hypobiosis and the periparturient rise in sheep. Vet Clin N Amer: Food Anim Prac 1986;2:345–53.

52. Eysker M. Experiments on inhibited development of *Haemonchus contortus* and *Ostertagia circumcincta* in sheep in The Netherlands. Res Vet Sci 1981;30:62–5.

53. Eysker M. Some aspects of inhibited development of trichostrongylids in ruminants. Vet Parasitol 1997;72:265–83.

54. Zajac AM, Moore GA. Treatment and control of gastrointestinal nematodes in sheep. Compend Contin Educ Pract 1993;15. 1099-1011.

55. Grosz DD, Eljaki AA, Holler LD, et al. Overwintering strategies of a population of anthelmintic-resistant *Haemonchus contortus* within a sheep flock from the United States Northern Great Plains. Vet Parasitol 2013;196:143–52.

56. Chartier C, Hoste H, Bouqet W, et al. Peripartrient rise in fecal egg counts associated with prolactin concentration increase in French Alpine dairy goats. Parasitol Res 1998;84:806–10.

57. Mandonnet N, Bachand M, Mahieu M, et al. Impact on productivity of peri-parturient rise in fecal egg counts in Creole goats in the humid tropics. Vet Parasitol 2005;134:249–59.

58. Morgan ER, van Dijk J. Climate and the epidemiology of gastrointestinal nematode infections of sheep in Europe. Vet Parasitol 2012;189:8–14.

59. Vineer HR, Steiner J, Knapp-Lawitzke F, et al. Implications of between-isolate variation for climate change impact modelling of *Haemonchus contortus* populations. Vet Parasitol 2016;229:144–9.

60. Rose H, Wang T, van Dijk J, et al. GLOWORM-FL: a simulation model of the effects of climate and climate change on the free-living stages of gastro-intestinal nematode parasites of ruminants. Ecol Model 2015;297:232–45.

61. Fox NK, Marion G, Davidson RS, et al. Climate-driven tipping-points could lead to sudden, high-intensity parasite outbreaks. R Soc Open Sci 2015;2:140296.

62. Rose H, Caminade C, Bolajoko MB, et al. Climate-driven changes to the spatio-temporal distribution of the parasitic nematode, *Haemonchus contortus,* in sheep in Europe. Global Change Biol 2016;22:1271–85.

63. van Dijk J, David G, Baird G, et al. Back to the future: developing hypotheses on the effect of climate change on ovine parasitic gastroenteritis from historical data. Vet Parasitol 2008;158:73–84.

64. Emery DL, Hunt PW, LeJambre LF. *Haemonchus contortus:* the then and now, and where to from here? Int J Parasitol 2016;46:755–69.

65. Howell SB, Burke JM, Miller JE, et al. Prevalence of anthelmintic resistance on sheep and goat farms in the southeastern United States. JAVMA 2008;233: 1913–9.

66. Falzon LC, Menzies PI, Vanleeuwen J, et al. A survey of farm management practices and their associations with anthelmintic resistance in sheep flocks in Ontario, Canada. Small Rumin Res 2013;114:41–5.

67. Crook EK, O'Brien DJ, Howell SB, et al. Prevalence of anthelmintic resistance on sheep and goat farms in the mid-Atlantic region and comparison of *in vivo and in vitro* detection methods. Small Rumin Res 2016;143:89–96.

68. Lanusse C, Sallovitz J, Bruni S, et al. Antinematodal drugs. In: Reviere J, Papich M, editors. Veterinary pharmacology and therapeutics. 10th edition. Hobeken (NJ): John Wiley& Sons; 2018. p. 1035–80.

69. Lifschitz A, Lanusse C, Alvarez L. Host pharmacokinetics and drug accumulation of anthelmintics within target helminth parasites of ruminants. NZ Vet J 2017;65: 176–84.

70. Howell S, Park B, Vidyashankar A, et al. A 16-year retrospective analysis of anthelmintic resistance in Haemonchus contortus on small ruminant farms in the United States. Proceedings of the 27th Conference of the World Association

for the Advancement of Veterinary Parasitology. Madison, WI, July 7–11, 2019. p. 116–7.

71. Lanusse C, Imperiale F, Lifschitz A. Macrocyclic lactones endectocide compounds. In: Reviere J, Papich M, editors. Veterinary pharmacology and therapeutics. 10th edition. Hobeken (NJ): John Wiley& Sons; 2018. p. 1102–27.

72. Lanusse C, Alvarez L, Lifschitz A. Gaining insights into the pharmacology of anthelmintics using *Haemonchus contortus* as a model nematode. Adv Parasitol 2016;93:466–515.

73. Sales N, Love S. Resistance of *Haemonchus* sp to monepantel and reduced efficacy of a derquantel/abamectin combination confirmed in sheep in NSW, Australia. Vet Parasitol 2016;228:193–6.

74. Hodgkinson JE, Kaplan RM, Kenyon F, et al. Refugia and anthelmintic resistance: concepts and challenges. Int J Parasitol: Drugs and Drug Resistance 2019; 10:51–7.

75. Lanusse C, Lifschitz A, Alverez. Basic and clinical pharmacology contribution to extend anthelmintic molecules lifespan. Vet Parasitol 2015;212:35–46.

76. Lespine A, Chartier C, Hoste H, et al. Endectocides in goats: pharmacology, efficacy and use conditions in the context of anthelmintics resistance. Small Rumin Res 2012;103:10–7.

77. Geary TG, Hosking BC, Skuce PJ, et al. World Association for the Advancement of Veterinary Parasitology (W.A.A.V.P.) guideline: anthelmintic combination products targeting nematode infections of ruminants and horses. Vet Parasitol 2012; 190:306–16.

78. Leathwick DM. Modelling the benefits of a new class of anthelmintic in combination. Vet Parasitol 2012;186:93–100.

79. Burke JM, Kaplan RM, Miller JE, et al. Accuracy of FAMACHA© system for on farm use by sheep and goat producers in the southeastern United States. Vet Parasitol 2007;147:89–95.

80. Burke JM, Miller JE, Terrill TH, et al. Examination of commercially available copper oxide wire particles in combination with albendazole for control of gastrointestinal nematodes in lambs. Vet Parasitol 2016;215:1–4.

81. Burke JM, Miller JE, Olcott D, et al. Effect of copper oxide wire particles dosage and feed supplement level on *Haemonchus contortus* infection in lambs. Vet Parasitol 2004;123:235–43.

82. Terrill TH, Miller JE, Burke JM, et al. Experiences with integrated concepts for the control of *Haemonchus contortus* in sheep and goats in the United States. Vet Parasitol 2012;186:28–37.

83. Singh P, Scott I, Jacob A. Pharmacokinetics of abamectin in sheep, goat and deer. Small Rumin Res 2018;165:30–3.

84. Hennessy D. The disposition of antiparasitic dugs in relation to the development of resistance by parasites of livestock. Acta Trop 1994;56:125–41.

85. Martin KL, Clapham MO, Davis JL, et al. Extralabel drug use in small ruminants. JAVMA 2018;253:1001–9.

86. Leathwick DM, Miller CM, Atkinson DS, et al. Drenching adult ewes: implications of anthelmintic treatments pre- and post-lambing on the development of anthelmintic resistance. New Zealand Vet J 2006;54:297–304.

87. Westers T, Jones-Bitton A, Menzies P, et al. Identification of effective treatment criteria for use in targeted selective treatment programs to control haemonchosis in periparturient ewes in Ontario Canada. Prev Vet Med 2016;134:49–57.

Sustainable Approaches to Parasite Control in Ruminant Livestock

Joan M. Burke, PhD[a],*, James E. Miller, DVM, MPVM, PhD[b]

KEYWORDS

- Condensed tannins • Copper oxide wire particles • *Duddingtonia flagrans*
- Genetics

KEY POINTS

- Because of the high prevalence of anthelmintic resistance, there is a need to integrate alternatives to anthelmintics for sustainable pasture-based ruminant livestock production.
- Copper oxide wire particles can perform like an anthelmintic, and can be integrated into a control program for *Haemonchus contortus*, even in organic production.
- Secondary plant compounds including condensed tannins can reduce numbers of abomasal nematodes and egg output, especially of *H contortus*.
- Nematode-trapping fungi fed to livestock kill developing larvae in the feces, thereby reducing pasture contamination.
- Host-based resistance to parasites is a heritable trait that, when selected for, can lead to reduced levels of parasitism in the flock or herd over time.

INTRODUCTION

Most of this article is focused on small ruminants, but alternative approaches for use in cattle are also presented as appropriate. Multiple-drug anthelmintic resistance in gastrointestinal nematode (GIN) parasites of small ruminants is highly prevalent in the United States,[1–3] and complete anthelmintic resistance is a growing concern. Anthelmintic resistance in GINs of cattle is an increasing problem, but remains less prevalent[4,5] than in small ruminants. In addition, pathogenicity of GINs is lower in cattle than in small ruminants, with most impact being subclinical.[6] New classes of anthelmintics are unlikely to offer lasting solutions because resistance can develop quickly, as occurred with monepantel in sheep and goats.[7,8]

Alternative approaches for control of GINs are necessary because of anthelmintic resistance but also because of a desire by consumers for reduced use of

a USDA ARS Dale Bumpers Small Farms Research Center, 6883 South State Highway 23, Booneville, AR 72927, USA; b Department of Pathobiological Sciences, School of Veterinary Medicine, Louisiana State University, Skip Bertman Drive, Baton Rouge, LA 70803, USA
* Corresponding author.
E-mail address: Joan.burke@usda.gov

Vet Clin Food Anim 36 (2020) 89–107
https://doi.org/10.1016/j.cvfa.2019.11.007
0749-0720/20/Published by Elsevier Inc.

pharmaceuticals in meat animals, and reduced chemical residues in food and the environment. This need is reflected in high consumer demand for organic and grass-fed livestock products.[9] Some alternative methods of control for *Haemonchus contortus* in both conventional and organic production are good nutrition, rotational grazing, multispecies grazing, and use of resistant breeds[10] or genetic resistance.[11] Copper oxide wire particles (COWPs) have been shown to effectively reduce *H contortus* infection in small ruminants and are readily available to producers. Condensed tannin–rich plants and plants with secondary plant compounds can be used as a tool to reduce fecundity of worms, primarily of *H contortus*, and improve anemia, but are unlikely to offer complete control and are useful combined with other methods of control. The nematode-trapping fungus *Duddingtonia flagrans* recently became available in the United States and has been available in Australia and several other countries for a longer period. The fungus targets developing GIN larvae in the feces, reducing numbers of larvae on pasture and subsequent uptake from the pasture by the animals. These practical modes of GIN control are discussed in detail primarily as they apply to small ruminants, and to cattle when applicable.

COPPER OXIDE WIRE PARTICLES

Commercial COWPs were developed to alleviate copper deficiency associated with grazing on copper-deficient pastures; however, early nutrition studies inadvertently discovered a benefit for control of GINs.[12] Since then, numerous studies have shown that COWPs (**Fig. 1**) can be effectively used as a component of integrated GIN control programs for small ruminants, specifically to control *H contortus*.[13–17]

Mode of Action

Administration of COWPs results in substantial reduction in fecal egg counts (FECs) within 7 days[14] (**Fig. 2**). Initially, COWPs administered as a bolus or in the feed[18,19] quickly move through the rumen to the abomasum, where many of the particles are retained in abomasal folds where *H contortus* reside. The bioavailability of copper in the gastrointestinal tract is sensitive to pH; the acid pH in the abomasum causes the slow release of copper ions. Bang and colleagues[20] determined that free copper ions from COWPs in the abomasum were not eluted at pH greater than 3.4. This finding may have biological implications because abomasal pH in lambs infected with *H contortus* can reach as high as 6,[21,22] whereas the pH of uninfected lambs is less than 1.

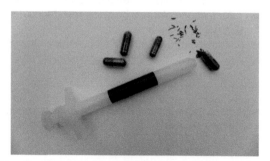

Fig. 1. Copper oxide wire particles are repackaged into gelatin capsules of lower doses (1 g and 2 g) for control of *H contortus* to minimize risk of copper toxicity. Suggested dosing apparatus shown. (*Courtesy of* Joan M. Burke, PhD, Booneville, AR.)

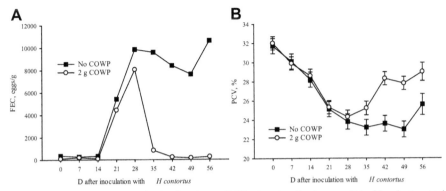

Fig. 2. Mean FEC (*A*) and packed cell volume (PCV) plus standard errors (*B*) of lambs treated with 2 g of COWP on day 28 (*open circles*) or left untreated (*closed squares*). Lambs were inoculated with 10,000 *H contortus* L3 on day 0. (*Modified from* Burke JM, Miller JE, Olcott DD et al. Effect of copper oxide wire particles dosage and feed supplement level on *Haemonchus contortus* infection in lambs. Vet Parasitol 2004; 123:235-243; with permission.)

Bang and colleagues[20] postulated that COWPs were indirectly acting on adult nematodes through the increased copper status of the host, or directly because of increased copper in the abomasum, which could potentially damage and penetrate the cuticle of *H contortus*.[20] Moscona and colleagues[23,24] found evidence of a direct effect of COWPs on *H contortus*. Examination of *H contortus* by transmission electron microscopy recovered from lambs between 12 and 84 hours after COWP administration showed lesions of the cuticle, as well as a greater concentration of copper in the worms. Thus, evidence suggests that COWPs affect *H contortus* directly, rather than through increased copper status of the host.

Efficacy Against Gastrointestinal Nematodes

Bang and colleagues[25] reported a 96% reduction in adult *H contortus* and 56% reduction in *Teladorsagia circumcincta* in lambs administered COWPs. However, Chartier and colleagues[26] reported a 75% reduction in *H contortus* and little effect against *T circumcincta* or *Trichostrongylus colubriformis* in goats administered COWPs. In some studies, there was limited or no effect on worm counts or FECs when COWPs were administered at the time of initial *H contortus* infection or on incoming larvae.[16,27,28] In contrast, Knox[29] observed a 37% reduction in *H contortus* when COWPs were administered 7 days before infection, and Galindo-Barboza and colleagues[30] observed a 46% to 73% reduction in worms when sheep were administered COWPs 7 or 14 days, respectively, before an artificial infection. Soli and colleagues[31] determined that efficacy of COWPs against *H contortus* was similar between lambs and kids.

Doses of COWPs as low as 0.5 g administered to lambs[13] or kids[16] were effective in reducing FECs of *H contortus* by 90%, and the lower doses reduced the risk of copper toxicity. Interpretation of changes in FECs reported in various studies should consider the proportion of abomasal to intestinal genera measured in coprocultures, because there is essentially no efficacy against intestinal nematode species.

The effectiveness of COWPs may be greater in combination with feeding or grazing sericea lespedeza, a forage rich in condensed tannins,[16,32] and this points to the usefulness of using different strategies in an integrated fashion. To increase efficacy of COWPs or anthelmintics (albendazole or levamisole), a combination can be used, which is especially important in the presence of anthelmintic resistance. COWPs alone target H contortus, but, in combination, efficacy on intestinal GINs improved[15] (Burke and Miller, unpublished data, 2019). In these studies, the genera of GINs included a mix of predominantly H contortus and Trichostrongylus spp.

Even though particles can be found in the abomasum for several weeks,[14,33] anthelmintic activity may not persist more than 21 days[16] or 41 days[34] in goats, and 35 days in artificially infected lambs.[30] However, in naturally infected grazing lambs, anthelmintic activity did not last more than 28 days.[13] Persistence and efficacy of COWPs may be enhanced with good nutrition[35] and combination with other alternatives, such as sericea lespedeza.[16] In addition, digesta passes through the abomasum more quickly during an intense new H contortus infection,[36] and could affect retention of COWPs in the abomasum at that time, failing to reduce FECs of H contortus in a small number of lambs (Burke, unpublished observations, 2019). It is suggested that, if small ruminants are determined to be heavily infected (ie, FAMACHA [Faffa Malan chart] score of 4 or 5), then COWPs should be coupled with an anthelmintic.

Evidence does not support efficacy of COWPs for control of Ostertagia ostertagi or Cooperia spp in cattle[37] (Miller, unpublished data, 2008), but few studies have been published. More research is needed in this area.

Copper Sulfate

Copper sulfate, often mixed with other compounds such as sodium arsenite or nicotine sulfate, was used as an anthelmintic before synthetic modern anthelmintics were developed.[38,39] However, no value was found in including copper sulfate in the mineral or feed of growing goats for control of H contortus.[40] Because a copper drench could substantially increase the risk of copper toxicity in sheep and possibly goats, it is not recommended in a holistic approach to GIN management.

Risks

It is well established that administration of COWPs increases the copper concentrations in the liver of sheep and goats. There was a linear increase in concentrations of copper in the liver of lambs relative to dose of COWPs.[14,41–43] The liver enzyme aspartate aminotransferase (AST) can be used as an indicator of copper toxicity, although with low doses (0.5 or 1 g) plasma enzyme activity remained low.[13] Copper concentrations increased in the liver of goats treated with COWPs,[16,26,35] but less is known about a threshold to induce copper toxicity in goats compared with sheep. When 4 g of COWPs were administered to pregnant Katahdin ewes, there was an initial increase in plasma AST activity of offspring, and body weight of twin-born lambs from dams treated with 2 or 4 g of COWPs may have been reduced.[44] Given these risks, it is recommended that COWPs be used only under veterinary guidance and that liver copper levels be monitored, particularly when used in sheep.

SECONDARY PLANT COMPOUNDS

Medicinal plants or plants with secondary plant compounds have been used as anthelmintics for centuries.[45,46] Numerous plants worldwide have been used, both singly and in combination, but few have been scientifically validated for effectiveness against helminths, and even fewer against GINs in ruminant livestock. Secondary plant compounds with anthelmintic activity include tannins, lactones, alkaloids, saponins, terpines, glycosides, and phenolic compounds, some of which can have detrimental effects on the animal, such as reducing feed intake, inducing nutritional deficiencies, and triggering neurologic effects.[47] These compounds are thought to protect the plant from pests, drought, excess moisture, and grazing animals. When used in moderation or when restricted to high-risk exposure to GINs, a few secondary plant compounds have shown potential for controlling GINs in small ruminants, with the most widely studied being condensed tannins.

Plants rich in condensed tannins with demonstrated activity against GINs in sheep and goats include *Lespedeza cuneata* (sericea lespedeza), *Onobrychis viciifolia* (sainfoin), *Hedysarum coronarium* (sulla), *Lotus pedunculatus* (big trefoil), and *Lotus corniculatus* (bird's foot trefoil) (reviewed by Hoste and colleagues[47]). Condensed tannins or proanthocyanidins are heterogeneous complexes of oligomers and polymers of flavonoid units linked by carbon-carbon bonds.[48] The concentration of condensed tannins in sericea lespedeza are higher than in other plants studied, and comprised 97% prodelphinidins of high molecular weight and a high proportion of cis-flavanols.[49] Condensed tannins are able to bind to proteins in the rumen (reviewed by Min and Hart[50]; Waghorn[51]), which then disassociate in the abomasum and the small intestine.[52,53] Thus, this can result in greater protein availability to the animal, which can lead to increased animal performance measured by weight gains. In addition, condensed tannins produce direct effects on worms in the abomasum.

Visible damage to the cuticle of adult *H contortus* collected from goats fed sericea lespedeza[54] or when in contact with extracts of *Lysiloma latisiliquum* (a condensed tannin–rich browse species[47]) was detected using electron microscopy. In addition, extract aggregates were found around the buccal area of worms.[47] In some studies, numbers of adult worms recovered from animals fed condensed tannin were similar to numbers in control fed animals[54–56]; however, in other studies, numbers of adult worms were significantly reduced.[49,57]

Grazing or feeding condensed tannin–containing plants can be used in an integrated management system to control GIN.[58–60] Sericea lespedeza, either grazed or fed as hay or pellets, reduced FECs of primarily *H contortus*. The plant may reduce worm burdens and, in some cases, negatively affect larval development and survival in the feces.[55,57–62] Although FECs have been reduced during feeding, often counts increase or rebound after removal of condensed tannins in the diet[57,55] (**Fig. 3**). A weekly drench of condensed tannin–rich *Acacia mearnsii* aqueous extract reduced *H contortus* FECs of goats for 120 days during the dry season, but no differences were observed between the *Acacia* group and control during 80 days of the wet season.[63] When feeding sericea lespedeza for more than 4 to 6 weeks, growth rate of lambs and kids slows[32,56,64] and reductions in trace minerals such as molybdenum, selenium, and zinc occur.[65] Thus, recommendations to control *H contortus* are to limit feeding during periods of highest GIN susceptibility, such as around the time of weaning or during the periparturient period.

There is little reported on the anthelmintic effects of condensed tannin plants on GINs in cattle, but extracts of tannins from sainfoin, bird's foot trefoil, and big trefoil reduced in vitro activity of cattle parasites *Cooperia oncophora* and *O ostertagi*.[66–68] In Louisiana, pelleted sericea lespedeza leaf meal was fed to naturally infected yearling heifers in confinement for 21 days. FECs of sericea lespedeza compared with control fed heifers were reduced by 52%, 64%, and 15% on days 7, 14, and 21 of feeding (J.E. Miller, unpublished observations, 2014).

Hydrolyzable tannins such as those found in *Epilobium angustifolium*, *Quercus robur*, *Rubus idaeus*, and *Rosa rugosa* showed in vitro anthelmintic activity against *H contortus*.[69] In vitro contact with plant solutions led to changes in the surface of the cuticle, the cephalic region of L1 and L2 stages, and the unhatched eggs, along with aggregates located at the buccal capsule and the anterior amphidial channels.

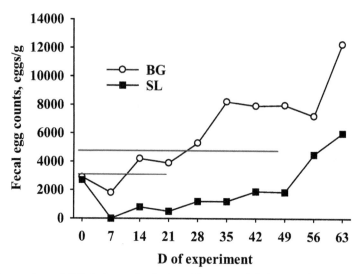

Fig. 3. Comparison of FECs between lambs (n = 6/treatment) fed Bermuda grass (BG) or ser-icea lespedeza (SL) between days 0 (first day of experiment) and 49 (*green line*). Lambs were administered *H contortus* between days 0 and 21 (1000 L3 3 times a week for 3 weeks; *red line*). On day 49, SL hay feeding switched to BG hay feeding. Treatments differed over time (*P*<.05) based on log transformed data. (*Modified from* Lange K, Olcott DD, Miller JE, et al. Effect of sericea lespedeza (*Lespedeza cuneata*) fed as hay, on natural and experimental *Haemonchus contortus* infections in lambs. Vet Parasitol 2006; 141:273-278; with permission.)

More research is needed on in vivo activity and potential toxicity in sheep and goats, which readily consume some of these plant species.

The success of growing condensed tannin–rich plant species depends on climate and soils, and specific species should match suitable agronomic sites. Sericea lespe-deza, a warm season perennial, grows well in the southeastern United States, but not in cooler climates, and can tolerate poor soils.[70,71] The forage responds well to added nutrients such as phosphorus and potassium, but, as a legume, does not need addi-tional nitrogen. More details about planting and parasite control can be found at www. wormx.info.

NEMATODE-TRAPPING FUNGI

Nematode-trapping fungi, also known as predatory or nematophagous fungi, have po-tential as a biological control agent against the free-living larval stages of GINs in live-stock feces. These fungi are found worldwide and occur at low levels naturally in soil and other environments that are rich in organic matter, where they normally feed on a variety of nonparasitic soil nematodes.[72] The fungi range in feeding habits from sapro-phytic fungi to fungi classified as obligate parasites.[73] These fungi trap and destroy developing parasitic larvae in feces, by producing a variety of trapping structures such as constricting rings, nonconstricting rings, adhesive knobs, adhesive hyphae, adhesive branches, and adhesive networks on the mycelium (bundle of hyphae).[74]

Trapping structures formed depend on the species and the environment, which in-cludes both abiotic and biotic factors. Some members of the predatory fungi group form traps spontaneously, whereas others depend on environmental factors (eg, nem-atode presence) to induce trap formation. The most important biotic factor is the presence of larvae, because they can induce trap formation by touching the mycelium, and they serve as a food source.[73] Once a nematode is secured by the trapping structures, tropic hyphae penetrate the cuticle and grow, filling the body of the nematode, digesting the contents.[75,76]

In livestock, spores of the fungus must be fed orally. Of the various species of fungi tested, *D flagrans* spores have the best ability to survive passage through the gastrointestinal tract of ruminants.[77] This ability is important because active spores of the fungi must be present in the feces when deposited to have activity against the developing larvae. These fungi have rapid growth rates and high affinity for trapping and digesting larvae.[78] After the animal defecates, the spores germinate and grow in the feces to form the sticky, sophisticated traps/loops that trap the developing larval stages of GINs in the fecal environment (**Fig. 4**). This process of producing sticky networks happens concomitantly with egg hatching and development of GIN larvae in the feces.[79] Once trapped, larvae are unable to migrate out of the fecal mass and onto forage; thus, fewer larvae are available for consumption by a grazing ruminant host.[80] The nematode-trapping loops may be present within the first 9 to 10 hours after defecation and a mucilaginous substance is present where contact with the larvae occurs, followed by cuticle penetration within 48 hours from nematode-fungal contact[81] (see **Fig. 4**).

Importantly, *D flagrans* does not seem to have adverse effects on native free-living nematodes that inhabit the soil, and the fungus was no longer detectable in the environment 2 months following treatment.[82] This form of control has been successfully applied under field conditions and is an environmentally safe biological approach for forage-based (not confinement) feeding systems.[83]

The primary delivery system is thorough mixing of the fungal spore material into supplement feedstuffs for daily feeding[84] (**Fig. 5**). Daily feeding is necessary to provide a continuous source of fungus in the feces. This approach requires a management system that can accommodate daily feeding in which each animal has the opportunity to consume an adequate amount of the feed/spore mixture. To achieve adequate control of larvae in the feces during the transmission season (June to September for most US areas), spores need to be fed for a period of 60 to 120 days, usually starting at the beginning of the grazing season (especially young after weaning). Feeding spores to dams during the periparturient period (late pregnancy and lactation) also helps to reduce pasture contamination caused by the periparturient increase in FECs. Numerous studies with sheep, goats, and cattle have shown high reductions in

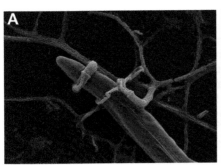
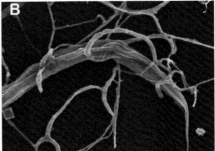

Fig. 4. Scanning electron microscopic image of trichostrongylid L3 trapped in sticky loops of *D flagrans* after 8 hours (*A*) or 48 hours (*B*) of interaction. (Image of Duddingtonia flagrans IAH 1297 as supplied by International Animal Health Products Pty Ltd.)

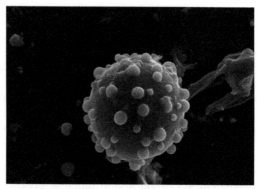

Fig. 5. Scanning electron microscopic image of spherical mature chlamydospore of *D fla-grans*. (Image of Duddingtonia flagrans IAH 1297 as supplied by International Animal Health Products Pty Ltd.)

numbers of larvae both in feces and on pasture following the feeding of *D flagrans* fungus.[80,85–93] During the dry season or other low transmission periods, it would not be necessary to feed fungal spores because natural processes prevent the development and survival of GIN larvae.

Two formulations of *D flagrans* recently became commercially available in the United States: BioWorma, and Livamol with BioWorma (International Animal Health Products, Huntingwood, NSW, Australia). Livamol is a protein supplement. Bio-Worma is available through veterinarians, premix companies, and feed mills, whereas Livamol with BioWorma is available through consumer outlets. These products are the only GIN control method that specifically targets the nematode population on pasture, where most (estimated at more than 90%) of the total worm population resides during periods of high transmission. However, these products are expensive; consequently, the practicality of their use in an integrated parasite management program varies from farm to farm. It is expected that, over time, the cost of these products will decline, making them more cost-effective. In addition, it is important to emphasize that these products are just 1 component of an integrated control program, and should not be relied on as a sole method for GIN control.

GENETICS

Taking advantage of host genetics for resistance and resilience to infection represents a promising and sustainable means to minimize GIN infection in a herd or flock. Host resistance is the ability of the host animal to initiate and maintain an immune response to suppress establishment or eliminate the parasite.[94] Host resilience is the ability of the host animal to remain healthy and productive even when parasitized. Resistance, and perhaps also resilience, are likely caused by the inheritance of genes that function in the expression of host immunity.[95] Both resistance and resilience to GINs are moderately heritable, and therefore are expected to respond to genetic selection.[94,96–102] The advantage of having genetic resistance to GINs in an individual or flock/herd is that there will be fewer interventions for worm control, and, within a resistant flock, fewer infective larvae on pasture. Breeds of tropical or African origin (eg, St Croix, Barbados Blackbelly, Gulf Coast Native, Santa Ines) generally show greater resistance as measured by FECs than breeds of temperate origins.[98,103–107]

Breeding for Gastrointestinal Nematode Resistance and Resilience

Natural selection against susceptibility to GINs is an ecological and evolutionary process that has been happening for millions of years, long before anthelmintics were available. It still occurs in wild populations of small ruminants and is considered essential in maintaining a healthy herd. However, in domestic populations, since the first use of modern anthelmintic drugs more than 50 years ago, this process has been inhibited by the killing of worms with drugs. However, given the high levels of anthelmintic resistance and the increasing concerns for animal welfare, it is highly desirable and important to select against GIN susceptibility in animals.

Traditional breeding programs and selection for traits such as GIN resistance have been used successfully to establish flocks of sheep with high levels of resistance to GINs in Australia and New Zealand.[11,96,106–110] These selection programs were considered long term, and achieving a satisfactory outcome required 10 to 20 years.[111] The National Sheep Improvement Program (NSIP) in the United States provides predictable, economically important genetic evaluation information as estimated breeding values (EBVs) to sheep producers by converting performance records into relevant decision-making tools (http://nsip.org). NSIP offers weaning and postweaning FEC EBVs as indicators of parasite resistance in sheep and goats. Selection using FAMA-CHA, a measure of resilience, could be used, but is not currently offered.[112]

Progress can be tracked by NSIP genetic trends. As an example, the US Department of Agriculture, Agricultural Research Service flock in Booneville, Arkansas, reduced the flock average EBVs from more than +40% to −60% in 10 years. An animal with +40% has the genetic potential to have a 40% higher FEC than an individual with 0%, whereas an animal with −60% would have a 60% lower FEC. Selecting for a ram on the top end of the scale for resistance, −100%, would predict his offspring to have 50% lower FECs because his lambs inherit half of his genetics.[113]

Other programs that provide EBVs for parasite resistance for sheep and/or goats include Signet (Agriculture and Horticulture Development Board, Warwickshire, United Kingdom), Sheep Genetics (Meat and Livestock Australia, 2004), and Sheep Improvement Limited (New Zealand). The NSIP provides EBVs related to GIN resistance based on collection of fecal samples for FECs in lambs at weaning (between 42 and 90 days of age) and postweaning (usually between 91 and 150 days of age) to assess variations in innate and acquired resistance to GINs.[114] In the Katahdin breed, FECs reached a maximum at 121 days of age and declined thereafter.[100,112] In general, older lambs with prior exposure to parasites are more resistant than younger lambs.[104] It is important to use offspring from multiple sires in a common contemporary group. It is also important that lambs or kids have an adequate pasture challenge so that, according to NSIP, the mean FEC is more than 500 eggs per gram of feces to achieve phenotypic variability among the group. However, even the lower means of FECs were heritable in the Katahdin breed of sheep.[99]

Goat breeds within the United States are not considered resistant, but Spanish and Kiko seem to be more tolerant than Boers.[115] However, within a breed, heritability of GIN resistance was reported to be as high as 0.37 in Creole goats using FEC at weaning as an indicator trait, and 0.33 using blood packed cell volume.[116] Data for goat herds in the United States can be entered into NSIP to generate GIN resistance EBVs following the same guidelines as sheep (www.nsip.org), but procedures and outcomes have not been validated.

In cattle, heritability of resistance to GINs, including *C oncophora*, was moderate as determined through FECs.[117,118] Similar to EBVs, breed associations in the United States and Canada calculate estimated progeny differences for GIN resistance.

Resistance may not be equal across genera of GINs in cattle.[119] Little information is available in the literature on breed resistance to GINs for selection programs to improve genetic resistance in cattle. However, the same principles apply.

The periparturient period for the ewe represents a time when the dam's immune system relaxes and she becomes more susceptible to GIN infection. Selection for resistance during the periparturient increase in the ewe has the potential to reduce pasture contamination, especially important if using a susceptible terminal sire breed in which offspring will be more susceptible to GINs. The periparturient increase of FEC is moderately heritable[100,106,112,120–122] and correlated between the dam and her lambs.[100,112] In the United States, FECs of lambs of the Katahdin breed peaked at approximately 28 days postlambing, thus it is recommended to collect and evaluate FEC between 0 and 30 days postlambing and make future culling decisions on these values.

For low-resource farms without access to technology such as NSIP or FEC analyses, use of the FAMACHA system offers an easily implementable approach for making genetic progress.[102] During periods of high worm transmission, stress of weaning, or periparturient increase of ewes, FAMACHA should be checked at least every 2 weeks (see recommendations on www.wormx.org). Anemic animals (sheep, goats, camelids) with FAMACHA scores of 4 or 5, and sometimes 3, should be dewormed. Farmers should keep records of animals that need to be dewormed, and then cull those animals that consistently need deworming.

OTHER METHODS

Optimal nutrition is an important factor in tolerance to GINs.[123–125] Increased dietary protein is associated with reduced FECs and reduced worm burdens, and modulates inappetence related to GIN infection.[126] Increased protein enhances immune function, which regulates the establishment, fecundity, and survival of GINs.[126,127] Increased energy in the diet often led to increased body weight, but did not always influence GIN infection measures.[127] Effects of higher protein levels in the diet may be more important for parasite-susceptible than parasite-resistant breeds.[128] Increased protein can be sourced from supplements or high-quality forages.

Grazing management can influence GIN infection of livestock. Use of browse for goats to minimize grazing decreases the numbers of infective larvae that are ingested, and use of plant species with more complex leaf structure and higher-protein forages or legumes helps reduce GIN infection. Multispecies grazing and/or alternate grazing of cattle or horses with sheep or goats offers important benefits to GIN control because parasite species differ between host species.[129–131]

Rotational grazing is another strategy that can reduce exposure to GIN larvae on pasture.[132–135] Rotational grazing of animals among forage plots, with return to previously grazed plots after variable time periods depending on land availability and forage quality, can have multiple benefits. Rotation of lambs to new grass plots every 3 to 7 days, with return to the original grass plots 28 to 35 days later, led to a reduced incidence of deworming (based on FAMACHA) and lower worm infections in tracer lambs compared with continuously grazed grass plots.[133,134] When animals were dewormed at the beginning of the rotational grazing scheme, rotational compared with continuous grazing reduced FEC and need for deworming for the 52 weeks studied,[132,134] and combining with D flagrans greatly reduced FEC and worm burden.[134] In 1 study performed with cattle, rotational grazing systems forced closer grazing to fecal pats and no benefit to GIN control was realized.[131] However, when rotational grazing was combined with other measures, such as strategic deworming or D flagrans, benefits were seen.[37,93]

Table 1	
Sustainable approaches to gastrointestinal nematode control in ruminant livestock	
Method	**Target**
COWP	Adult *H contortus*
Secondary plant compounds	Adult *H contortus* and other GIN dependent on plant species; possibly also developing larvae
Nematophagous fungi	Free-living stages of GIN larvae
Host genetics	All parasitic stages of GIN

Diatomaceous earth (DE) is a natural siliceous substance that is formed from the skeletal remains of unicellular organisms. It is soft to the touch but, microscopically, the diatom particles have sharp edges. When DE is ingested by livestock, the microscopic shards are thought to use mechanical movements within the gut to cause injury to the cuticle of nematodes and ultimately lead to the dehydration then death of the adult parasites. However, there is no real evidence that DE has any beneficial effects on GINs. The literature is nearly void of studies on DE against livestock GINs, but Ahmed and colleagues[136] observed no reduction in FEC after feeding 2% of diet as DE for 7 days. Other unpublished studies that the authors are aware of showed similar lack of effect. However, despite the evidence, many farmers swear by the use of DE for parasite control.

Similarly, despite widespread use of herbal products and many anecdotal claims of benefits, studies have consistently failed to show any benefits for the control of GIN. Use of herbal products,[137,138] garlic,[139] papaya,[137] pumpkin seeds,[140] and ginger[140] all failed to reduce FECs or worms, or show improvements in anemia in small ruminants. Consequently, these products cannot be recommended for the control of GINs, and any apparent success in GIN control that farms using these products have are probably caused by other things the farms are doing (eg, good nutrition, good pasture management).

SUMMARY

In response to increasing levels of anthelmintic resistance, sustainable alternatives include use of COWPs alone or with an anthelmintic, secondary plant compounds, grazing systems, increased plane of nutrition, and genetic selection for increased parasite resistance and resilience. These approaches to control GIN are most effective when used in an integrated fashion together with selective use of anthelmintics. A summary of methods and their targets hints at why using tools together is more beneficial so as to target different stages of the GIN life cycle (**Table 1**) or biological processes of the host. As an example, a combination of host resistance through genetic selection and use of COWPs as needed in sheep allows organic producers to meet certification requirements, which do not allow use of anthelmintics for slaughter stock or fiber production. Similarly, in cattle, good pasture management that could include rotational grazing (information found at www.wormx.info) combined with use of breeds more tolerant to infection, such as tropical breeds, should yield sustainable GIN control.

Fact sheets describing these technologies and how to use then in an integrated parasite control program are available at www.wormx.info (American Consortium for Small Ruminant Parasite Control), and more information on BioWorma can be found at www.iahp.com.au (International Animal Health Products).

DISCLOSURE

This work was supported by the U.S. Department of Agriculture, Agricultural Research Service.

REFERENCES

1. Crook EK, O'Brien DJ, Howell SD, et al. Prevalence of anthelmintic resistance on sheep and goat farms in the mid-Atlantic region and comparison of in vivo and in vitro detection methods. Small Rumin Res 2016;143:89–96.

2. Howell SB, Burke JM, Miller JE, et al. Anthelmintic resistance on sheep and goat farms in the southeastern United States. J Am Vet Med Assoc 2008;233:1913–9.

3. Kaplan RM. Drug resistance in nematodes of veterinary importance: a status report. Trends Parasitol 2004;20:477–81.

4. Gasbarre LC. Anthelmintic resistance in cattle nematodes in the US. Vet Parasitol 2014;204:3–11.

5. Sutherland IA, Leathwick DM. Anthelmintic resistance in nematode parasites of cattle: a global issue? Trends Parasitol 2011;27:176–81.

6. Waller PJ. The development of anthelmintic resistance in ruminant livestock. Acta Trop 1994;56:233–43.

7. Hamer K, Bartley D, Jennings A, et al. Lack of efficacy of monepantel against trichostrongyle nematodes in a UK sheep flock. Vet Parasitol 2018;257:48–53.

8. Scott I, Pomroy WE, Kenyon PR, et al. Lack of efficacy of monepantel against *Teladorsagia circumcincta* and *Trichostrongylus colubriformis*. Vet Parasitol 2013;198:166–71.

9. USDA, National Agricultural Statistics Service. Certified organic survey, 2016 summary. Washington, DC: US Department of Agriculture; 2017.

10. Terrill TH, Miller JE, Burke JM, et al. Experiences with integrated concepts for the control of *Haemonchus contortus* in sheep and goats in the United States. Vet Parasitol 2012;186:28–37.

11. Baker RL, Watson TG, Bisset SA, et al. Breeding sheep in New Zealand for resistance to internal parasites: research results and commercial application. In: Gray GD, Woolaston RR, editors. Breeding for disease resistance in sheep. Melbourne (Australia): Australian Wool Corporation; 1991. p. 19–32.

12. Judson GJ, Brown TH, Gray D, et al. Oxidized copper wire particles for copper therapy in sheep. Aust J Agric Res 1982;33:1073–83.

13. Burke JM, Miller JE. Evaluation of multiple low dose copper oxide wire particles compared with levamisole for control of *Haemonchus contortus* in lambs. Vet Parasitol 2006;139:145–9.

14. Burke JM, Miller JE, Olcott DD, et al. Effect of copper oxide wire particles dosage and feed supplement level on *Haemonchus contortus* infection in lambs. Vet Parasitol 2004;123:235–43.

15. Burke JM, Miller JE, Terrill TH, et al. Examination of commercially available copper oxide wire particles in combination with albendazole for control of gastrointestinal nematodes in lambs. Vet Parasitol 2016;215:1–4.

16. Burke JM, Terrill TH, Kallu RR, et al. Use of copper oxide wire particles to control gastrointestinal nematodes in goats. J Anim Sci 2007;85:2753–61.

17. Spickett A, de Villiers JF, Boomker J, et al. Tactical treatment with copper oxide wire particles and symptomatic levamisole treatment using the FAMACHA© system in indigenous goats in South Africa. Vet Parasitol 2012;184:48–58.

18. Burke JM, Orlik S, Miller JE, et al. Using copper oxide wire particles or sericea lespedeza to prevent a peri-parturient gastrointestinal nematode infection in sheep and goats. Livest Sci 2010;132:13–8.
19. Burke JM, Soli F, Miller JE, et al. Administration of copper oxide wire particles in a capsule or feed for gastrointestinal nematode control in goats. Vet Parasitol 2010;168:346–50.
20. Bang KS, Familton AS, Sykes AR. Effect of ostertagiasis on copper status in sheep: a study involving use of copper oxide wire particles. Res Vet Sci 1990; 49:306–14.
21. Christie MG, Brambell MR, Mapes CJ. Effect of young *Haemonchus contortus* on abomasal pH in sheep. Vet Rec 1967;80:207–8.
22. Nicholls CD, Hayes PR, Lee DL. Physiological and microbiological changes in the abomasum of sheep infected with large doses of *Haemonchus contortus*. J Comp Pathol 1987;97:299–308.
23. Moscona AK. Copper oxide wire particles used to control *Haemonchus* infections: efficacy in giraffe (*Giraffa camelopardalis*) at Busch Gardens Tampa and potential mechanism of action [Master's Thesis]. Baton Rouge (LA): Louisiana State University; 2013.
24. Moscona AK, Borkhsenious O, Sod GA, et al. Mechanism of action of copper oxide wire particles (COWP) as an anthelmintic agent. Proc 53rd Ann Meet Amer Assoc Vet Parasitol 2008; 39 (Abstr), July 19-22, 2008, New Orleans, LA, USA.
25. Bang KS, Familton AS, Sykes AR. Effect of copper oxide wire particle treatment on establishment of major gastrointestinal nematodes in lambs. Res Vet Sci 1990;49:132–7.
26. Chartier C, Etter E, Hoste H, et al. Efficacy of copper oxide needles for the control of nematode parasites in dairy goats. Vet Res Commun 2000;24:389–99.
27. Vatta AF, Waller PJ, Githiori JB, et al. The potential to control *Haemonchus contortus* in indigenous South African goats with copper oxide wire particles. Vet Parasitol 2009;162:306–13.
28. Waller PJ, Bernes G, Rudby-Martin L, et al. Evaluation of copper supplementation to control *Haemonchus contortus* infections of sheep in Sweden. Acta Vet Scand 2004;45:149–60.
29. Knox MR. Effectiveness of copper oxide wire particles for *Haemonchus contortus* control in sheep. Aust Vet J 2002;80:224–7.
30. Galindo-Barboza AJ, Torres-Acosta JFJ, Cámara-Sarmiento R, et al. Persistence of the efficacy of copper oxide wire particles against Haemonchus contortus in sheep. Vet Parasitol 2011;176:201–7.
31. Soli F, Terrill TH, Shaik SA, et al. Efficacy of copper oxide wire particles against gastrointestinal nematodes in sheep and goats. Vet Parasitol 2010;168:93–6.
32. Burke JM, Miller JE, Mosjidis JA, et al. Use of a mixed sericea lespedeza pasture system for control of gastrointestinal nematodes lambs and kids. Vet Parasitol 2012;186:328–36.
33. Judson GJ, Brown TH, Gray D, et al. Oxidized copper wire as a copper supplement for sheep: a study of some variables which may alter copper availability. Aust Vet J 1984;61:294–5.
34. Vatta AF, Waller PJ, Githiori JB, et al. Persistence of the efficacy of copper oxide wire particles against *Haemonchus contortus* in grazing South African goats. Vet Parasitol 2012;190:159–66.
35. Martínez Ortiz de Montellano C, Vargas-Magaña JJ, Aguilar-Caballero AJ, et al. Combining the effects of supplementary feeding and copper oxide needles for

the control of gastrointestinal nematodes in browsing goats. Vet Parasitol 2007; 146:66–76.

36. Bueno L, Dakkak A, Fioramonti J. Gastro-duodenal motor and transit disturbances associated with *Haemonchus contortus* infection in sheep. Parasitology 1982;84:367–74.

37. Dimander S-O, Höglund J, Uggla A, et al. Evaluation of gastro-intestinal nematode parasite control strategies for first-season grazing cattle in Sweden. Vet Parasitol 2003;111:193–209.

38. Gordon HM. Anthelmintic efficiency against immature *Haemonchus contortus*. Aust Vet J 1939;15:57–66.

39. Wright WH, Bozicevich J. Control of gastrointestinal parasites of sheep by weekly treatments with various anthelmintics. J Agric Res 1931;43:1053–69.

40. Burke JM, Miller JE. Dietary copper sulfate for control of gastrointestinal nematodes in goats. Vet Parasitol 2008;154:289–93.

41. Judson GJ, Trengove CL, Langman MW, et al. Copper supplementation of sheep. Aust Vet J 1984;61:40–3.

42. Langlands JP, Bowles JE, Donald GE, et al. Copper oxide particles for grazing sheep. Aust J Agric Res 1983;34:751–65.

43. Suttle NF. Safety and effectiveness of cupric oxide particles for increasing liver copper stores in sheep. Res Vet Sci 1987;42:219–23.

44. Burke JM, Miller JE, Brauer DK. The effectiveness of copper oxide wire particles as an anthelmintic in pregnant ewes and safety to offspring. Vet Parasitol 2005; 131:291–7.

45. Athanasiadou S, Kyriazakis I. Plant secondary metabolites: antiparasitic effects and their role in ruminant production systems. Proc Nutr Soc 2004;63:631–9.

46. Sandoval-Castro CA, Torres-Acosta JFJ, Hoste H, et al. Using plant bioactive materials to control gastrointestinal tract helminths in livestock. Anim Feed Sci Technol 2012;176:192–201.

47. Hoste H, Martinez-Ortiz-De-Montellano C, Manolaraki F, et al. Direct and indirect effects of bioactive tannin-rich tropical and temperate legumes against nematode infections. Vet Parasitol 2012;186:18–27.

48. Hagerman AE, Butler LG. The specificity of proanthocyandin-protein interactions. J Biol Chem 1991;256:4494–7.

49. Mechineni A, Kommuru DS, Gujja S, et al. Effect of fall-grazed sericea lespedeza (*Lespedeza cuneata*) on gastrointestinal nematode infections of growing goats. Vet Parasitol 2014;204:221–8.

50. Min BR, Hart SP. Tannins for suppression of internal parasites. J Anim Sci 2003; 81:102–9.

51. Waghorn G. Beneficial and detrimental effects of dietary condensed tannins for sustainable sheep and goat production – Progress and challenges. Anim Feed Sci Tech 2008;147:116–39.

52. Barry TN, Manley TR. Interrelationships between the concentrations of total condensed tannin, free condensed tannin and lignin in *Lotus* sp. And their possible consequences in ruminant nutrition. J Sci Food Agric 1986;37:248–54.

53. Waghorn GC, Ulyatt JJ, John A, et al. The effect of condensed tannins on the site of digestion of amino acids and other nutrients in sheep fed on *Lotus corniculatus* L. Br J Nutr 1987;57:115–26.

54. Iqbal Z, Sarwar M, Jabbar A, et al. Direct and indirect anthelmintic effects of condensed tannins in sheep. Vet Parasitol 2007;144:125–31.

55. Min BR, Pomroy WE, Hart SP, et al. The effect of short-term consumption of a forage containing condensed tannins on gastro-intestinal nematode parasite infections in grazing wether goats. Small Rumin Res 2004;51:279–83.

56. Niezen JH, Robertson HA, Waghorn GC, et al. Production faecal egg counts and worm burdens of ewe lambs which grazed six contrasting forages. Vet Parasitol 1998;80:15–27.

57. Kommuru DS, Whitley NC, Miller JE, et al. Effect of sericea lespedeza leaf meal pellets on adult female *Haemonchus contortus* in goats. Vet Parasitol 2015;207: 170–5.

58. Lange K, Olcott DD, Miller JE, et al. Effect of sericea lespedeza (*Lespedeza cuneata*) fed as hay, on natural and experimental *Haemonchus contortus* infections in lambs. Vet Parasitol 2006;141:273–8.

59. Moore DA, Terrill TH, Kouakou B, et al. The effects of feeding sericea lespedeza hay on growth rate of goats naturally infected with gastrointestinal nematodes. J Anim Sci 2008;86:2328–37.

60. Shaik SA, Terrill TH, Miller JE, et al. Sericea lespedeza hay as a natural deworming agent against gastrointestinal nematode infection in goats. Vet Parasitol 2006;139:150–7.

61. Min BR, Hart SP, Miller D, et al. The effect of grazing forage containing condensed tannins on gastro-intestinal parasite infection and milk composition in Angora does. Vet Parasitol 2005;130:105–13.

62. Terrill TH, Mosjidis JA, Moore DA, et al. Effect of pelleting on efficacy of sericea lespedeza hay as a natural dewormer in goats. Vet Parasitol 2007;146:117–22.

63. Costa-Júnior LM, Costa JS, Lôbo ICPD, et al. Long-term effects of drenches with condensed tannins from *Acacia mearnsii* on goats naturally infected with gastro-intestinal nematodes. Vet Parasitol 2014;205:725–9.

64. Burke JM, Miller JE, Terrill TH, et al. The effects of supplemental sericea lespedeza pellets in lambs and kids on growth rate. Livest Sci 2014;159:29–36.

65. Acharya M, Burke JM, Coffey KP, et al. Changes in concentrations of trace minerals in lambs fed sericea lespedeza leaf meal pellets with or without dietary sodium molybdate. J Anim Sci 2016;94:1592–9.

66. Desrues O, Fryganas C, Ropiak HM, et al. Impact of chemical structure of flavanol monomers and condensed tannins on in vitro anthelmintic activity against bovine nematodes. Parasitology 2016;143:444–54.

67. Novobilský A, Mueller-Harvey I, Thamsborg SM. Condensed tannins act against cattle nematodes. Vet Parasitol 2011;182:213–20.

68. Novobilský A, Stringano E, Hayot Carbonero C, et al. In vitro effects of extracts and purified tannins of sainfoin (*Onobrychis viciifolia*) against two cattle nematodes. Vet Parasitol 2013;196:532–7.

69. Engström MT, Karonen M, Ahern JR, et al. Chemical structures of plant hydrolyzable tannins reveal their in vitro activity against egg hatching and motility of *Haemonchus contortus* nematodes. J Agric Food Chem 2016;64:840–51.

70. Ball DM, Hoveland CS, Lacefield GD. Southern forages. Modern concepts for forage crop management. 5th edition. Peachtree Corners (GA): Int. Plant Nutr. Inst.; 2015.

71. Terrill TH, Whitley N. Sericea Lespedeza. 2018. Available at: www.wormx.info. Accessed November 14, 2019.

72. Jackson F, Miller JE. Alternative approaches to control—Quo vadit? Vet Parasitol 2006;139:371–84.

73. Nordbring-Hertz B, Jansson HB, Tunlid A. Nematophagous fungi. Wiley, Chichester, UK: Encyclopedia of Life Sciences; 2006. Available at: http://www.onlinelibrary.wiley.com/doi/10.1002/9780470015902.a0000374.pub3.

74. Grønvold J, Wolstrup J, Nansen P, et al. Nematode-trapping fungi against parasitic cattle nematodes. Parasitol Today 1993;9:137–40.

75. Grønvold J, Henriksen SA, Larsen M, et al. Aspects of biological control—with special reference to arthropods, protozoans and helminthes of domesticated animals. Vet Parasitol 1996;64:47–64.

76. Grønvold J, Nansen P, Henriksen SA, et al. Induction of traps by Ostertagia ostertagi larvae, chlamydospore production and growth rate in the nematode-trapping fungus Duddingtonia flagrans. J Helminthol 1996;70:291–7.

77. Hoste H, Torres-Acosta JFJ. Non chemical control of helminthes in ruminants: adapting solutions for changing worms in a changing world. Vet Parasitol 2011;180:144–54.

78. Waller PJ, Thamsborg SM. Nematode control in 'green' ruminant production systems. Trends Parasitol 2004;29:493–7.

79. Ketzis JK, Vercruysse J, Strombert BE, et al. Evaluation of efficacy expectations for novel and non-chemical helminth control strategies in ruminants. Vet Parasitol 2006;139:321–35.

80. Fontenot ME, Miller JE, Peña MT, et al. Efficiency of feeding Duddingtonia flagrans chlamydospores to grazing ewes on reducing availability of parasitic nematode larvae on pasture. Vet Parasitol 2003;118:203–13.

81. Campos A, Araújo J, Guimarães M. Interaction between the nematophagous fungus Duddingtonia flagrans and infective larvae of Haemonchus contortus (Nematoda: Trichostrongyloidea). J Helminthol 2008;82:337–41.

82. Saumell CA, Fernández AS, Echevarria F, et al. Lack of negative effects of the biological control agent Duddingtonia flagrans on soil nematodes and other nematophagous fungi. J Helminthol 2016;90:706–11.

83. Healey K, Lawlor C, Knox MR, et al. Field evaluation of Duddingtonia flagrans IAH 1297 for the reduction of worm burden in grazing animals: tracer studies in sheep. Vet Parasitol 2018;253:48–54.

84. Waller PJ. Management and control of nematode parasites of small ruminants in the face of total anthelmintic failure. Trop Biomed 2004;21:7–13.

85. Knox MR, Faedo M. Biological control of field infections of nematode parasites of young sheep with Duddingtonia flagrans and effects of spore intake on efficacy. Vet Parasitol 2001;101:155–60.

86. Larsen M, Faedo M, Waller PJ, et al. The potential of nematophagous fungi to control the free-living stages of nematode parasites of sheep: studies with Duddingtonia flagrans. Vet Parasitol 1998;76:121–8.

87. Mendoza de Gives P, Crespo JF, Rodriguez DH, et al. Biological control of Haemonchus contortus infective larvae in ovine faeces by administering an oral suspension of Duddingtonia flagrans chlamydospores to sheep. J Helminthol 1998;72:343–7.

88. Terrill TH, Larsen M, Samples O, et al. Capability of the nematode-trapping fungus Duddingtonia flagrans to reduce infective larvae of gastrointestinal nematodes in goat feces in the southeastern United States: dose titration and dose time interval studies. Vet Parasitol 2004;120:285–96.

89. Waghorn TS, Leathwick DM, Chen L-Y, et al. Efficacy of the nematode trapping fungus Duddingtonia flagrans against three species of gastro-intestinal nematodes in laboratory faecal cultures from sheep and goats. Vet Parasitol 2003;118:227–34.

90. Waller PJ, Knox MR, Faedo M. The potential of nematophagous fungi to control the free-living stages of nematode parasites of sheep: feeding and block studies with *Duddingtonia flagrans*. Vet Parasitol 2001;102:321–30.

91. Waller PJ, Ljungström B-L, Schwan O, et al. Biological control of sheep parasites using *Duddingtonia flagrans*: trials on commercial farms in Sweden. Acta Vet Scand 2006;47:23–32.

92. Peña MT, Miller JE, Fontenot ME, et al. Evaluation of Duddingtonia flagrans in reducing infective larvae of Haemonchus contortus in feces of sheep. Vet Parasitol 2013;103:259–65.

93. Dimander S-O, Höglund J, Waller PJ. Seasonal translation of infective larvae of gastrointestinal nematodes of cattle and the effect of Duddingtonia flagrans: a 3-year plot study. Vet Parasitol 2003;117:99–116.

94. Woolaston RR, Baker RL. Prospects of breeding small ruminants for resistance to internal parasites. Int J Parasitol 1996;26:845–55.

95. Miller JE, Horohov DW. Immunological aspects of nematode parasite control in sheep. J Anim Sci 2006;84(Suppl 13):E124–32.

96. Albers GAA, Gray GD, Piper LR, et al. The genetics of resistance and resilience to *Haemonchus contortus* in young Merino sheep. Int J Parasitol 1987;17:1355–63.

97. Bisset SA, Morris CA, McEwan JC, et al. Breeding sheep in New Zealand that are less reliant on anthelmintics to maintain health and productivity. N Z Vet J 2001;49:236–46.

98. Miller JE, Bishop SC, Cockett NE, et al. Segregation of natural and experimental gastrointestinal nematode infection in F2 progeny from susceptible Suffolk and resistant Gulf Coast Native sheep and its usefulness in assessing genetic variation. Vet Parasitol 2006;140:83–9.

99. Ngere L, Burke JM, Morgan JLM, et al. Genetic parameters for fecal egg counts and their relationship with body weights in Katahdin lambs. J Anim Sci 2018;96:1590–9.

100. Notter DR, Burke JM, Miller JE, et al. Factors affecting fecal egg counts in periparturient Katahdin ewes and their lambs. J Anim Sci 2017;95:103–12.

101. Piper LR. Genetic variation in resistance to internal parasite. In: McGuirk VJ, editor. Merino improvement programs in Australia. Sydney (Australia): Australian Wool Corp; 1987. p. 351–63.

102. Riley DG, Van Wyk JA. Genetic parameters for FAMACHA© score and related traits for host resistance/resilience and production at differing severities of worm challenge in a Merino flock in South Africa. Vet Parasitol 2009;164:44–52.

103. Amarante AFT, Bricarello PA, Rocha RA, et al. Resistance of Santa Ines, Suffolk and Ile de France sheep to naturally acquired gastrointestinal nematode infections. Vet Parasitol 2004;120:91–106.

104. Courtney CH, Parker CF, McClure KE, et al. Resistance of exotic and domestic lambs to experimental infection with *Haemonchus contortus*. Int J Parasitol 1985;15:101–9.

105. Gamble HR, Zajac AM. Resistance of St. Croix lambs to *Haemonchus contortus* in experimentally and naturally acquired infections. Vet Parasitol 1992;41:211–25.

106. Vanimisetti HB, Andrew SL, Zajac AM, et al. Inheritance of fecal egg count and packed cell volume and their relationship with production traits in sheep infected with *Haemonchus contortus*. J Anim Sci 2004;82:1602–11.

107. Vanimisetti HB, Greiner SP, Notter DR. Performance of hair sheep composite breeds: resistance of lambs to Haemonchus contortus. J Anim Sci 2004;82: 595–604.

108. Windon RG, Dineen JK. Parasitological and immunological competence of lambs selected for high and low responsiveness to vaccination with irradiated *Trichostrongylus colubriformis* larvae. In: Dineen JK, Outteridge PM, editors. Immunogenetic approaches to the control of endoparasites. Melbourne (Australia): CSIRO; 1984. p. 13–28.

109. Windon RG. Selective breeding for the control of nematodiasis in sheep. Rev Sci Tech 1990;2:555–76.

110. Windon RG. Resistance mechanisms in the *Trichostrongylus* selection flocks. In: Gray GD, Woolaston RR, editors. Breeding for disease resistance in sheep. Melbourne (Australia): Australian Wool Corporation; 1991. p. 77–86. Available at: http://hdl.handle.net/102.100.100/250532?index=1.

111. Albers GAA, Gray GD. Breeding for worm resistance: a perspective. Int J Parasitol 1986;17:559–66.

112. Notter DR, Burke JM, Miller JE, et al. Association between FAMACHA scores and fecal egg counts in Katahdin lambs. J Anim Sci 2017;95:1118–23.

113. Bowdridge S, Weaver A. Genetic selection. Using crossbreeding and estimated breeding values American Consortium for Small Ruminant Parasite Control. Keedysville (MD): University of Maryland; 2019. Available at: www.wormx.info.

114. Notter DR. Selection for parasite resistance. Proc. XL Reunión de la Asociación Mexicana para la Producción Animal y la Seguridad Alimentaria y IX Seminario Internacional de Producción de Ovinos en el Trópico, Villahermosa, Tabasco, Mexico, May 22–24, 2013. Universidad Juárez Autónoma de Tabasco, Villahermosa. p. 3–12. Available at: https://www.researchgate.net/publication/315772264_Selection_ for_ parasite _resistance_Seleccion_para_ resistencia_parasitaria.

115. Browning R Jr, Leite-Browning ML, Byars M Jr. Reproductive and health traits among Boer, Kiko, and Spanish meat goat does under humid, subtropical pasture conditions of the southeastern United States. J Anim Sci 2011;89: 648–60.

116. Mandonnet N, Aumont G, Fleury J, et al. Assessment of genetic variability of resistance to gastrointestinal nematode parasites in Creole goats in the humid tropics. J Anim Sci 2001;79:1706–12.

117. Mackinnon MJ, Meyer K, Hetzel DJS. Genetic variation and covariation for growth, parasite resistance and heat tolerance in tropical cattle. Livest Prod Sci 1991;27:105–22.

118. Gasbarre LC, Leighton EA, Davies CJ. Genetic control of immunity to gastrointestinal nematodes of cattle. Vet Parasitol 1990;37:257–72.

119. Gasbarre LC, Leighton EA, Sonstegard T. Role of the bovine immune system and genome in resistance to gastrointestinal nematodes. Vet Parasitol 2001; 98:51–64.

120. Brown DJ, Fogarty NM. Genetic relationships between internal parasite resistance and production traits in Merino sheep. Anim Prod Sci 2017;57:209–15.

121. Goldberg V, Ciappesoni G, Aguilar I. Genetic parameters for nematode resistance in periparturient ewes and post-weaning lambs in Uruguayan Merino sheep. Livest Sci 2012;147:181–7.

122. Safari E, Fogarty NM, Gilmour AR. A review of genetic parameter estimates for wool, growth, meat and reproduction traits in sheep. Livest Prod Sci 2005;92: 271–89.

123. Coop RL, Holmes I. Nutrition-parasite interaction. Int J Parasitol 1996;26: 951–62.
124. Coop RL, Kyriazakis I. Nutrition-parasite interaction. Vet Parasitol 1999;84: 187–204.
125. Houdijk JGM, Kyriazakis I, Kidane A, et al. Manipulating small ruminant parasite epidemiology through the combination of nutritional strategies. Vet Parasitol 2012;186:38–50.
126. Strain SAJ, Steer MJ. The influence of protein supplementation on the immune response to *Haemonchus contortus*. Parasite Immunol 2001;23:527–31.
127. Houdijk JGM. Differential effects of protein and energy scarcity on resistance to nematode parasites. Small Rumin Res 2012;103:41–9.
128. Steel JW. Effects of protein supplementation of young sheep on resistance development and resilience to parasitic nematodes. Austr J Exp Agric 2003; 43:1469–76.
129. Fernanadez LH, Seno MCZ, Amarante AFT, et al. Efeito do pastejo rotacionado e alternado com bovinos adultos no controle da verminose em ovelhas. Arq Bras Med Vet Zootec 2004;56:733–40.
130. Rocha RA, Bresciani KDS, Barros TFM, et al. Sheep and cattle grazing alternately: nematode parasitism and pasture decontamination. Small Rumin Res 2008;75:135–43.
131. Stromberg BE, Averbeck GA. The role of parasite epidemiology in the management of grazing cattle. Int J Parasitol 1999;29:33–9.
132. Barger IA, Siale K, Banks DJD, et al. Rotational grazing for control of gastrointestinal nematodes of goats in a wet tropical environment. Vet Parasitol 1994;53: 109–16.
133. Burke JM, Miller JE, Terrill TH. Impact of rotational grazing on management of gastrointestinal nematodes in weaned lambs. Vet Parasitol 2009;163:67–72.
134. Chandrawathani P, Jamnah O, Adnan M, et al. Field studies on the biological control of nematode parasites of sheep in the tropics, using the microfungus *Duddingtonia flagrans*. Vet Parasitol 2004;120:177–87.
135. Colvin AF, Walkden-Brown SW, Knox MR, et al. Intensive rotational grazing assists control of gastrointestinal nematodosis of sheep in a cool temperate environment with summer-dominant rainfall. Vet Parasitol 2008;153:108–20.
136. Ahmed MA, Laing MD, Nsahlai IV. Studies on the ability of two isolates of Bacillus thuringiensis, an isolate of Clonostachys rosea f. rosea and a diatomaceous earth product to control gastrointestinal nematodes of sheep. Biocontrol Sci Technol 2013;23:1067–82.
137. Burke JM, Wells A, Casey P, et al. Herbal dewormer fails to control gastrointestinal nematodes in goats. Vet Parasitol 2009;160:168–70.
138. Luginbuhl JM, Pietrosemoli S, Howell JM, et al. Alternatives to traditional anthelmintics to control gastrointestinal nematodes in grazing meat goats. Arch Latinoam Prod Anim 2010;18:113–22.
139. Burke JM, Wells A, Casey P, et al. Garlic and papaya lack control over gastrointestinal nematodes in goats and lambs. Vet Parasitol 2009;159:171–4.
140. Matthews KK, O'Brien DJ, Whitley NC, et al. Investigation of possible pumpkin seeds and ginger effects on gastrointestinal nematode infection indicators in meat goat kids and lambs. Small Rum Res 2016;136:1–6.

The Epidemiology and Control of Liver Flukes in Cattle and Sheep

Alison K. Howell, BVSc, MSc, MRes, PhD, MRCVS*,
Diana J.L. Williams, BSc, PhD

KEYWORDS

- Liver fluke • Fasciola • Hepatica • F gigantica • Fascioloides magna • Cattle
- Sheep

KEY POINTS

- *Fasciola hepatica, F gigantica*, and *Fascioloides magna* are liver flukes causing disease of economic and welfare importance in cattle and sheep worldwide.
- Their life cycle involves a snail intermediate host and thus requires suitable moisture and temperature conditions for at least 3 months of the year.
- Drug treatment is the mainstay of control and needs to be applied with an understanding of the life cycle and epidemiology of the parasites concerned.

INTRODUCTION

The liver flukes are digenean trematode parasites that cause economically important disease of domestic livestock. This article discusses 3 of the most important species of liver fluke: *Fasciola hepatica* (the common liver fluke or cattle fluke), *F gigantica* (the tropical fluke), and *Fascioloides magna* (the giant liver fluke or deer fluke). The 2 *Fasciola* species are best documented as infecting domesticated ruminants, although wild herbivores and most mammals can also be infected. In terms of zoonotic importance, 17 million people are estimated to be infected with these parasites in more than 70 countries worldwide.[1]

Conversely, *F magna* is primarily a parasite of wild ungulates, but can infect sheep and cattle as dead end or aberrant hosts.

F hepatica is the most widespread species, occurring in 70 countries worldwide in temperate climates, including parts of Latin America, the Caribbean, Europe, the Middle East, Africa, Asia, and Oceania. In the United States, *F hepatica* is limited to areas of high rainfall and poorly drained pasture within Texas, the Gulf Coast, Great Lakes, and northwestern states.

Institute of Infection and Global Health, University of Liverpool, Leahurst Campus, Chester High Road, Neston CH64 7TE, UK
* Corresponding author.
E-mail address: ahowell@liverpool.ac.uk

Vet Clin Food Anim 36 (2020) 109–123
https://doi.org/10.1016/j.cvfa.2019.12.002
0749-0720/20/© 2019 Elsevier Inc. All rights reserved.

F gigantica is present in tropical regions of Africa and Asia. The 2 *Fasciola* species coexist in areas of North Africa, the highlands of east Africa, and Asia, and there is evidence of hybridization in some regions.[2,3]

F magna originated in North America, and is currently endemic in 5 parts of the United States and southern Canada: the north Pacific Coast, Rocky Mountain trench, Great Lakes region, northern Quebec, and Labrador, and the area comprising the Gulf Coast, lower Mississippi, and southern Atlantic seaboard.[4] It has been introduced into parts of Central Europe through imported game animals and is now present with 1 population in northern Italy, and a genetically distinct population that originated in Czech Republic and southwestern Poland, and has since spread to forests in Austria, Slovakia, Hungary, Croatia, Serbia, and Germany.[5]

Recent increases in cattle movements and climate change have led to liver flukes expanding their range[6]: in the United States, *F hepatica* and/or *F magna* are now found in 26 states and in 24% of slaughtered cattle. Similarly in Europe, *F hepatica* is now found in areas that were once considered free of flukes.[7–9]

The liver flukes exert a considerable economic burden on livestock farming, with subclinical losses contributing a large proportion of the cost. Reduced milk yield and fertility, slower growth rates, and reduced feed conversion are seen even with low burdens.[10,11] Emerging resistance to flukicide drugs is a challenge to control in Europe and Australia.[12,13]

LIFE CYCLE

The life cycle of all 3 fluke species involves a definitive (mammalian) host and an intermediate (snail) host. The life cycle is dependent on suitable habitat, moisture, and temperature to sustain the intermediate host. The life cycle of *F hepatica* is described below, with species variations described afterward.

Fluke eggs are passed into the environment with feces, via the gall bladder. If suitably mild and moist conditions exist, embryonation occurs. Moisture is essential for egg survival and embryonation, with eggs quickly dessicating in dry conditions. Embryonation takes 6 months at 10°C, decreasing to 8 days at 30°C.[14] At higher temperatures, viability periods are decreased.[15] At temperatures between 0°C and 10°C, eggs remain viable for at least 2 years, but they are killed if exposed to temperatures below −5°C for longer than 2 weeks.[16] Aerobic conditions and a pH of between 4.2 and 9 are also required.[15]

Eggs must be liberated from feces to create the correct conditions for hatching to occur, a process that is aided by water or mechanical disturbance. An active miracidium hatches from the egg and swims energetically for up to 24 hours to find an intermediate snail host.[17] The miracidium penetrates the body of the snail and becomes a sporocyst, from which, following parthenogenic multiplication, up to 200 rediae burst.[18] Each redia then gives rise to around 20 cercariae. This final larval stage then migrates out of the snail, around 4 to 7 weeks after infection. Following a short active phase of up to 2 hours, the cercariae encyst on nearby plant matter or on the surface of water as metacercariae, the infective stage. A proportion of metacercariae may survive on pasture for up to a year, although the infective load will decrease during this time. Survival relies on suitable moisture and temperature levels, with the heat and drought of a typical Australian or US summer, or temperatures below −10°C causing mortality.[16,19,20] Metacercariae may survive in damp hay for a short time; however, they will not survive in silage under anaerobic conditions (B. John, unpublished results, 2019).

Once inside the host, excystation occurs and the newly excysted juvenile flukes migrate through the walls of the small intestines, and into the abdominal cavity within a few hours. Penetration of the liver capsule takes up to a week, and juvenile flukes then burrow through the liver parenchyma for up to 6 weeks before reaching the bile ducts where they remain. Fluke can survive for several years in sheep. Fluke are hermaphrodites although they reproduce mainly by cross-fertilization,[21] with eggs being produced from 10 to 12 weeks postinfection. Therefore, the complete life cycle takes at least 16 weeks, although it may take much longer.

For the tropical liver fluke, *F gigantica*, the life cycle is similar except that the temperatures required for the host snail species and parasite development are higher, and the time scales are longer. The prepatent period is 12 to 16 weeks, and the time for the full life cycle is at least 20 weeks.

F magna also has a similar life cycle, with requires temperature and moisture levels being similar to *F hepatica*, but with considerably longer time required. The prepatent period is at least 30 weeks and the full life cycle takes around 7 months to complete. Fluke migrate through the liver until they encounter another fluke, where, in deer, the immune system of the host leads to the formation of a fibrous capsule in which the hermaphrodite flukes mature and remain for up to 5 years.[22,23] In deer, eggs are able to pass out of the pseudocyst and reach the environment.[24] However, in cattle, eggs remain trapped within the pseudocyst and therefore cattle do not contribute to the completion of the life cycle. In sheep, the formation of the pseudocyst is not effective and eggs can be excreted, if the sheep survives for long enough.[25,26]

Intermediate Hosts

Lymnaeid snails are the intermediate host species for all the liver flukes. *Galba truncatula* (**Fig. 1**) is the preferred host of *F hepatica* in most parts of the world, and has been found in parts of Africa, North and South America, and Asia. *G cubensis* and *G bulimoides* are the main host species in North America.[27,28] These snails live in semiaquatic habitats on the banks of streams or ponds, wet flushes, and drainage ditches, or anywhere exposed wet mud allows algae to grow. Damage to pasture caused by trampling by livestock or tractor tyres, combined with wet conditions, can cause snail habitats to expand. The snails are small, measuring 1 to 10 mm in length, and can survive periods of drought by estivation. Where *F hepatica* and *F magna* coexist, they share intermediate snail species.

Members of *Lymnaea auriculara sensu lato* are the preferred host of *F gigantica*.[29] In Africa this is predominantly *L a natalensis*, whereas in the Indian subcontinent *L a rufescens* is the main host species.[30] *L auriculara* are less able to estivate and therefore live in permanent water bodies, being found deep in rivers and lakes.

EFFECT ON THE HOST
Clinical Signs

For the 2 *Fasciola* species, 2 main forms of disease are seen: acute fasciolosis, caused by migration of juvenile flukes through the liver parenchyma, and chronic fasciolosis, caused by adult flukes in the bile ducts. Acute fasciolosis occurs 6 to 8 weeks after ingestion of large numbers of infective metacercariae.[31] Liver damage and blood loss caused by migrating flukes leads to anemia, proteinemia, weight loss, and frequently in sheep, death. Sheep are more susceptible to acute fasciolosis, although sudden death can occasionally be seen in cattle.

Chronic fasciolosis is seen 4 to 5 months after ingestion of smaller numbers of metacercariae[31] and is associated with adult flukes in the bile ducts. Typical signs include loss of condition, anemia, submandibular edema, ascites, decreased milk yield, and fibrosis, and, in cattle, calcification of the bile ducts may be seen at postmortem

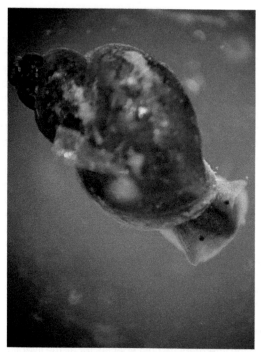

Fig. 1. *Galba truncatula* seen under the dissecting microscope.

examination. In addition, subclinical infections in cattle are common, and may result in considerable reduction in growth rates and milk production. For *F hepatica*, reductions in milk production of 3% to 15%, reduced growth rates in cattle of 6% to 9%, and negative effects on reproduction have been reported.[32–37]

F magna in cattle are contained within a pseudocyst[25,26] and usually do not cause clinical signs.[22,38] In sheep, the pseudocyst does not form effectively and the mature fluke migrates throughout the liver and other tissues, such as lungs, causing hemorrhage and death in most cases.[22]

Liver damage caused by flukes can allow *Clostridium novyi* bacteria to enter and result in sudden death from infectious necrotic hepatitis (Black disease).

Immunology

Most immunologic research on flukes has been on *F hepatica*. Cattle and sheep can become infected at any age, and do not develop protective immunity.[39,40] The predominant immune response in naturally infected animals is Th2/regulatory,[41] which is likely to be a host adaptation to chronic infections, to avoid excessive tissue damage resulting from inflammatory Th1 cytokines, and is also induced by fluke antigens.[42,43] Antibodies are detectable from 2 to 3 weeks after infection and levels remain high throughout the period of infection.[44,45] However, these Th2/regulatory responses do not give protective immunity against liver flukes. *F hepatica* has the ability to modulate the immune system to promote its own survival, and this has been shown to have bystander effects on coinfecting pathogens, such as *Mycobacterium bovis*, although the practical implications are still unclear.[46–50] Conversely, some sheep breeds and rats have an innate immunity to *F gigantica* and others can acquire it. This may be due to differences in antigen expression between the 2 parasites, or because *F hepatica* is able to suppress the protective response.[51]

DIAGNOSIS

Diagnostic methods include fecal egg count, antibody detection in milk or serum, and antigen detection in feces (**Table 1**). Premortem diagnosis of *F magna* in cattle and sheep is difficult as eggs are not usually produced. For all methods, sensitivity tends to be worse in animals harboring only a light infection, where a missed diagnosis is likely to be of least importance.[52]

For *F hepatica* and *F gigantica*, fecal egg detection is easy and cheap, although it has the disadvantage that only patent infections can be diagnosed. Using traditional sedimentation methods, 10 to 50 g of feces per animal can be tested and eggs identified with a dissecting microscope (see **Fig. 2**, **Table 2**). Taking 5 g from 10 sheep in a group to make 50 g is a convenient way of testing a pooled sample.[59] For cattle, taking 10×10-g samples, mixing well, and testing a 10-g subsample is equally sensitive.[60] For individuals, Flukefinder (Richard Dixon, ID, USA) is a convenient way of rapidly testing 2 to 3 g per animal. Flukefinder is a unit made up of 2 sieves and uses the same principle as sedimentation. Despite the smaller volume of feces, the sensitivity is comparable with traditional sedimentation[61] and offers a considerable time saving.

Commercial enzyme-linked immunosorbent assays are currently only validated and marketed for *F hepatica*, but it is likely that these cross-react with the other 2 species, which could limit their use in areas where more than 1 species coexist.[65,66] Antibodies can be detected from 2 to 4 weeks postinfection.[44,65] Antibody tests are more sensitive than egg detection in the early stage of infection, and can remain high for several weeks after treatment. Antibody levels do not directly correlate with parasite burden, but do give an indication.[11] On dairy farms, bulk milk antibody detection is a convenient way of screening the whole herd for *F hepatica*.[44,55,67] A positive result suggests that approximately 25% of the herd is seropositive.

Coproantigen detection can detect infections slightly earlier than fecal egg counting, but performance has been variable, with a different cutoff from that recommended by the manufacturer needed to increase the sensitivity to acceptable levels.[11,68]

All 3 parasites can be diagnosed postmortem by identification of parasites in the liver. In sheep and cattle with *F hepatica* or *F gigantica* infection (**Fig. 2**), thickened bile ducts, liver fibrosis, and scarring may be seen with either current or previous infection. In *F magna* infection, black pigmentation in the hepatic parenchyma, lymph nodes, and other tissues, and necrosis and hemorrhage due to migration; in cattle, white fibrous capsules are seen.[23]

EPIDEMIOLOGY AND CONTROL
Effects of Climate and Environment

Liver flukes only occurs in regions where conditions support the intermediate snail host, and suitable moisture and temperature levels are needed for at least 3 months for completion of parasite development within the snail. As a result, in many areas with cooler climates, only 1 complete life cycle takes place each year and fasciolosis is a seasonal disease. In contrast, in warm climates, such as the US Gulf Coast states, transmission can occur for 6 months of more, and only ceases once the weather becomes too hot and dry for the snails in the late spring or early summer. Because of the time required for the parasite to mature within the snail, the peak infectious period begins when high numbers of metacercariae reach the pasture, which, assuming animals are present and excreting eggs onto the pasture, occurs around 10 to 12 weeks after the snails become active. In the United States, *F hepatica* is found in the Gulf Coast and western states, where high rainfall, poorly drained pastures, and soil types that can support the intermediate host snail are found.[69–71] Several states in the

Table 1
A summary of the performance of some of the tests commonly used to diagnose liver fluke infection in cattle

Test	Sensitivity (%)	Specificity (%)	Comments	Suitable for	References
Fecal egg count (traditional sedimentation or Flukefinder)	43–65	90–100	Prepatent period is 8–12 wk following infection (F hepatica) or 13–16 wk (F gigantica). Sensitivity depends on egg count and weight of feces used. Most methods are based on sedimentation	F hepatica and F gigantica, individuals or pooled samples for groups	11
Serology	79–95	80–93	Can detect infection 2–4 wk postinfection Remains positive for several weeks after cure	Validated for F hepatica. Likely to cross-react with other species	11,44
Milk antibody detection	92 / 96	88 / 80	Individual Herd	Validated for F hepatica. Individual or herds. Likely to cross-react with other species	44,53
Coproantigen enzyme-linked immunosorbent assay	40–98	92–94	Detects infection 6–8 wk postinfection, Returns to negative 1–2 wk posttreatment	Validated for F hepatica. Likely to cross-react with other species individuals or pooled samples for groups	11,54–57
Postmortem diagnosis	63–93	100	Sensitivity varies: lower at meat inspection, higher if liver is sliced up and soaked	All 3 species	58

Data from Refs. [11,44,53–58]

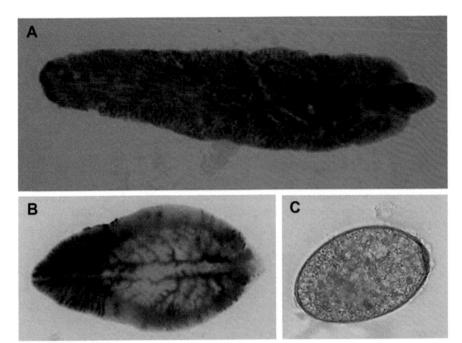

Fig. 2. (*A*) *F. gigantica* adult. (*B*) *F. hepatica* adult. (*C*) *F. hepatica* egg seen under dissecting microscope. It is morphologically indistinguishable from the eggs of *F. gigantica* and *F. magna.* (*Courtesy of* [*A, B*] E. James LaCourse, BSc, PhD, Liverpool, UK; and [C] John Graham-Brown, BVSc, MSc, PhD, MRCVS, Liverpool, UK.

mountainous northwestern region also are enzootic for *F hepatica* as a consequence of pasture irrigation. The weather conditions in the US Gulf Coast translate into the snails being most active during the relatively warm winters, and hence the peak infectious period is in the late winter and spring, before snail numbers decline due to hot dry summer conditions.[69,72] Counterintuitively, however, drought conditions can lead to higher infection levels as livestock congregate around the few remaining drinking and grazing areas. In the northwestern mountain states of the United States, and in northern European climates where cold winter weather is the limiting factor, snails are most active during the warm summer months and infectious metacercariae on pasture peak in late summer to early autumn.

Table 2
Morphology of *F hepatica*, *F gigantica*, and *F magna* and their eggs

	Egg		Adult Parasite	
	Appearance	Length (μm)	Appearance	Length (mm)
F hepatica	Oval, operculated,	120–164[62]	Leaf-shaped,	10–30[63]
F gigantica	orange. Eggs cannot be reliably distinguished	129–204[64]	dorsoventrally flattened, *F gigantica* more elongated	30–55[63]
F magna		109–175[24]	Similar but lacking anterior cone	30–80[22]

Data from Refs.[22,24,62–64]

Snail numbers and hence infectious levels on pasture also vary largely between years, with wetter, milder conditions leading to more severe fasciolosis outbreaks. Changes to farming systems, such as increases in pasture irrigation can introduce liver flukes to new areas.[71]

In tropical regions where *F gigantica* is present, conditions are generally limited by moisture. In areas where the main snail habitat is rivers and lakes, peak numbers of infected snails are found at the end of the rainy season. As habitats dry out and water levels drop, oxygen concentrations can become too low to support snails, but infection levels rise as animals congregate in these areas.

Man-made water supplies, such as irrigation canals, and reservoirs, can be an ideal snail habitat, for example, in the Andean highlands, Pakistan, and Cambodia.[73–75] Irrigation alters the seasonality of the liver fluke life cycle by enabling a longer period of snail activity than would otherwise have occurred, or enabling 2 periods per year. In other cases where rainfall is very low, irrigation is the only source of water and leads to new areas of snail activity.[29]

Aspects to Consider in F hepatica Control

Localized risk factors

Grazing management can reduce exposure of animals to liver fluke risk pastures.[76] On some farms, it may be possible to fence off or drain high-risk areas, although this is often challenging as snail habitats can be localized, temporary, and difficult to identify, or too widespread throughout the available pasture. As an alternative, avoiding grazing the high-risk pastures during the most risky times of year may be possible.[77] Snail control using molluscicides is currently banned in most countries due to adverse environmental effects.

The local climate and/or timing of crop irrigation determines when the peak transmission periods are likely to be and thus when the optimal time for treatment is. In some countries, forecasting systems are available to help farmers decide when to treat. Wet weather leading to standing water during the time of year when temperatures are above 10°C but below 30°C is the key feature of high-risk years.[69]

The species and production type of animals present on farms

Sheep are at risk of acute fasciolosis, therefore a drug active against immature stages may be needed at around 8 weeks after the peak snail season; however, in the United States none of the available anthelmintics have activity against the immature stages, therefore, this would not be possible. An anthelmintic treatment in spring using a product effective against mature stages may help to reduce pasture contamination from mature flukes that have built up in the animals over winter. The lack of anthelmintics that target the immature stages makes raising sheep a challenge in the areas of the United States where *F hepatica* is highly prevalent.

Cattle are unlikely to suffer from acute fasciolosis, therefore treatment should be aimed at killing mature parasites to control chronic disease that may affect production, and to reduce pasture contamination. In warmer climates, such as in the southern United States, the optimal time for treatment is late summer or autumn.[69,70] This is the earliest time at which the parasites that infected the animals during the peak transmission time of winter and spring are likely to have reached maturity, and thus are susceptible to the available treatments. Treating at this time has the added benefit of preventing egg shedding at the time of year when snail populations are re-establishing themselves; this then greatly decreases fluke transmission in the next cycle. In northern Europe, where infection occurs mainly during the summer, the most efficient time to treat is during the late autumn and winter. If animals are housed for winter, a treatment several weeks posthousing can be given. A single annual treatment may be enough if timed correctly, because after the intermediate host snails become inactive, infection pressure decreases until the following season. Restrictions of treatment in dairy animals mean that treatment may only be possible during the dry period, which may not fall at an ideal time of year. Therefore, where there are several animal types present on 1 farm, it may be preferable to graze dairy cattle and sheep on drier land at high-risk times, and allow beef suckler cattle to graze the wetter areas, as they can more easily be treated and are at less risk of acute fascioliasis.

Animals coming onto the farm

All incoming animals, including sheep, cattle, bulls, rams, and seasonal sheep should be included in the control program, to avoid bringing in animals harboring heavy burdens or drug-resistant flukes. These animals should be quarantined, tested, and treated to reduce the risk. This practice is especially important in areas where drug-resistant flukes are known to exist.

Effective use of drugs

Abattoir returns or diagnostic testing should be used to inform the need for and frequency of treatment. Several drugs are available to treat liver flukes, and these vary both in terms of the life stages of the parasite killed and availability in different countries (**Table 3**). Accurate dosing is important and overuse of a single product should be avoided to delay the development of resistance.

Drug resistance

Triclabendazole resistance is now widespread in much of Europe and there also are reports of closantel resistance.[13,81–83] This is a great problem on sheep units because of the risk of acute fasciolosis. In the event of suspected treatment failure, a fecal egg count reduction test should be performed. This has only been validated in sheep and for triclabendazole,[84] but the same principle applies for cattle and for other drugs. Although at present there is no internationally recognized standard protocol for diagnosing resistance in flukes, the following protocol has worked well in Europe. Samples (20 × 5 g) are taken from a penned group of sheep, before treating them with triclabendazole. The samples are tested as 2 pools of 50 g each using the sedimentation method. The same group is then resampled 3 weeks later. A reduction in egg count of less than 90% between the first and second testing indicates resistance is present. An alternative is to use the coproantigen test to check drug efficacy.[85]

Table 3 Flukicide drugs and their availability		
Drug Name	**Fluke Life Stage Treated**	**Availability in North America**
Albendazole	10 wk onward	United States and Canada
Clorsulon	10 wk onward (can be effective from 8 wk but a higher dose required)	United States
Closantel	7–8 wk onward	Canada
Nitroxynil	8 wk onward	No
Oxyclosanide	10 wk onward	No
Rafoxanide	4 wk onward	No
Triclabendazole	2 wk onward (cattle), 2 d onward (sheep)	No

Data from Refs.[78–80]

F gigantica Control

Although the same drugs are effective, in many countries where F gigantica is endemic they are unavailable or prohibitively expensive. Little evidence exists for the beneficial effect of these drugs on productivity. In terms of timing of treatment in areas where snail habitats are water bodies in pastoral areas the same principles apply as for F hepatica, in terms of treating 8 to 10 weeks after the end of the rainy season when peak snail activity occurs. In areas where irrigated rice fields exist, treatment in advance of planting has been suggested to ensure that cattle dung used as fertilizer is free of eggs and therefore does not cause infection of snails. Treatment of cattle after they have grazed rice stubble may be most effective time to prevent chronic fasciolosis. Regarding F hepatica, the timing of this postexposure treatment depends on whether the product is effective against immature flukes or only adults.[29]

F magna Control

In cattle, F magna is not usually associated with any clinical signs, and eggs are not shed as they are unable to escape the fibrous capsule within which the parasite is contained.[38] Losses are usually confined to condemnation of the liver at slaughter. Therefore, treatment is not needed.

In sheep, albendazole (7.5 mg/kg), triclabendazole (20 mg/kg), clorsulon (21 mg/kg), and closantel (15 mg/kg) are reported to be at least partially effective against mature and late-stage immature (from 8–10 weeks) F magna.[79,86–89] Of these, albendazole is approved for this purpose in the United States. Treatment should be given 8 to 10 weeks after peak snail activity to kill the maximum number of flukes at the earliest possible stage. As a single F magna can be fatal in sheep, and none of these drugs are completely effective, the mortality rate can be high even when treatment is given in a timely fashion. Drug treatment of wild deer has proved ineffective at preventing infection in livestock, and preventing access of deer to pasture is likely to be impractical.[72,90]

SUMMARY

The 3 liver fluke species present a considerable burden to cattle and sheep farming worldwide. As a consequence of the complex life cycles of these parasites, including the dependence on an intermediate host that is very sensitive to environmental conditions, effective control depends on a good understanding of their life cycles and local epidemiology.

DISCLOSURE

The authors have nothing to disclose.

REFERENCES

1. Mas-Coma S, Valero MA, Bargues MD. Fasciola, lymnaeids and human fascioliasis, with a global overview on disease transmission, epidemiology, evolutionary genetics, molecular epidemiology and control. Adv Parasitol 2009;69:41–146.
2. Afshan K, Valero MA, Qayyum M, et al. Phenotypes of intermediate forms of Fasciola hepatica and F. gigantica in buffaloes from Central Punjab, Pakistan. J Helminthol 2014;88(4):417–26.
3. Periago MV, Valero MA, El Sayed M, et al. First phenotypic description of Fasciola hepatica/Fasciola gigantica intermediate forms from the human endemic area of the Nile Delta, Egypt. Infect Genet Evol 2008;8(1):51–8.

4. Králová-Hromadová I, Juhásová L, Bazsalovicsová E. The giant liver fluke, *Fascioloides magna*: past, present and future research. SpringerBriefs in animal sciences. Cham (Switzerland): Springer; 2016. https://doi.org/10.1007/978-3-319-29508-4_4.

5. Králová-Hromadová I, Bazsalovicsová E, Štefka J, et al. Multiple origins of European populations of the giant liver fluke *Fascioloides magna* (Trematoda: Fasciolidae), a liver parasite of ruminants. Int J Parasitol 2011;41(3–4):373–83.

6. Pybus MJ, Butterworth EW, Woods JG. An expanding population of the giant liver fluke (*Fascioloides magna*) in elk (*Cervus canadensis*) and other ungulates in Canada. J Wildl Dis 2015;51(2):431–45.

7. Beesley NJ, Caminade C, Charlier J, et al. *Fasciola* and fasciolosis in ruminants in Europe: identifying research needs. Transbound Emerg Dis 2017. https://doi.org/10.1111/tbed.12682.

8. Caminade C, Van Dijk J, Baylis M, et al. Modelling recent and future climatic suitability for fasciolosis in Europe. Geospat Health 2015;9(2):301.

9. Pritchard GC, Forbes AB, Williams DJL, et al. Emergence of fasciolosis in cattle in East Anglia. Vet Rec 2005;157(19):578–82.

10. Mazeri S, Rydevik G, Handel I, et al. Estimation of the impact of *Fasciola hepatica* infection on time taken for UK beef cattle to reach slaughter weight. Sci Rep 2017; 7(1):7319.

11. Charlier J, De Meulemeester L, Claerebout E, et al. Qualitative and quantitative evaluation of coprological and serological techniques for the diagnosis of fasciolosis in cattle. Vet Parasitol 2008;153(1–2):44–51.

12. Brockwell YM, Elliott TP, Anderson GR, et al. Confirmation of *Fasciola hepatica* resistant to triclabendazole in naturally infected Australian beef and dairy cattle. Int J Parasitol Drugs Drug Resist 2014;4(1):48–54.

13. Gordon D, Zadoks R, Skuce P, et al. Confirmation of triclabendazole resistance in liver fluke in the UK. Vet Rec 2012;171(6):159–60.

14. Clunies Ross I, McKay AC. The bionomics of *Fasciola hepatica* in New South Wales and of the intermediate host *Limnea brazieri* (Smith). Melbourne(Australia): Council for Scientific and Industrial Research; 1929. Available at: https://catalogue.nla.gov.au/Record/169654. Accessed May 20, 2019.

15. Rowcliffe SA, Ollerenshaw CB. Observations on the bionomics of the egg of *Fasciola hepatica*. Ann Trop Med Parasitol 1960;54(2):172–81.

16. Boray JC. Experimental fascioliasis in Australia. Adv Parasitol 1969;7:95–210.

17. Hope Cawdery MJ, Gettinby G, Grainger JNR. Mathematical models for predicting the prevalence of liver-fluke disease and its control from biological and meteorological data [sheep]. Geneva (Switzerland): Tech Note - World Meteorol Organ; 1978. Available at: http://agris.fao.org/agris-search/search.do?recordID=XF7900170. Accessed May 20, 2019.

18. Krull W. The number of cercariae of *Fasciola hepatica* developing in snails infected with a single miracidium. In: Christie J, editor. Proceedings of the Helminthological Society of Washington. Washington, DC: The Helminthological Society of Washington; 1941. p. 55–8.

19. Boray JC, Enigk K. Laboratory studies on the survival and infectivity of *Fasciola hepatica*- and *F. gigantica*-metacercariae. Z Tropenmed Parasitol 1964;15:324–31. Available at: http://www.ncbi.nlm.nih.gov/pubmed/14316630. Accessed May 22, 2019.

20. Olsen OW. Longevity of Metacercariae of *Fasciola hepatica* on pastures in the upper coastal region of Texas and its relationship to liver fluke control. J Parasitol 1947;33(1):36.

21. Beesley NJ, Williams DJL, Paterson S, et al. *Fasciola hepatica* demonstrates high levels of genetic diversity, a lack of population structure and high gene flow: possible implications for drug resistance. Int J Parasitol 2017;47(1):11–20.

22. Foreyt WJ, Todd AC. Development of the large American liver fluke, *Fascioloides magna*, in white-tailed deer, cattle, and sheep. J Parasitol 1976;62(1):26–32.

23. Foreyt WJ, Samuel WM, Todd AC. *Fascioloides magna* in White-Tailed Deer (*Odocoileus virginianus*): observations on the pairing tendency. J Parasitol 1977;63(6):1050.

24. Swales WE. The life cycle of *Fascioloides magna* (Bassi, 1875), the large liver fluke of ruminants, in Canada: with observations on the bionomics of the larval stages and the intermediate hosts, pathology of Fascioloidiasis magna, and control measures. Can J Res 1935;12(2):177–215.

25. Foreyt WJ. Domestic sheep as a rare definitive host of the large American liver fluke *Fascioloides magna*. J Parasitol 1990;76(5):736.

26. Campbell WC, Todd AC. Natural infections of *Fascioloides magna* in Wisconsin sheep. J Parasitol 1954;40(1):100.

27. Cruiz-Reyes A, Malek EA. Suitability of six lymnaeid snails for infection with *Fasciola hepatica*. Vet Parasitol 1987;24(3–4):203–10.

28. Zukowski SH, Wilkerson GW, Malone JB. Fascioliasis in cattle in Louisiana. 2. Development of a system to use soil maps in a geographic information-system to estimate disease risk on Louisiana Coastal marsh rangeland. Vet Parasitol 1993;47(1–2):51–65.

29. Spithill TW, Smooker PM, Copeman DB. *Fasciola gigantica*: epidemiology, control, immunology and molecular biology. In: Dalton JP, editor. Fiasciolosis. Oxford (England): CABI Publishing; 1999. p. 465–525.

30. Kendall SB. Relationships between the species of *Fasciola* and their molluscan hosts. Adv Parasitol 1965;3:59–98.

31. Behm CA, Sangster NC. Pathology, pathophysiology and clinical aspects. In: Dalton JP, editor. Fasciolosis. New York: CABI Publishing; 1999. p. 185–224.

32. Charlier J, Duchateau L, Claerebout E, et al. Associations between anti-*Fasciola hepatica* antibody levels in bulk-tank milk samples and production parameters in dairy herds. Prev Vet Med 2007;78(1):57–66.

33. Charlier J, Hostens M, Jacobs J, et al. Integrating fasciolosis control in the dry cow management: the effect of closantel treatment on milk production. PLoS One 2012;7(8). https://doi.org/10.1371/journal.pone.0043216.

34. Howell A, Baylis M, Smith R, et al. Epidemiology and impact of *Fasciola hepatica* exposure in high-yielding dairy herds. Prev Vet Med 2015;121(1–2):41–8.

35. Mezo M, Gonzalez-Warleta M, Antonio Castro-Hermida J, et al. Association between anti-*F. hepatica* antibody levels in milk and production losses in dairy cows. Vet Parasitol 2011;180(3–4):237–42.

36. Sanchez-Vazquez MJ, Lewis FI. Investigating the impact of fasciolosis on cattle carcase performance. Vet Parasitol 2013;193(1–3):307–11.

37. Schweizer G, Braun U, Deplazes P, et al. Estimating the financial losses due to bovine fasciolosis in Switzerland. Vet Rec 2005;157(7):188–93. Available at: http://www.scopus.com/inward/record.url?eid=2-s2.0-20544464957&partnerID=40&md5=a82fe6020531614a8e13d8c3a3245d37.

38. Conboy GA, Stromberg BE. Hematology and clinical pathology of experimental *Fascioloides magna* infection in cattle and guinea pigs. Vet Parasitol 1991;40(3–4):241–55.

39. Clery D, Torgerson P, Mulcahy G. Immune responses of chronically infected adult cattle to *Fasciola hepatica*. Vet Parasitol 1996;62(1–2):71–82.

40. McCole DF, Doherty ML, Baird AW, et al. T cell subset involvement in immune responses to *Fasciola hepatica* infection in cattle. Parasite Immunol 1999; 21(1):1–8.
41. Graham-Brown J, Hartley C, Clough H, et al. Dairy heifers naturally exposed to *Fasciola hepatica* develop a type 2 immune response and concomitant suppression of leukocyte proliferation. Infect Immun 2017;86(1) [pii:e00607-17].
42. Spellberg B, Edwards JE. Type 1/type 2 immunity in infectious diseases. Clin Infect Dis 2001;32(1):76–102.
43. Moreau E, Chauvin A. Immunity against helminths: interactions with the host and the intercurrent infections. J Biomed Biotechnol 2010. https://doi.org/10.1155/2010/428593.
44. Salimi-Bejestani MR, McGarry JW, Felstead S, et al. Development of an antibody-detection ELISA for *Fasciola hepatica* and its evaluation against a commercially available test. Res Vet Sci 2005;78(2):177–81.
45. Ortiz PL, Claxton JR, Clarkson MJ, et al. The specificity of antibody responses in cattle naturally exposed to *Fasciola hepatica*. Vet Parasitol 2000;93(2):121–34. Available at: http://www.ncbi.nlm.nih.gov/pubmed/11035230. Accessed September 15, 2016.
46. Claridge J, Diggle P, McCann CM, et al. *Fasciola hepatica* is associated with the failure to detect bovine tuberculosis in dairy cattle. Nat Commun 2012;3. https://doi.org/10.1038/ncomms1840.
47. Flynn RJ, Mannion C, Golden O, et al. Experimental *Fasciola hepatica* infection alters responses to tests used for diagnosis of bovine tuberculosis. Infect Immun 2007;75(3):1373–81.
48. Flynn RJ, Mulcahy G, Welsh M, et al. Co-infection of cattle with *Fasciola hepatica* and *Mycobacterium bovis*—immunological consequences. Transbound Emerg Dis 2009;56(6–7):269–74.
49. Byrne AW, Graham J, Brown C, et al. Bovine tuberculosis visible lesions in cattle culled during herd breakdowns: the effects of individual characteristics, trade movement and co-infection. BMC Vet Res 2017;13(1):400.
50. Byrne AW, McBride S, Graham J, et al. Liver fluke (*Fasciola hepatica*) co-infection with bovine tuberculosis (bTB) in cattle: a retrospective animal-level assessment of bTB risk in dairy and beef cattle. Transbound Emerg Dis 2019. https://doi.org/10.1111/tbed.13083.
51. Spithill TW, Piedrafita D, Smooker PM. Immunological approaches for the control of fasciolosis. Int J Parasitol 1997;27(10):1221–35.
52. Vercruysse J, Claerebout E. Treatment vs non-treatment of helminth infections in cattle: defining the threshold. Vet Parasitol 2001;98(1–3):195–214.
53. Salimi-Bejestani MR, Daniel R, Cripps P, et al. Evaluation of an enzyme-linked immunosorbent assay for detection of antibodies to *Fasciola hepatica* in milk. Vet Parasitol 2007;149(3–4):290–3.
54. Brockwell YMM, Spithill TW, Anderson GR, et al. Comparative kinetics of serological and coproantigen ELISA and faecal egg count in cattle experimentally infected with *Fasciola hepatica* and following treatment with triclabendazole. Vet Parasitol 2013;196(3–4):417–26.
55. Duscher R, Duscher G, Hofer J, et al. *Fasciola hepatica*—monitoring the milky way? The use of tank milk for liver fluke monitoring in dairy herds as base for treatment strategies. Vet Parasitol 2011;178(3–4):273–8.
56. Valero MA, Ubeira FM, Khoubbane M, et al. MM3-ELISA evaluation of coproantigen release and serum antibody production in sheep experimentally infected with *Fasciola hepatica* and *F. gigantica*. Vet Parasitol 2009;159(1):77–81.

57. Kajugu P-E, Hanna REB, Edgar HW, et al. Specificity of a coproantigen ELISA test for fasciolosis: lack of cross-reactivity with *Paramphistomum cervi* and *Taenia hydatigena*. Vet Rec 2012;171(20):502.

58. Rapsch C, Schweizer G, Grimm F, et al. Estimating the true prevalence of *Fasciola hepatica* in cattle slaughtered in Switzerland in the absence of an absolute diagnostic test. Int J Parasitol 2006;36(10–11):1153–8.

59. Williams DJL, Howell A, Graham-Brown J, et al. Liver fluke—an overview for practitioners. Cattle Pract 2014;22:238–44. Available at: https://www.researchgate.net/publication/285998125_Liver_fluke_-_An_overview_for_practitioners.

60. Graham-Brown J, Williams DJL, Skuce P, et al. Composite *Fasciola hepatica* faecal egg sedimentation test for cattle. Vet Rec 2019;184(19):589.

61. Faria RN, Cury MC, Lima WS. Evaluation of two available methods to detect eggs of *Fasciola hepatica* in cattle faeces. Arq Bras Med Vet Zootec 2008;60(4):1023–5.

62. Abrous M, Comes a M, Gasnier N, et al. Morphological variability in *Fasciola hepatica* eggs in ruminants, rodents and lagomorphs. J Helminthol 2009;72(4):313.

63. Shaldoum FM, Muhammad AA, Sadek AG, et al. Advanced and classical diagnosis of *Fasciola* spp. in Egypt. J Am Sci 2015;11(5):1003–545.

64. Valero MA, Perez-Crespo I, Periago MV, et al. Fluke egg characteristics for the diagnosis of human and animal fascioliasis by *Fasciola hepatica* and *F. gigantica*. Acta Trop 2009;111(2):150–9.

65. Novobilský A, Kašný M, Mikeš L, et al. Humoral immune responses during experimental infection with *Fascioloides magna* and *Fasciola hepatica* in goats and comparison of their excretory/secretory products. Parasitol Res 2007;101(2):357–64.

66. Young ND, Jex AR, Cantacessi C, et al. A portrait of the transcriptome of the neglected trematode, *Fasciola gigantica*—biological and biotechnological implications. PLoS Negl Trop Dis 2011;5(2):e1004. Ghedin E, ed.

67. Bennema S, Vercruysse J, Claerebout E, et al. The use of bulk-tank milk ELISAs to assess the spatial distribution of *Fasciola hepatica*, *Ostertagia ostertagi* and *Dictyocaulus viviparus* in dairy cattle in Flanders (Belgium). Vet Parasitol 2009;165(1–2):51–7.

68. Gordon DK, Zadoks RN, Stevenson H, et al. On farm evaluation of the coproantigen ELISA and coproantigen reduction test in Scottish sheep naturally infected with *Fasciola hepatica*. Vet Parasitol 2012;187(3–4):436–44.

69. Malone JB, Loyacano AF, Hugh-Jones ME, et al. A three-year study on seasonal transmission and control of *Fasciola hepatica* of cattle in Louisiana. Prev Vet Med 1984;3(2):131–41.

70. Malone J, Loyacano A, Armstrong D, et al. Bovine fascioliasis: economic impact and control in gulf coast cattle based on seasonal transmission. Bov Pract 1982;17:126–33.

71. Kaplan RM. *Fasciola hepatica*: a review of the economic impact in cattle and considerations for control. Vet Ther 2001;2(1):40–50. Available at: http://www.ncbi.nlm.nih.gov/pubmed/19753697. Accessed June 13, 2019.

72. Craig TM, Bell RR. Seasonal transmission of liver flukes to cattle in the Texas Gulf Coast. J Am Vet Med Assoc 1978;173(1):104–7.

73. Esteban JG, González C, Bargues MD, et al. High fasciliasis infection in children linked to a man-made irrigation zone in Peru. Trop Med Int Health 2002;7(4):339–48. Available at: http://www.ncbi.nlm.nih.gov/pubmed/11952950. Accessed June 13, 2019.

74. Afshan K, Fortes-Lima CA, Artigas P, et al. Impact of climate change and man-made irrigation systems on the transmission risk, long-term trend and seasonality of human and animal fascioliasis in Pakistan. Geospat Health 2014;8(2):317.

75. Tum S, Puotinen M, Copeman D. A geographic information systems model for mapping risk of fasciolosis in cattle and buffaloes in Cambodia. Vet Parasitol 2004;122(2):141–9.

76. Knubben-Schweizer G, Torgerson PPR. Bovine fasciolosis: control strategies based on the location of *Galba truncatula* habitats on farms. Vet Parasitol 2015;208(1–2):77–83. Available at: https://linkinghub.elsevier.com/retrieve/pii/S0304401714006530. Accessed November 24, 2017.

77. Knubben-Schweizer G, Ruegg S, Torgerson PR, et al. Control of bovine fasciolosis in dairy cattle in Switzerland with emphasis on pasture management. Vet J 2010;186(2):188–91.

78. Anon. Flukicide products for cattle. Control worms sustain. 2017. Available at: https://www.cattleparasites.org.uk/app/uploads/2018/04/Flukicide-product-table.pdf. Accessed June 13, 2019.

79. Foreyt WJ. Evaluation of clorsulon against immature *Fascioloides magna* in cattle and sheep. Am J Vet Res 1988;49(7):1004–6. Available at: http://www.ncbi.nlm.nih.gov/pubmed/3421522. Accessed June 14, 2019.

80. Trematodocidal drugs. In: Mehlhorn H, editor. Encyclopedia of parasitology. Berlin: Springer Berlin Heidelberg; 2008. p. 1442–65.

81. Novobilský A, Höglund J. First report of closantel treatment failure against *Fasciola hepatica* in cattle. Int J Parasitol Drugs Drug Resist 2015;5(3):172–7.

82. Moll L, Gaasenbeek CP, Vellema P, et al. Resistance of *Fasciola hepatica* against triclabendazole in cattle and sheep in The Netherlands. Vet Parasitol 2000;91:153–8. Available at: http://helminto.inta.gob.ar/Foro 07/ResistMoll.pdf. Accessed June 14, 2019.

83. Kamaludeen J, Graham-Brown J, Stephens N, et al. Lack of efficacy of triclabendazole against *Fasciola hepatica* is present on sheep farms in three regions of England, and Wales. Vet Rec 2019;184(16):502.

84. Daniel R, van Dijk J, Jenkins T, et al. Composite faecal egg count reduction test to detect resistance to triclabendazole in *Fasciola hepatica*. Vet Rec 2012;171(6):153, 1-5.

85. Flanagan A, Edgar H, Forster F, et al. Standardisation of a coproantigen reduction test (CRT) protocol for the diagnosis of resistance to triclabendazole in *Fasciola hepatica*. Vet Parasitol 2011;176(1):34–42.

86. Ballweber L. *Fascioloides magna* in ruminants. Kenilworth (NJ): MSD Vet Man; 2019.

87. Stromberg B, Schlotthauer J, Conboy G. Efficacy of albendazole against *Fascioloides magna* in sheep. Am J Vet Res 1984;45(1):80–2.

88. Stromberg B, Schlotthauer J, Conboy G. The efficacy of closantel against *Fascioloides magna* in sheep. J Parasitol 1984;70(3):446–7.

89. Foreyt WJ. Efficacy of triclabendazole against experimentally induced *Fascioloides magna* infections in sheep. Am J Vet Res 1989;50(3):431–2.

90. Slavica A, Florijančić T, Janicki Z, et al. Treatment of fascioloidosis (*Fascioloides magna*, Bassi, 1875) in free ranging and captive red deer (*Cervus elaphus* L.) at eastern Croatia. Vet Arh 2006;76:9–18. Available at: http://vetarhiv.vef.unizg.hr/papers/2006-76-7-1.pdf. Accessed June 14, 2019.

Diagnostic Methods for Detecting Internal Parasites of Livestock

Guilherme G. Verocai, DVM, MSc, PhD[a],*,
Umer N. Chaudhry, DVM, MSc, PhD[b],
Manigandan Lejeune, BVSc, MSc, PhD[c]

KEYWORDS

- Diagnostic parasitology • Molecular diagnostics • Immunodiagnostics
- Fecal egg count • Nematodes • Tapeworms • Flukes • Coccidia

KEY POINTS

- Time-tested classical parasitology techniques remain the mainstay of parasite diagnosis, and diagnostic laboratories across North America continue to offer these techniques to assist livestock veterinarians.
- Increased awareness of the pros and cons of the various available techniques can guide veterinarians to make the most appropriate decisions when performing or requesting laboratory tests for parasite diagnosis.
- Routine use of parasite diagnostics is key for implementing effective parasite control programs and for monitoring the success of these programs.

INTRODUCTION

Internal parasites (or endoparasites) of various taxonomic groups, including helminths (nematodes, trematodes, and cestodes) and protozoans (coccidians, flagellates) infect ruminant livestock.[1] Some of these parasites are of major concern because they can affect the health and well-being of production animals clinically and subclinically, and ultimately cause significant economic loss.[2,3] Therefore, diagnostic tests for parasites of livestock are an integral part of management practices, and for assessing individual and herd health. In this review, we focus on the tests that are commonly and

---

[a] Parasitology Diagnostic Laboratory, Department of Veterinary Pathobiology, Texas A&M University, College of Veterinary Medicine and Biomedical Sciences, College Station, TX, USA; [b] University of Edinburgh Royal (Dick) School of Veterinary Studies, The Roslin Institute, Easter Bush Veterinary Centre, Roslin, Midlothian EH25 9RG, Scotland; [c] Clinical Parasitology, Department of Population Medicine and Diagnostic Sciences, Cornell University, College of Veterinary Medicine, Animal Health Diagnostic Center, 240 Farrier Drive, Ithaca, NY 14853, USA
* Corresponding author.
E-mail address: gverocai@cvm.tamu.edu
Twitter: @guiverocai (G.G.V.)

Vet Clin Food Anim 36 (2020) 125–143
https://doi.org/10.1016/j.cvfa.2019.12.003
0749-0720/20/© 2019 Elsevier Inc. All rights reserved.

routinely performed by veterinarians and diagnostic laboratories for detecting the most relevant parasitic infections of livestock in North America. In addition, we highlight the most recent advancement in the diagnosis of parasitic infections in livestock, including molecular and immunologic tests.

Generalities and Types of Diagnostic Techniques

Fecal examination is foremost for detecting parasites of the gastrointestinal tract, which make up most of the most economically and clinically relevant parasites of livestock. In addition, parasites of other body systems may also shed their eggs or larvae in feces.[4] Therefore, most diagnostic tests covered herein are microscopy-based fecal diagnostic tests. These are routinely performed by practicing veterinarians and diagnostic laboratories across North America.

Fecal parasitology tests are broadly classified as either qualitative or quantitative. The former identifies a particular parasite taxa based on distinctive morphology of their diagnostic stages, such as eggs, oocysts, cysts, or larvae; the latter aims to quantify the occurrence of targeted parasite taxa by counting their diagnostic stages. The quantitative tests are the most widely used diagnostics in livestock parasites because they relate to infection intensity, which consents informed management decision and control strategies. Results generated by quantitative tests are referred as eggs or oocysts per gram of feces (EPG and OPG, respectively).[4]

In contrast, qualitative diagnostic tests focus on the presence (positive) or absence (negative) of certain parasites. Qualitative tests may be interpreted as semiquantitative tests, when the sample tested is classified as demonstrating "few," "moderate," or "many" parasite stages. Alternatively, they are described as 1+, 2+, or 3+ based on reporting conventions established by a laboratory. Qualitative tests are not designed to be quantitative; therefore, applying semiquantitative interpretations to qualitative results often are poorly accurate as compared with properly performed quantitative tests. Furthermore, it should be understood that even quantitative (or semiquantitative) results are only estimates that may assist in treatment decisions by veterinarians or producers, but should not be interpreted as a direct indication of the number of parasites present in that animal.

GASTROINTESTINAL NEMATODES

Gastrointestinal nematodes (GIN) are among the most common and economically important parasites of livestock worldwide (**Fig. 1**).[3] Among North American livestock, the most common GIN genera and species are: *Haemonchus* spp (the barber pole worm, its predilection is the abomasum of various ruminants), *Ostertagia ostertagi* (the brown stomach worm, it resides in the abomasum of cattle), *Teladorsagia circumcincta* (in the abomasum of small ruminants), *Trichostrongylus axei* (in the abomasum of various ruminants), *Cooperia* spp and *Trichostrongylus* spp (in the small intestine of various ruminants), and *Oesophagostomum* spp (also known as the nodular worm, it resides in the large intestine of various ruminants). A recent review has covered the biology and veterinary importance of various GIN in depth,[2] and Christine B. Navarre's article, "Epidemiology and Control of Gastrointestinal Nematodes of Cattle in Southern Climates,"; Johannes Charlier and colleagues' article, "Biology and Epidemiology of Gastrointestinal Nematodes in Cattle,"; Michael B. Hildreth and John B. McKenzie's article, "Epidemiology and Control of Gastrointestinal Nematodes of Cattle in Northern Climates,"; Anne M. Zajac and Javier Garza's article, "Biology, Epidemiology, and Control of Gastrointestinal Nematodes of Small Ruminants," within this issue bring more detailed and relevant information on some of these parasites.

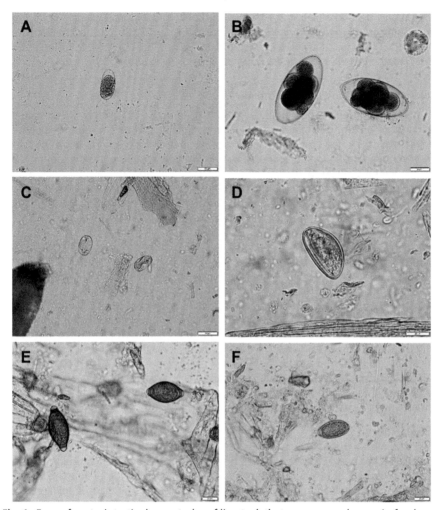

Fig. 1. Eggs of gastrointestinal nematodes of livestock that are commonly seen in fecal samples. (*A*) Strongyle-type egg. (*B*) *Nematodirus* sp eggs. (*C*) *Strongyloides* sp eggs. (*D*) *Skrjabinema* sp egg. (*E*) *Trichuris* sp eggs. (*F*) Capillarid-type egg.

Infections by GIN are most commonly subclinical, or cause subtle clinical disease in their livestock hosts. However, some GIN, such *Haemonchus* and *Ostertagia*, are capable of causing fatal infections. More commonly, disease can also be attributed to the combined deleterious effects of different genera and species at individual or at herd level, causing a condition called parasitic gastroenteritis.[5] Nevertheless, in most cases, the concern about levels of infection by GIN is the main driver for performing routine microscopy-based, quantitative diagnostic parasitology tests.

The most important GIN of livestock are taxonomically included in the superfamilies Trichostrongyloidea and Strongyloidea; therefore, the results of fecal egg count (FEC) techniques are given in numbers of trichostrongyle or strongyle EPG of feces. Morphometry of the eggs of different GIN largely overlaps across genera and species, preventing a genus or species-level identification. The eggs of most GINs are ellipsoidal (65–100 × 34–50 µm), have a thin shell, and contain a morula of developing cells when freshly passed in feces.[1,4] However, morphologically distinguishable strongyle eggs, such as eggs of *Nematodirus* spp (152–260 × 67–120 μm, football-shaped, larger cells in morula) and of *Marshallagia* (160–200 × 75–100 μm, with more parallel sides, smaller cells in morula), are counted separately in an FEC.[1,6]

Quantitative Fecal Egg Count Techniques

The diagnostic methods commonly used for the detection of GIN eggs are based on the principle of flotation; therefore, all of these FEC techniques include the use of a flotation solution in the protocol. These flotation solutions are used to allow the parasite developmental stages to float on a solution whose specific gravity is greater than that of buoyant densities of the parasitic stage. Different laboratories and clinics adopt solutions of their choice, but the most commonly used solutions are sodium nitrate (1.25–1.3 specific gravity [spg]), Sheather's or saturated sucrose (1.24–1.33 spg), and sodium chloride (1.2 spg). Information on flotation solutions and diagnostic techniques is found in **Tables 1** and **2**, respectively.

Among the most commonly used microscopy-based techniques for quantitative diagnosis of GIN and coccidians in livestock are: the modified McMaster (including its highly sensitive version) and the recently developed Mini-FLOTAC. Both of these techniques are based on the principle of "dilution egg count." In contrast, various iterations of the concentration-flotation method including the modified Wisconsin double-centrifugation method, that work on the principle of "concentration egg count" are also widely used. The result of any of these diagnostic tests may inform targeted treatment decisions, parasite management and control strategies, and can also be used to assess the anthelmintic resistance status of a given herd or flock as part of a fecal egg count reduction test (FECRT) (See Ray M. Kaplan's article, "Biology, Epidemiology, Diagnosis, and Management of Anthelmintic Resistance in Gastrointestinal Nematodes of Livestock," in this issue).

McMaster technique

The McMaster (or more accurately, the modified McMaster) is the most widely used dilution FEC method.[7] Protocols differ among various laboratories and clinics depending on the amount of feces used and the volume of and the type of flotation solution used. As a quantitative technique, the amount of feces and volume of solution used for dilution directly impacts the detection sensitivity of the test.[4] Briefly, a fecal slurry is made by mixing a known amount of feces and a known volume of flotation solution. Often, this slurry is sieved through cheesecloth and the liquid is used to fill a counting slide chamber, which contains two gridded areas. Strongyle eggs present in the gridded areas are counted and multiplied by 25, 50, or 100, depending on the protocol. The McMaster slide chamber or a complete McMaster kit are commercially available. A modification of the traditional McMaster method is the high sensitivity McMaster, which uses a three-chamber slide and has higher sensitivity than the McMaster (8 EPG vs 25, 50, or 100 EPG).[8] It is generally assumed that every livestock animal is parasitized by GIN, thus not seeing an egg during an FEC test does not mean that the animal is not infected, but rather that the level of egg shedding is below the detection threshold of the method used.

Mini-FLOTAC technique

The Mini-FLOTAC is a recently developed dilution FEC method that is user-friendly, and offers a high detection sensitivity.[9] The Mini-FLOTAC apparatus consists of two devices: the Fill-FLOTAC, which is a self-enclosed system that permits homogenization of the fecal solution and then direct filling of the counting chamber with

Table 1
Flotation solutions routinely used for quantitative and qualitative diagnostic methods of fecal stages of livestock parasites

Solution	Specific Gravity	Methods	Pros	Con
Sodium nitrate (NaNo₃)	1.25–1.3	McMaster, Mini-FLOTAC	Detection of most nematode eggs, *Moniezia* eggs, and Coccidia oocysts Commercially available	Distorts *Giardia* cysts Does not float fluke eggs May not float unusual nematode or tapeworm eggs Faster crystallization than sugar, not ideal for centrifugation
Saturated sodium chloride (NaCl)	1.2	McMaster	Detection of most nematode eggs, *Moniezia* eggs, and Coccidia oocysts	Does not float fluke eggs May not float unusual nematode or tapeworm eggs Faster crystallization than sugar, not ideal for centrifugation
Zinc sulfate 33% (ZnSo₄)	1.18	Wisconsin double-centrifugation for *Giardia*	Commercially available Does not distort *Giardia* cysts Allows Lugol iodine staining of *Giardia* cysts	Does not float nematode or fluke eggs well May not float unusual nematode or tapeworm eggs Faster crystallization than sugar, slides must be read quickly
Sheather's sucrose	1.25	Wisconsin double-centrifugation	Floats most nematode eggs, *Moniezia* eggs, and Coccidia oocysts Slides do not crystalize as fast as salt solutions	Distorts *Giardia* cysts Does not float fluke eggs It creates a sticky surface on benchtop and equipment
Saturated sugar	1.33	Wisconsin double-centrifugation	Floats most nematode eggs, *Moniezia* eggs, and Coccidia oocysts Floats *Dicrocoelium* eggs	Distorts *Giardia* cysts Distorts *Fasciola* eggs It creates a sticky surface on benchtop and equipment

Note: All solutions distort lungworm larvae, often impairing adequate morphologic identification. Baermann is the diagnostic method of choice.

Table 2
Routine microscopy-based diagnostic methods[a] for GIN and other internal parasites of livestock using feces

Technique	Main Purpose	Amount of Feces Large Ruminant	Amount of Feces Small Ruminant	Results
Quantitative				
McMaster	GIN counts, *Eimeria* oocyst counts	4 g	2–4 g	Eggs and/or oocysts per gram of feces, other parasites noted
High sensitivity McMaster	GIN counts, *Eimeria* oocyst counts	4 g	2–4 g	Same as above
Mini-FLOTAC	GIN counts, *Eimeria* oocyst counts	5 g	2–5 g	Same as above
Wisconsin double-centrifugation[a]	GIN counts (adult cattle, bison), *Eimeria* oocyst counts Detection of other helminths and protozoans	3–5 g	2–5 g	Same as above, often other parasites may be also quantified
Coproculture[c]	Genus-level identification of strongyle/trichostrongyle third-stage larvae	5–10 g/animal, usually pooled	2–10 g/animal, usually pooled	Percentage of different genera (and rarely species) Higher level of training/expertise required for identification
Qualitative				
Direct or stained smear	Detection of *Cryptosporidium* oocysts	<1 g; or air-dried fecal smear on slide	<1 g; or air-dried fecal smear on slide	Presence/absence Not sensitive

Wisconsin double-centrifugation with zinc[b]	Detection of *Giardia* cysts	2–5 g	2–3 g	Presence/absence
Sedimentation/Flukefinder	*Fasciola hepatica*	3–10 g	3–5 g	Larger amount of feces would yield higher sensitivity It can be made semiquantitative
Baermann	Lungworms larvae: *Dictyocaulus* in all ruminant livestock *Muellerius* and *Protostrongylus* in small ruminants	5–10 g	3–5 g	Presence/absence It can be made semiquantitative

[a] Diagnostic laboratories have a few basic requirements for sample submission. Because these may vary according to the laboratory or tests requested, it is recommended to contact the laboratory before submission. In general, laboratories recommend samples to be as fresh as possible, and to be stored in sealed, clean, and properly labeled bags, vials, or palpation gloves. Expressing the excess air from bags to create an anaerobic environment prevents undesired development and hatching of GIN eggs. It is also recommended to ship samples overnight on cold packs or ice (not directly touching the sample), accompanied by a filled submission form. Note that if multiple tests are requested on the same sample, account for the amount necessary for each of the tests (minimum amounts found in table; varies among laboratories).

[b] Certain diagnostic laboratories recommend running two Wisconsin-type double centrifugations in each sample, one with sucrose solution (1.25–1.33) and one with zinc sulfate (1.18) for maximizing the diagnosis of different parasites. In this case, double the amount of sample is required.

[c] Most often performed after individual fecal egg count; therefore, it should be submitted enough for sample for both tests.

filtration; and a counting chamber with two gridded areas that are examined under the microscope. The Fill-FLOTAC is a container with a conical bottom into which the fecal sample is added and weighted. Once the flotation solution is added, the screw top has a built-in pumping device that allows for thorough homogenization. The top lid also has a built-in sieve and a spout attachment that is used to fill the counting chamber.[9]

In North America, the Mini-FLOTAC has been used mainly for research purposes and by a few academic diagnostic laboratories, but in the future should find increased use in veterinary practices, particularly for conducting FECRT. The detection threshold of the regular protocol of the Mini-FLOTAC is five EPG; however, as for all other dilution techniques, the detection threshold may be adjusted according to the amount of feces and volume of flotation solution used. A recent study demonstrated that the Mini-FLOTAC was more accurate and more precise for performing FEC on cattle and sheep fecal samples than the high sensitivity McMaster and the modified Wisconsin method.[8]

Concentration-flotation techniques

The most notable example of a concentration FEC method is the modified Wisconsin double-centrifugation method. This protocol consists of a first centrifugation step performed in a fecal slurry made up of feces and water, and a second centrifugation step where the sediment of the previous step is homogenized with the flotation solution. Variations in concentration-flotation protocols exist across laboratories.[4,8] It depends on the initial amount of feces used, volume and type of flotation solution, and time of each centrifugation step. Because there is no dilution step, the Wisconsin double-centrifugation technique permits high detection sensitivity (one EPG or even less). It is sometimes recommended by parasitologists for use in older large ruminants, such as cattle and bison, which normally have lower EPGs.[2] Logistically, it may be more challenging for practitioners to implement this method in their clinics, because it requires a centrifuge, and requires considerably more time to perform than the other methods. Additionally, the Wisconsin method had much lower accuracy and precision in sheep and cattle than did the McMaster or mini-FLOTAC methods.[8] Consequently, unless EPG are extremely low, then the other methods are preferred. But if EPG are extremely low, then the usefulness of performing FEC is limited making the Wisconsin method rarely an optimal choice for performing FEC.

Coproculture technique

The coproculture method is used for genus or species-level identification of third-stage larvae (L3) based on larval morphology, because the eggs of strongyles/trichostrongyles are virtually morphologically indistinguishable. The coproculture is also recommended during the precollection and postcollection for FECRT, because these data can indicate which genus/genera are resistant to the anthelmintic drug used. Coproculture protocols vary among diagnostic laboratories in North America. Most often, coprocultures are performed using pooling of samples, with the same or approximately the same amount of feces from each animal used for each of the pooled samples.[10] Feces are mixed with vermiculite, which helps in retaining moisture and keeping the fecal matter and parasite eggs and larvae oxygenated. The mixture of feces and vermiculite are kept at room temperature, or incubator with controlled temperature for 7 to 21 days, with 10 to 14 days being the most common time frame for recovery of L3. The protocols used to recover L3s from a coproculture also vary among laboratories, although the Baermann method (described later) is the most commonly used technique. After recovery, collected L3s are killed and stained with Lugol iodine, which enhances morphologic features used for identification. These features include length of the L3, shape and structures of the cephalic extremity, and length of tail and cuticular sheath, among others.[4,10] Typically, 100 L3 are identified, or if less than 100 L3 are available then all L3 in the sample are examined, and results are reported as percentage of each genus/species found.

Molecular diagnostic tools

Recent research has focused on the development and validation of novel molecular methods for identifying GIN to species-level using eggs or larvae recovered from coproculture. Sequence variations in the coding and noncoding regions of the nuclear ribosomal DNA have been the most commonly used genetic markers for parasitic nematode species identification to date. In the case of GIN, the internal transcribed spacer ribosomal DNA (ITS-1 and ITS-2) generally provide an appropriate level of interspecies variation for reliable species identification.[11–13]

The nemabiome is a recently developed molecular diagnostic method that accurately identifies and provides relative quantification of the community of GIN species infecting livestock hosts.[14] Currently, this method has been validated for GIN of cattle and bison,[14–17] with potential for application in other domestic livestock species, and wild ungulates. The use of barcoded primers allows a large number of samples to be pooled and sequenced in a single Mi-Seq run, making the technology suitable for high throughput analysis.[14] By multiplexing the barcoded primer combinations, it is possible to run 384 samples at once on a single Illumina Mi-Seq flow cell (San Diego, CA), helping to reduce the cost. This methodology is a promising tool to be implemented in routine diagnostics of GIN in livestock, and in the future, it may serve as a preferred option over the coproculture and microscopic identification.

OTHER GASTROINTESTINAL NEMATODES

Many other nematodes that do not belong to the superfamilies Trichostrongyloidea or Strongyloidea also reside in the gastrointestinal tract of livestock, and are commonly diagnosed when performing FEC (**Fig. 2**).[2,4] Among these nematodes are *Trichuris* spp (whipworms), which are characterized by eggs that are barrel-shaped, golden-brown, bipolar plugged ($70–80 \times 30–42$ μm), and *Aonchotheca* spp (= *Capillaria*), whose eggs are similar to those of *Trichuris* but smaller and less symmetric ($45–50 \times 22–25$ μm). *Strongyloides* spp (threadworms) are characterized by eggs that are ellipsoidal, thin shelled, smaller than GIN, and larvated in fresh feces ($40–60 \times 32–40$ μm) and are often found in young animals of various ruminant species. *Toxocara vitulorum* (roundworm) of cattle and bison shed dark-brown, thick-shelled, round eggs ($75–95 \times 60–75$ μm). *Skrjabinema* (pinworm) is only found in small ruminants and shed small, asymmetrical eggs ($47–63 \times 27–36$ μm). The eggs of these different parasites are distinguishable based on a combination of morphologic features, including dimensions, color, and special structures. Most often, veterinarians and diagnosticians note the presence of these in a fecal sample, but it is not usual to quantify them as is done for trichostrongyle/strongyle eggs.

LUNGWORMS

Nematode species that infect the lungs of ruminants shed either larvated eggs or first-stage larvae (L1) in feces, and are occasionally diagnosed in diagnostic laboratories. *Dictyocaulus viviparus* infects cattle and bison, whereas *Dictyocaulus filaria* infects small ruminants.[1,18] Small ruminants are also infected with *Muellerius capillaris*[19] and *Protostrongylus rufescens*.[20]

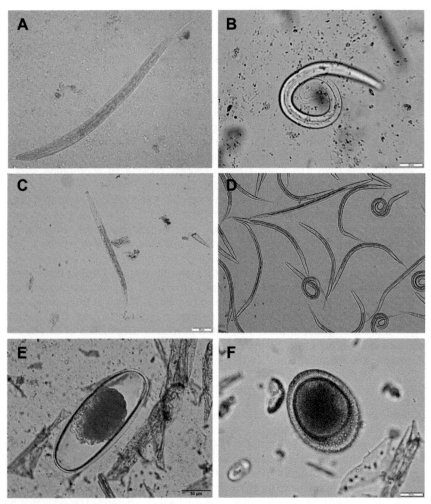

Fig. 2. Diagnostic stages of less common nematodes of livestock. (*A*) *Protostrongylus* sp larva. (*B*) *Muellerius capillaris* larva. (*C*) *Dictyocaulus viviparus* larva. (*D*) Strongyle, third-stage larvae. (*E*) *Marshallagia* sp egg. (*F*) *Toxocara vitulorum* egg.

Baermann and its Modifications

The Baermann technique relies on the migration of live larvae out of a fecal sample into water. This technique is most often used for detection of lungworm larvae but can also be used to recover any motile larvae including the recovery of trichostrongyle/strongyle larvae from coproculture. Lungworms shed larvae in feces or larvated eggs that hatch in contact with lukewarm water in a given period of time.[4] These larvae sediment overnight (16–24 hours) at room temperature and are recovered using the Baermann apparatus, which consist of a suspended funnel attached with a clamped tubing. Various adaptations exist that replace the traditional Baermann apparatus.[4,21,22] The amount of feces used directly impacts the sensitivity of the test (see **Table 2**).[4] The sediment is assessed under a compound microscope for the presence of L1, whose genus and/or species may be distinguished based on morphology. Larvae of *Dictyocaulus* have an intestine filled with large food granules, and have a short and pointy tail. L1s of bovine *D viviparus* are shorter (300–360 μm) than *D filaria* of small ruminants (550–580 μm). Larvae of *M capillaris* (300–320 μm) have a dorsal spine at the base of a kinky, segmented tail, whereas larvae of *P rufescens* (340–400 μm) have an elongate, pointy tail, and lack food granules and a dorsal spine.[4,23]

Other Diagnostic Methods for Dictyocaulus

Despite not being routinely used or commercially available in North America, some immunodiagnostic techniques are often used for detecting *Dictyocaulus* infection in cattle.[24,25] These include a serologic enzyme-linked immunosorbent assay (ELISA) test, which uses the major sperm protein from adult male lungworms expressed as recombinant antigen,[24,26] and pooled or bulk milk-ELISA.[25] *Dictyocaulus* and other lungworm larvae may be detected using bronchoalveolar lavage.[26] Practitioners are more likely to perform a bronchoalveolar lavage than a Baermann, because the former allows also for eosinophil count.

CESTODES (TAPEWORMS)

Moniezia spp are the most common cestode that infects the small intestine of domestic ruminants (**Fig. 3**). It is considered nonpathogenic, but high-intensity infections, especially in young animals, may cause obstruction. *Moniezia* eggs are embryonated (approximately 65–75 μm), and have a peculiar shape and pyriform apparatus in their interior.[4] Eggs of *Moniezia benedeni* of cattle and bison are more square-shaped, whereas eggs of *Moniezia expansa* of small ruminants have a diamond or triangular shape. Two additional tapeworm species, less commonly found infecting domestic ruminants in western North America, are the fringed tapeworm *Thysanosoma actinoides* and *Wyominia tetoni*, both found in the bile ducts.[27] These are occasionally observed while performing FEC or at necropsy.

TREMATODES (FLUKES)
Fasciola hepatica

The common liver fluke, *Fasciola hepatica*, is patchily distributed across North America, including some states along the Gulf Coast, the Pacific Northwest, and the inland Northwest.[28,29] Adult flukes are found in the bile ducts of cattle, sheep, goat, camelids, and various other animals. The ruminant host becomes infected by ingesting the metacercaria, which is an encysted larval form, found on the vegetation. More information on the biology, epidemiology, economic importance, and control of liver flukes is found in Joan M. Burke and James E. Miller's article, "Sustainable Approaches to Parasite Control in Ruminant Livestock," in this issue. Although eggs may not be detected during the acute phase of infection, fecal testing using a sedimentation technique can be performed to detect eggs.

Sedimentation and Flukefinder Sedimentation

Traditional fecal sedimentation for diagnosing *F hepatica* is infrequently offered by diagnostic laboratories across North America; however, a modified version of the sedimentation method that uses a commercially available device called the Flukefinder is often used to detect fluke infection in domestic and wild ruminants.[4,30] The method consists of sieving a fecal sample (3–10 g) through a pair of sieves: the first separates larger debris, and the second retains the eggs while letting smaller debris pass. The material retained in the second sieve is collected into test tubes, and undergoes a series of sedimentation and washing steps. The final material is assessed in a Petri

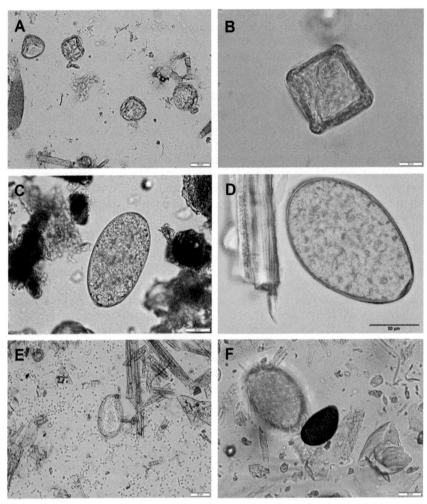

Fig. 3. Diagnostic stages of common cestodes and trematodes of livestock. (*A*) *Moniezia expansa* egg, (*B*) *Moniezia benedeni* egg, (*C*) *Fasciola hepatica* egg, (*D*) *Fascioloides magna* egg, (*E*) Amphistome egg, and (*F*) *Dicrocoelium dendriticum* egg. (*Courtesy of* [*C*] Yoko Nagamori, DVM, MS, DACVM, Stillwater, OK; and [*D*] Paul Gajda, Calgary, Canada.)

dish under a dissection microscope, after addition of a drop of methylene blue, which stains the fecal debri/fiber blue-green, making the large, golden-brown, operculate *F hepatica* eggs (130–150 × 63–90 μm) easier to see.[4] Chronic fascioliasis is the most common presentation in infected ruminants, and in such cases it is likely that eggs are seen in the sedimentation test. However, it is important to stress that hosts affected by acute fasciolosis likely do not shed eggs in feces, because the major damage is caused by migrating juvenile flukes. In such cases microscopy-based sedimentation methods may not be reliable, and immunodiagnostic tests are preferred. To assess cost-benefit for producers, a recent study showed that composite fecal sample (pooling samples from more than one animal) was a useful method for detecting *F hepatica* in cattle, but negative results should be followed up by a second test because of limitations related to the diagnostic sensitivity.[31]

Beyond microscopy-based detection of *F hepatica* eggs, there has been strong emphasis on the development and validation of improved diagnostics of fasciolosis using DNA-based molecular methods and immunodiagnostics.[32] Commercial ELISA tests for detection of *F hepatica* antibodies in serum and milk samples, and ELISA tests for detection of coproantigens are available in the Europe and other parts of the world, and have been used in epidemiologic studies in various continents, but not in the United States or Canada.[24,33] Overall, immunodiagnostic tests have several advantages over microscopy-based tests, including increased sensitivity; suitability for high throughput formats that are used for a variety of biologic samples; and the ease for implementation in large-scale, herd-level epidemiologic studies.

Fascioloides magna

The giant liver fluke or deer fluke, *Fascioloides magna*, is a parasite of North American cervids, including deer, elk, and caribou.[6,34] In cervids, eggs passed in feces are indistinguishable from those of *F hepatica*, and are detected using sedimentation methods described previously.[35] Domestic ruminants may get infected with *F magna* in various regions of North America, and infection can be fatal. In cattle, these flukes form a thick-walled cyst in the liver, and in sheep and goats these undergo extensive migration and cause significant liver damage. Infection in domestic livestock can be fatal.[36,37] Domestic livestock are dead-end host and do not shed eggs in feces; therefore, sedimentation techniques do not detect infection in these hosts.

There are no commercial antemortem diagnostics available to confirm fascioloidosis in domestic ruminants, although antibody testing based on ELISA methodology has been developed in research laboratories to study animal exposure to *F magna*.[38] In the absence of antemortem tests in domestic ruminants, postmortem observation of *F magna* specimens, migration tracks, or cysts remain as the only definitive diagnostic.

Amphistomes

Amphistomes are pear-shaped flukes belonging to various genera (*Paramphistomum*, *Cotylophoron*, *Calicophoron*) and found in the rumen of cattle and other bovids. The adults are mainly considered nonpathogenic, but their migrating larval forms may cause production loss and mortality.[39] Amphistome eggs are large, transparent, and operculate (114–175 × 65–100 μm), and are detected in feces by the same techniques used for diagnosing *F hepatica*.[4] Therefore, veterinarians, and diagnosticians must be familiar with the morphologic differences between liver fluke and amphistome eggs.

Dicrocoelium dendriticum

Dicrocoelium dendriticum, popularly known as the lancet liver fluke, infects the bile ducts of cattle, sheep and goat, and some wild cervids in areas of North America. The range of distribution of *D dendriticum* seems to have expanded in North America, especially in the eastern United States, Atlantic Provinces of Canada, and in Alberta, from its limited range known in early 1950s.[40] Heavy infestations by *D dendriticum* may be associated with cirrhosis, which may lead to anemia and weight loss. In most cases in cattle, the disease is asymptomatic and does not warrant fecal assessment for parasite stages. However, condemnation of liver at slaughter makes a case for routine fecal checking for this small fluke in animals from endemic areas. The eggs are much smaller than those of other flukes (38–45 × 22–30 μm), brown, and operculate, and contain a fully formed miracidium that appears as two eyes.[4] Double-centrifugation Wisconsin using sucrose solution (1.33 spg) is ideal to recover *D dendriticum* eggs in feces. Eggs can also be detected using sedimentation techniques,[4] but excessive debris and the brown color of the egg makes it difficult to read the test. Some effort has been made toward identifying potential serologic markers for dicrocoeliosis.[41]

POSTMORTEM DIAGNOSTIC TESTS FOR HELMINTHS
Specimen Identification

Morphologic identification of helminth specimens collected at necropsy permits species-specific diagnosis. Specimens are observed under dissecting scope, and may be mounted on a glass slide with clearing agents for observation on a compound microscope. This process usually requires great expertise in classical parasitology, and is time consuming. The correct identification of worm specimens is informative to anatomic pathologists and veterinarians. Submitting specimens in 70% ethanol is ideal, because it allows for further molecular characterization of specimens if necessary. However, pathologists most often use buffered formalin, which may impact its use for molecular tests.

Abomasal Worm Count

This postmortem diagnostic technique is mostly restricted to research applications; however, it is offered by some diagnostic laboratories for quantifying the number of abomasal nematodes, and identification of these to genus or species level. Most often, worm counts are requested by anatomic pathologists as an ancillary test, for assisting cases in which haemonchosis or ostertagiosis are considered as potential cause of death. The abomasum together with its content are submitted to the laboratory on ice packs. A subsample of the contents is then examined under a dissecting microscope and worms are counted and recovered. Specimens can then be cleared with lactophenol to facilitate morphologically identification under a compound microscope.

GASTROINTESTINAL PROTOZOANS
Eimeria spp

Various species of coccidian protozoans of the genus *Eimeria* are found in the gastrointestinal tract of domestic livestock and the host gets infected by ingesting sporulated oocysts while grazing (**Fig. 4**). *Eimeria* spp cause destruction of the intestinal mucosa, leading to malabsorption of nutrients, and diarrhea particularly in young animals, and can cause production losses.

Oocysts of *Eimeria* spp are detected on any fecal flotation test.[4] Quantitative methods routinely used for determination of EPG of GIN, including McMasters and Mini-FLOTAC, are useful for counting oocysts, and results are expressed as OPG.[42,43]

Although *Eimeria* spp are host-specific, coinfections with different species are common in livestock hosts. However, many diagnostic laboratories are content with a broad identification of coccidia to the genus level rather than to species. This approach does not account for differences in pathogenicity among species, and may not be as informative for informing treatment decisions. Because coinfections with pathogenic and nonpathogenic species are common, ideally, species differentiation should be performed before any treatment plan is initiated. Morphologic differentiation of *Eimeria* oocysts poses a challenge because it requires considerable diagnostic expertise and the availability of microscopes with high-power objectives. There are a few definite morphologic keys available[44,45] that may aid species differentiation. Despite this limitation it is advisable to classically differentiate pathogenic

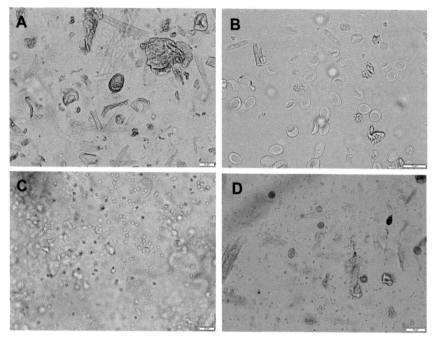

Fig. 4. Diagnostic stages of common protozoans of livestock. (*A*) *Eimeria bovis* oocyst. (*B*) *Giardia* sp cysts. (*C*) *Cryptosporidium parvum* oocysts. (*D*) *Cryptosporidium andersoni* oocysts.

Eimeria from the nonpathogenic ones. Recently, molecular techniques based on species-specific real-time polymerase chain reaction (PCR) assay have been developed for accurate *Eimeria* detection.[46] Nevertheless, it is doubtful that these tests will be commercially available in the near future.

Giardia duodenalis

Giardia duodenalis infection in ruminants is considered asymptomatic but diarrhea in young animals associated with this protozoan has been widely reported.[4] In an outbreak investigation, clinical and epidemiologic questions raised would determine whether classical techniques or molecular analysis is required for detecting *Giardia*. If one needs to relate the clinical sign (diarrhea) in a calf with that of *Giardia* infection, a double-centrifugation flotation test with $ZnSo_4$ would suffice (cysts are 9–13 × 7–9 μm). In contrast, to investigate the source of *Giardia* outbreak and its potential zoonotic implications to human handlers may necessitate detection by genotyping. Commercial fecal antigen capture ELISA are available for sensitive detection of *Giardia*, especially in situations where trained personnel is not available for classical detection. Most parasitology diagnostic laboratories also offer immunofluorescence antibody test and PCRs for diagnosing *Giardia*.

Cryptosporidium spp

Four species of *Cryptosporidium* namely, *Cryptosporidium parvum*, *Cryptosporidium bovis*, *Cryptosporidium ryanae*, and *Cryptosporidium andersoni*, have been reported in cattle and other domestic ruminants.[1] *C parvum* is the most pathogenic and commonly associated with diarrhea in young animals. Diagnosis is generally done by the double-centrifugation Wisconsin method using sucrose solution where the oocysts are refringent to light and assume a characteristic pink hue. Oocysts are small, making it challenging for an untrained eye to correctly detect them microscopically. Oocysts of most *Cryptosporidium* are not morphologically distinguishable (measures 4.6–5.4 × 3.8–4.7 μm), except for *C andersoni* (7.0–8.6 × 5.0–6.28 μm). Commercial ELISA tests based on antigen capture methodology are available for sensitive and accurate detection in fecal samples. Diagnostic laboratories often offer staining technique (Ziehl Neelsen) for detection of cryptosporidiosis, and immunofluorescence antibody test and PCR methods. PCR genotyping is the only option to identify *Cryptosporidium* to species.

SUMMARY

Microscopy-based fecal diagnostic techniques are the most widely used by veterinarians and offered as diagnostic service by veterinarians, producers, and laboratories across North America. Quantitative methods used for FEC are routinely performed for informing targeted anthelmintic treatment and control strategies, and FECRT. In addition, veterinarians may send out samples for Baermann for lungworms, and sedimentation for detection of liver fluke, among others. Choices on which test to perform or request from a service laboratory should be based on the accuracy of the test, and practicability and costs. Diagnostics for most other helminths, including flukes, and coccidian depend on a clinical case or outbreak, or are often associated with a certain age class or geographic locations within North America. Novel molecular tests for livestock parasites have been developed, but at this stage they are mainly used for research purposes. Immunodiagnostic tests targeting various nematodes have also been developed, but have not been implemented or are commercially available in North America.

DISCLOSURE

The authors have nothing to disclose.

REFERENCES

1. Bowman DD. Georgis' parasitology for veterinarians. 10th edition. St Louis (MO): Elsevier Saunders; 2014.
2. Craig TM. Gastrointestinal nematodes, diagnosis and control. Vet Clin North Am Food Anim Pract 2018;34(1):185–99.
3. Stromberg BE, Gasbarre LC. Gastrointestinal nematode control programs with an emphasis on cattle. Vet Clin North Am Food Anim Pract 2006;22(3):543–65.
4. Zajac AM, Conboy G. Veterinary clinical parasitology. 8th edition. West Sussex (UK): Wiley-Blackwell; 2012.
5. Armour A. Epidemiology of parasitic gastroenteritis in cattle and sheep. Vet Rec 1986;119:211.
6. Kutz SJ, Ducrocq J, Verocai GG, et al. Parasites of ungulates of arctic North America and Greenland: a view of contemporary diversity, ecology, and impact in a world under change. Adv Parasitol 2012;79:99–252.
7. Gordon HM, Whitlock HV. A new technique for counting nematode eggs in sheep faeces. J Counc Sci Industr Res 1939;12:50–2.
8. Paras KL, George MM, Vidyashankar AN, et al. Comparison of fecal egg counting methods in four livestock species. Vet Parasitol 2018;257:21–7.

9. Barda BD, Rinaldi L, Ianniello D, et al. Mini-FLOTAC, an innovative direct diagnostic technique for intestinal parasitic infections: experience from the field. PLoS Negl Trop Dis 2013;7(8):e2344.

10. van Wyk JA, Mayhew E. Morphological identification of parasitic nematode infective larvae of small ruminants and cattle: a practical lab guide. Onderstepoort J Vet Res 2013;80(1):539.

11. Chilton NB, Gasser RB. Sequence differences in the internal transcribed spacers of DNA among four species of hookworm (Ancylostomatoidea: Ancylostoma). Int J Parasitol 1999;29(12):1971–7.

12. Stevenson LA, Chilton NB, Gasser RB. Differentiation of *Haemonchus placei* from *H. contortus* (Nematoda: Trichostrongylidae) by the ribosomal DNA second internal transcribed spacer. Int J Parasitol 1995;25(4):483–8.

13. Zarlenga DS, Hoberg EP, Stringfellow F, et al. Comparisons of two polymorphic species of Ostertagia and phylogenetic relationships within the Ostertagiinae (Nematoda: Trichostrongyloidea) inferred from ribosomal DNA repeat and mitochondrial DNA sequences. J Parasitol 1998;84(4):806–12.

14. Avramenko RW, Redman EM, Lewis R, et al. Exploring the gastrointestinal "nemabiome": deep amplicon sequencing to quantify the species composition of parasitic nematode communities. PLoS One 2015;10(12):e0143559.

15. Avramenko RW, Redman EM, Lewis R, et al. The use of nemabiome metabarcoding to explore gastro-intestinal nematode species diversity and anthelmintic treatment effectiveness in beef calves. Int J Parasitol 2017;47(13):893–902.

16. Avramenko RW, Bras A, Redman EM, et al. High species diversity of trichostrongyle parasite communities within and between Western Canadian commercial and conservation bison herds revealed by nemabiome metabarcoding. Parasit Vectors 2018;11(1):299.

17. Scott H, Gilleard JS, Jelinski M, et al. Prevalence, fecal egg counts, and species identification of gastrointestinal nematodes in replacement dairy heifers in Canada. J Dairy Sci 2019;102(9):8251–63.

18. Panuska C. Lungworms of ruminants. Vet Clin North Am Food Anim Pract 2006; 22(3):583–93.

19. McCraw BM, Menzies PI. Treatment of goats Infected with the Lungworm *Muellerius capillaris*. Can Vet J 1986;27(8):287–90.

20. Mansfield LS, Gamble HR. Alveolar mastocytosis and eosinophilia in lambs with naturally acquired nematode infections of *Protostrongylus rufescens* and *Haemonchus contortus*. Vet Immunol Immunopathol 1995;49(3):251–62.

21. Verocai GG, Lejeune M, Finstad GL, et al. A Nearctic parasite in a Palearctic host: *Parelaphostrongylus andersoni* (Nematoda; Protostrongylidae) infecting semi-domesticated reindeer in Alaska. Int J Parasitol Parasites Wildl 2013;2: 119–23.

22. Hoggard KJ, Jarriel DM, Bevelock TJ, et al. Prevalence survey of gastrointestinal and respiratory parasites of shelter cats in northeastern Georgia, USA. Vet Parasitol Reg Stud Reports 2019;16:100270.

23. van Wyk JA, Cabaret J, Michael LM. Morphological identification of nematode larvae of small ruminants and cattle simplified. Vet Parasitol 2004;119(4): 277–306.

24. Frey CF, Eicher R, Raue K, et al. Apparent prevalence of and risk factors for infection with *Ostertagia ostertagi*, *Fasciola hepatica* and *Dictyocaulus viviparus* in Swiss dairy herds. Vet Parasitol 2018;250:52–9.

25. McCarthy C, Höglund J, Christley R, et al. A novel pooled milk test strategy for the herd level diagnosis of *Dictyocaulus viviparus*. Vet Parasitol X 2019;1: 100008.

26. Lurier T, Delignette-Muller ML, Rannou B, et al. Diagnosis of bovine dictyocaulosis by bronchoalveolar lavage technique: a comparative study using a Bayesian approach. Prev Vet Med 2018;154:124–31.

27. Craig TM, Shepherd E. Efficacy of albendazole and levamisole in sheep against *Thysanosoma actinioides* and *Haemonchus contortus* from the Edwards Plateau, Texas. Am J Vet Res 1980;41(3):425–6.

28. Kaplan RM. Fasciola hepatica: a review of the economic impact in cattle and considerations for control. Vet Ther 2001;2(1):40–50.

29. Malone JB. Fascioliasis and cestodiasis in cattle. Vet Clin North Am Food Anim Pract 1986;2(2):261–75.

30. Malone JB, Craig TM. Cattle liver flukes: risk assessment and control. Compend Contin Educ Vet 1990;12(5):747–54.

31. Graham-Brown J, Williams DJL, Skuce P, et al. Composite *Fasciola hepatica* faecal egg sedimentation test for cattle. Vet Rec 2019;184(19):589.

32. Charlier J, Vercruysse J, Morgan E, et al. Recent advances in the diagnosis, impact on production and prediction of *Fasciola hepatica* in cattle. Parasitology 2014;141(3):326–35.

33. Martinez-Sernandez V, Orbegozo-Medina RA, Gonzalez-Warleta M, et al. Rapid enhanced MM3-COPRO ELISA for detection of *Fasciola coproantigens*. PLoS Negl Trop Dis 2016;10(7):e0004872.

34. Samuel WM, Pybus MJ, Kocan AA. Parasitic diseases of wild mammals. Ames (IA): Iowa State University Press; 2001.

35. Pruvot M, Lejeune M, Kutz S, et al. Better alone or in ill company? The effect of migration and inter-species comingling on *Fascioloides magna* infection in Elk. PLoS One 2016;11(7):e0159319.

36. Wobeser BK, Schumann F. Fascioloides magna infection causing fatal pulmonary hemorrhage in a steer. Can Vet J 2014;55(11):1093–5.

37. Foreyt WJ, Leathers CW. Experimental infection of domestic goats with *Fascioloides magna*. Am J Vet Res 1980;41(6):883–4.

38. Schillhorn van Veen TW. Prevalence of *Fascioloides magna* in cattle and deer in Michigan. J Am Vet Med Assoc 1987;191(5):547–8.

39. Chaudhry U, van Paridon B, Lejeune M, et al. Morphological and molecular identification of *Explanatum* in domestic water buffalo in Pakistan. Vet Parasitol Reg Stud Reports 2017;8(Supplement C):54–9.

40. van Paridon BJ, Colwell DD, Goater CP, et al. Population genetic analysis informs the invasion history of the emerging trematode *Dicrocoelium dendriticum* into Canada. Int J Parasitol 2017;47(13):845–56.

41. Colwell DD, Goater CP. *Dicrocoelium dendriticum* in cattle from Cypress Hills, Canada: humoral response and preliminary evaluation of an ELISA. Vet Parasitol 2010;174(1–2):162–5.

42. Silva LMR, Vila-Viçosa MJM, Maurelli MP, et al. Mini-FLOTAC for the diagnosis of *Eimeria* infection in goats: an alternative to McMaster. Small Rumin Res 2013;114: 280–3.

43. Van Metre DC, Tyler JW, Stehman SM. Diagnosis of enteric disease in small ruminants. Vet Clin North Am Food Anim Pract 2000;16(1):87–115.

44. Florião MM, Lopes BB, Berto BP, et al. New approaches for morphological diagnosis of bovine *Eimeria* species: a study on a subtropical organic dairy farm in Brazil. Trop Anim Health Prod 2016;48(3):577–84.

45. Macedo LO, Santos MAB, Silba NMM, et al. Morphological and epidemiological data on *Eimeria* species infecting small ruminants in Brazil. Small Rumin Res 2019;171:37–41.
46. Kawahara F, Zhang G, Mingala CN, et al. Genetic analysis and development of species-specific PCR assays based on ITS-1 region of rRNA in bovine *Eimeria* parasites. Vet Parasitol 2010;174(1–2):49–57.

What Modeling Parasites, Transmission, and Resistance Can Teach Us

Hannah Rose Vineer, PhD Veterinary Parasitology

KEYWORDS

- Parasite • Ruminant • Modeling • Model • Climate change • Decision support
- Anthelmintic resistance • Disease

KEY POINTS

- Models are valuable for exploring complex parasite systems, especially when field trials would be costly or impossible.
- Research and development of novel approaches to parasite control can be model-guided, for example, vaccine development.
- Optimal control strategies can vary based on prevailing environmental conditions resulting from the impact of weather on the abundance of parasites, and modeling provides a means to compare the success of different strategies under such varying conditions.
- An array of model-based decision support tools is available for veterinary clinicians and farmers to facilitate sustainable parasite control practices.
- Modeling can provide evidence to guide and support policy on the sustainable control of parasites, especially the responsible use of new anthelmintics.

INTRODUCTION

Antiparasiticide resistance is widely reported in a range of ectoparasites and endoparasites[1,2] and is set against a backdrop of environmental change. Climate warming may have already changed the geographic distribution and seasonal abundance of some parasites,[3] and interannual climate variability could result in unexpected differences in the seasonal risk of parasitic infection between years.[4] These factors may also affect the local relevance of field studies performed decades ago before large-scale environmental changes.

Funded by: BBSRC. Grant number: BB/M003949/1 and the University of Liverpool's Institute of Infection and Global Health.

Veterinary Parasitology, Department of Infection Biology, Institute of Infection and Global Health, University of Liverpool, Institute of Veterinary Science, Chester High Road, Neston CH64 7TE, UK

E-mail address: hannah.vineer@liverpool.ac.uk

Twitter: @HannahVineer (H.R.V.)

Strategies that advocate more thoughtful and targeted applications of antiparasiticides promise to slow the development of resistance[2,5] while nonchemotherapeutic approaches offer promising alternatives.[2,6,7] However, host-parasite dynamics are complex, especially because of the diversity of ruminant livestock production systems used worldwide. Capturing this variability sufficiently using field trials alone would be prohibitively expensive and likely impossible. Furthermore, field trials can only be undertaken in the environmental conditions encountered during the trial and cannot capture interannual variability in weather patterns nor potential future climate change. Models offer an additional tool to complement and drive forward the development of novel approaches to parasite control, to further the understanding of host-parasite and epidemiologic processes and the development of drug resistance, and to generate decision support tools for veterinarians and farmers.

This article aims to provide veterinary practitioners with an understanding of what models are as well as their advantages and potential limitations, signpost model-based resources for assessing parasite disease and transmission risk, and highlight key areas where models are helping to shape the development of sustainable parasite control strategies.

WRONG, BUT USEFUL
What Are Models, and Why Do We Use Them?

Models are simplified, mathematical representations of real-world systems or events that either broadly describe the relationship between a variable of interest and a predictor variable (empirical model; **Box 1** and see **Fig. 1**A), or describe the system processes as a set of mathematical equations (mechanistic model; see **Box 1** and **Fig. 1**B).

While the process of developing a model can enhance understanding of parasites and epidemiologic processes, and focus attention onto specific topics for future research, models also allow rapid exploration of the impacts of change (eg, climate change[9]) or interventions (eg, the timing of antiparasiticide treatments[11]). To achieve this, usually the model input, such as climatic data representing different regions or time periods, or the values assigned to model components (parameters), are adjusted to represent the different scenarios of interest. Testing each of the scenarios in the "real world" would require a different field trial or controlled experiment, which can be prohibitively costly. In addition, the development of resistance to antiparasitic drugs can take years if not decades, so running field trials to compare the impact of different treatment strategies is challenging. The impacts of regional differences in climate on parasites and disease can also only feasibly be tested in the field at a limited number of locations and only over short time scales, thus usually representing a limited range of weather patterns over a 1- to 5-year period. It is also impossible to truly test parasites' responses to climate change in the field, as these conditions are not yet realized, or to monitor phenomena that are rare at present and cannot be measured, such as development of resistance to novel antiparasitic compounds. By contrast, models can rapidly explore large numbers of hypothetical scenarios and can be projected onto weather data for multiple regions or future climates, providing insight into parasite epidemiology that would otherwise be inaccessible without significant time and funding. As a result, models are applied in all fields of veterinary parasitology, including the management of drug resistance,[11] generating climate impact assessments,[9] informing vaccine development,[12] and informing selective breeding for nematode resistance.[10]

Box 1
Types of models

Models can be broadly described as either empirical or mechanistic. To understand the differences between these models, it is useful to first understand the model development process (**Fig. 1**).

Empirical modeling

The empirical modeling process (see **Fig. 1**A) typically involves relating parasite or disease data to independent variables (such as temperature, vegetation indices, farm characteristics, and parasite control strategies) using statistical models, to explain epidemiologic patterns or species' spatial distributions. The resulting model can be used to make predictions based on new independent variable data. Very little knowledge or understanding of the processes underlying the relationships is needed; therefore, the process is less data intensive than mechanistic modeling. However, care needs to be taken extrapolating the findings beyond the range of the data used to develop the model, because correlations between independent variables may change in time and space.

Empirical modeling example. Bryan and Kerr[8] developed an empirical model predicting gastrointestinal (GI) nematode larvae density on pasture (ie, an indirect measure of transmission risk) by relating monthly measures of larvae recovered from pasture in Queensland, Australia between 1975 and 1979, to temperature, rainfall, and dung beetle activity using a regression model. The model predicted that rainfall increased larval recovery from pasture while dung beetle activity reduced larval recovery. Based on the model, the authors made predictions to inform the optimal timing of anthelmintic treatments: they predicted that larval recovery would increase 92% following a 100-mm increase in rainfall, that beetle damage to pats could result in a reduction of between 57% and 94%, and therefore that treatments are best applied during the winter months when rainfall is high and beetles are inactive to reduce transmission risk. However, the effects of temperature could not be separated from the effects of dung beetles and rainfall, and the model may not be applicable to other regions nor beyond the late 1970s.

Mechanistic modeling

The mechanistic modeling process (see **Fig. 1**B) requires a detailed understanding of the processes underlying the epidemiology of parasite/disease dynamics to develop a conceptual framework (simplified representation of the processes) and mathematical equations representing the system processes, such as parasite establishment in the host. Model parameters such as death and transmission rates are then estimated using laboratory and field data. The models are usually validated using relevant independent variable data and parasite/disease data. If validation identifies significant discrepancies between the model predictions and these data, the model framework and parameter estimates are revisited and improved. Finally, the validated model can be applied to new independent variable data to make predictions. Mechanistic model development is usually much more data intensive than empirical model development, and as a result it is difficult to develop models for systems in which limited data exist (eg, understudied parasite species). However, as mechanistic models incorporate system processes and make fewer assumptions about correlations between independent variables, they are useful for projecting onto new conditions such as climate change.

For example, Rose and colleagues[9] developed a mechanistic model framework for the development, survival, and migration of ruminant gastrointestinal nematodes on pasture, based on current understanding of the life cycle and behavior of trichostrongylid nematodes (**Fig. 2**). Model parameters (death rates and transition rates such as development and migration) were estimated based on data in the literature (eg, the survival and development of eggs and larvae incubated in dung), and additional controlled field observations of larval migration from dung in response to rainfall. The model was validated using pasture larvae counts from a commercial farm and additional independent data sets from the literature. Adaptations of this model have been applied in a range of scenarios, for example to predict the potential epidemiologic benefits of breeding nematode-resistant ewes under climate-change scenarios,[10] and similar models have been used to identify optimal treatment strategies to delay the development of anthelmintic resistance.[11]

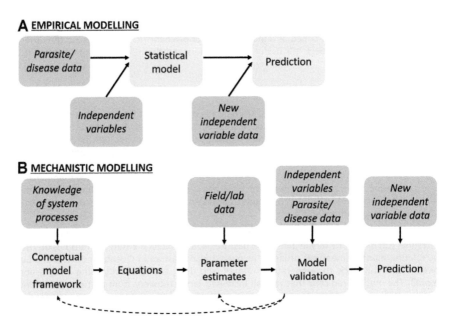

Fig. 1. Comparison of typical empirical (*A*) and mechanistic (*B*) modeling processes. Data inputs are shown in grey boxes (italicized font if viewing in grayscale) and key steps in the modeling process are shown in green boxes. The processes are described in detail in **Box 1**.

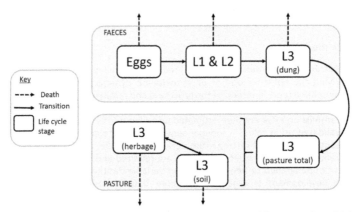

Fig. 2. Mechanistic model development is aided by conceptual frameworks, which visualize the current understanding of the system, help formulate mathematical equations, and identify key parameters. This conceptual framework details a model developed for the population dynamics of trichostrongylid gastrointestinal nematodes infecting ruminants.[9] Based on previous research, it is known that eggs are deposited in dung and develop (transition) through 2 larval stages (L1 ad L2) to reach the third, infective, larval stage (L3). L3 then migrate (transition) out of the dung onto pasture, where the total L3 on pasture is partitioned between the soil and the herbage. Data in the literature were available to estimate death rates for each life-cycle stage, development rates from egg to L3, and bidirectional migration between the soil and herbage, based on temperature. Further controlled observations were required to estimate the influence of moisture on the rate of migration between dung and pasture. Because trichostrongylid nematodes share the same life cycle, the model can be adapted for different species by simply adapting the death and transition rates.

Model Uncertainty and Validation

Since all models are wrong the scientist must be alert to what is importantly wrong.

—George Box (statistician), 1976[13]

George Box's words, which are widely paraphrased as "All models are wrong, but some are useful," highlight a fact that is easy to overlook: models will always produce predictions and output that are to some extent uncertain. They are imperfect representations of real-world observations, which themselves are imperfectly measured. How accurately a model represents the study system, and therefore how useful a model is likely to be, can be assessed by model validation. Usually this is done by comparing model output with field observations (see **Box 1**). Even fairly complex models can be validated through empirical testing of key findings, for example by designing field trials to specifically test model outcomes.[14,15]

The aim is not to perfectly reproduce the host-parasite system but to produce models that are useful; whereas it is impossible to eliminate uncertainty and avoid making assumptions, it is possible to produce useful models that replicate the system of interest in sufficient detail, or provide opportunities to compare scenarios. For example, the rate of development of anthelmintic resistance is difficult to measure in the field because it typically occurs over a period of years and is imprecisely measured using currently available technology. In this context, models provide an opportunity evaluate the relative impact of control strategies that may enhance or delay the development of resistance over extended time periods.[11]

Is Complex Always Better?

This then begs the question: are complex models always better? If 2 competing models produce equally useful and accurate output, the simplest model is preferable.[13] However, there are instances when additional complexity is beneficial and, in general, mechanistic models are preferred over empirical models if sufficient data are available for model development. The key requirement is that the models, as accurately as possible, represent the biology they are attempting to reproduce.

Different approaches to modeling *Fasciola hepatica* (liver fluke) risk illustrate this point. Empirical models have been developed since the 1950s to predict the risk of *F hepatica* infection by relating the incidence of fasciolosis (or measures of exposure) to environmental conditions. Although empirical models are useful to predict the risk of fasciolosis over time and space within the region where they were developed, care must be taken when extrapolating outside of these regions and into future climatic conditions because model accuracy under "new" environmental conditions is unknown. For example, Ollerenshaw and Rowlands[16] developed a model for risk of fasciolosis in Anglesey, United Kingdom. Because of its simplicity there is considerable potential for this model to be widely used to predict the seasonal risk of fasciolosis. However, the model was developed for the specific environmental conditions in Anglesey at the time of model development (temperate, with high rainfall year-round), and further validation would be necessary to assess its accuracy when applied outside of Anglesey or using current and future climatic data. Furthermore, the risk of parasite infection often varies at finer spatial scales than the available climatic data (eg, parasites clustered within a farm or field,[17] compared with several-km^2 resolution of climatic and weather data). This potentially limits the application of empirical models as decision support tools for farmers and veterinarians. In the case of *F hepatica*, mechanistic models[18] offer a solution to both of these limitations by explicitly modeling the processes underlying the relationships between the host, parasite, and environment **(Fig. 3)**.[16,18]

The implications of this are that veterinarians and their clients should ensure they are aware of the potential limitations of models so as to appreciate the uncertainty in model predictions. Model output should be interpreted in the context of farm management and local variation in weather/microclimate if the models are to be used to guide parasite control choices (used as decision support tools). For example, *Nematodirus battus* egg hatch predictions[4] based on a network of weather stations are provided in a Web-based tool alongside "rules of thumb" that can be used to adjust for local microclimate (aspect of fields and height above sea level) and farm management to assess risk **(Table 1)**.

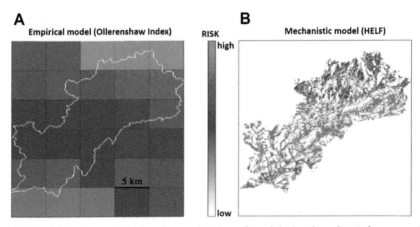

Fig. 3. One of the factors limiting the application of models developed to inform parasite control strategies for ruminant livestock is the availability of the data that can be used as model input. For example, weather stations may be some distance from the farm, and gridded weather data are often low resolution (eg, several km²) in comparison with the scale at which transmission takes place. Comparing output of an empirical model ("Ollerenshaw Index"[16]; *A*) and a mechanistic model ("HELF: Hydro-Epidemiological Liver Fluke model"[18]; *B*) for risk of *F hepatica* infection, for a river catchment area in Wales, UK, demonstrates how mechanistic modeling may provide a solution. High risk of infection is shown in orange, moderate risk is shown in gray, and low risk is shown in white. The empirical model output (*A*) may be useful to highlight larger regions at high risk of fasciolosis caused by high rainfall. However, a moderate to high risk was predicted throughout the catchment despite the fact that spatial risk often varies between and within fields owing to heterogeneity in suitable habitats for the snail intermediate host, which is determined in part by hydrologic processes. Beltrame and colleagues[18] coupled a mechanistic model of hydrologic processes with a simple mechanistic model of the population dynamics of *F hepatica* to predict metacercariae abundance depending on rainfall runoff and soil moisture (*B*; high abundance is shown as high risk). This mechanistic model used the same low-resolution weather data as the empirical model (*left*) but was able to predict risk at a finer spatial scale (25 m) by coupling this with high-resolution topography (elevation) data. The model predicted that much of the area predicted to be moderate to high risk using the empirical Ollerenshaw index (*A*) was actually likely to be low risk (*white, right*). These results could be used to plan grazing strategies to avoid infection. (*Adapted from* Beltrame L, Dunne T, Rose Vineer H, et al. A mechanistic hydro-epidemiological model of liver fluke risk. J Roy Soc Interface. 2018; 15(145).)

Table 1				
Ruminant parasite decision support systems implementing models				
DSS	Region	URL	Description	Model
Ask Bill	Australia	www.askbill.com.au	Predicts sheep well-being and productivity based on weather and farm management. Incorporates models of gastrointestinal nematode populations and blowfly strike risk	Kahn et al,[19] 2017
eggCounts	Global	http://shiny.math.uzh.ch/user/furrer/shinyas/shiny-eggCounts/	User interface to apply advanced analysis to fecal egg count and fecal egg count reduction test data	Wang et al,[20] 2017
Flyboss	Australia	www.flyboss.com.au	Predicts risk of blowfly strike to optimize treatment timing and compares multiple management options	Horton & Hogan,[21] 2010
LiceBoss	Australia	www.liceboss.com.au	Predicts the probability of infestation of sheep by *Bovicola ovis*, and the level of wool damage caused, to inform treatment decisions	Lucas & Horton,[22] 2014; Horton et al,[23] 2009
NADIS Blowfly alerts	UK	www.nadis.org.uk	Predicts *Lucilia sericata* abundance based on recent weather data	Wall et al,[24] 2000
Paracalc	Global	www.paracalc.be	Predicts the economic impact of nematode, liver fluke, and sheep scab infections in cattle, simulates the impact of treatment strategies on gastrointestinal nematodes, and provides decision support for liver fluke control	Charlier et al,[25] 2012
SCOPS *Nematodirus* alerts	UK	www.scops.org.uk	Predicts the timing of *Nematodirus battus* mass hatch in spring, depending on daily temperature data	Gethings et al,[4] 2015

URLs correct at June 14 2019.
Abbreviations: DSS, decision support systems; SCOPS, sustainable control of parasites in sheep.
Data from Refs.[4,19–25]

CONTRIBUTION OF MODELING TO ADVANCES IN RUMINANT PARASITOLOGY

Models of ruminant parasites and parasite transmission span several decades for both endoparasites[26] and ectoparasites.[24,27] These modeling efforts have contributed to several advances in ruminant parasitology, broadly categorized as advances that enhance the scientific understanding of epidemiology and disease processes, and advances that are of practical benefit to enhance parasite control capabilities.

Mechanistic models are indispensable as tools for testing and broadening epidemiologic understanding of host-parasite systems, driving forward research. For example, they have been used to identify the level of protection required from *F hepatica* vaccine candidates[12] and aid comprehension of endemic stability in bovine babesiosis, a complex epidemiologic process that depends on the balance of tick numbers, pathogen prevalence, and age structure of the host population.[27]

Table 2
Selected examples of model evaluation of sustainable parasite control practices

Parasite Control Strategy	Enhances (+) or Slows (−) Anthelmintic Resistance	Model
Treating ewes at lambing	+	Leathwick et al,[29] 1995; Leathwick et al,[30] 1997
Treating ewes in autumn	+	Leathwick et al,[29] 1995
Increasing treatment frequency	+	Leathwick et al,[29] 1995
Moving hosts to "clean" grazing (dose & move)	+	Leathwick et al,[29] 1995
Set stocking	+	Barnes & Dobson,[31] 1990
Grazing untreated ewes with treated lambs on same land after weaning (ewes follow lambs)	−	Leathwick et al,[29] 1995; Leathwick,[32] 2012
Targeted selective treatment/ Leaving a proportion of hosts untreated	−	Dobson et al,[33] 2011; Berk et al,[34] 2016
Single mid to late grazing season treatment with novel anthelmintic	−	Leathwick & Hosking,[11] 2009
Rotating anthelmintic classes annually	−	Learmount et al,[35] 2012
Persistent anthelmintics (includes long-acting and controlled-release devices)	+/−	Le Jambre et al,[36] 1999; Barnes & Dobson,[31] 1990; Leathwick et al,[30] 1997; Dobson et al,[37] 1996
Combination anthelmintics	+/−	Leathwick et al,[14] 2012; Learmount et al,[35] 2012; Leathwick,[32] 2012
Weather/climate	+/−	Dobson et al,[33] 2011

Whether the parasite control strategy is predicted to enhance or slow the development of anthelmintic resistance is shown as + or −, respectively. Predictions that vary by study or vary depending on interacting factors are shown as +/−.
    Data from Refs.[11,14,29–37]

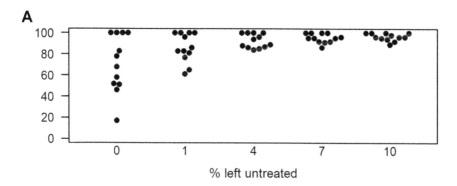

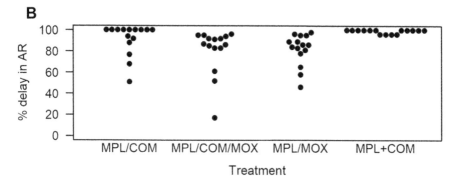

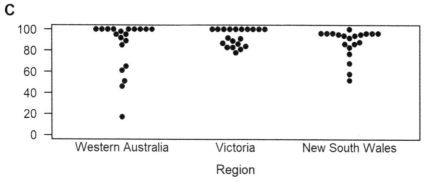

Fig. 4. Using models it is possible to simulate processes that are not easily measurable in the field (such as the development of anthelmintic resistance [AR]) over extended time scales. For example, Dobson and colleagues[33] simulated the population dynamics of multiple trichostrongylid nematode species infecting sheep in Australia, and the development of AR in these populations in response to a range of treatment strategies. The efficacy of each strategy was expressed as a percentage delay in the development of AR over a 20-year period compared with control scenarios whereby flocks were left untreated or treated exclusively with monepantel (MPL), moxidectin (MOX), or a combination (COM). Simulations varied the percentage of adult stock left untreated and the anthelmintic products used, and were replicated using weather data from 3 regions in Australia. Data shown were extracted from Tables S2–S4 of the original publication.[33] Points represent the output of model simulations. Simulations suggest that leaving even a small proportion of the flock untreated delays the development of resistance (*A*). However, how effective this strategy is in delaying AR was variable (eg, leaving 1% untreated results in approximately

Beyond broader scientific advances, there is now a plethora of models producing clinically relevant output, particularly to support and encourage more sustainable approaches to parasite control.

Reducing Reliance on Veterinary Medicines

Targeted treatment is a key aspect of sustainable parasite control, ensuring antiparasitic treatments are applied at the right time while avoiding unnecessary treatments.[2] Related to this is the potential to avoid infection by moving livestock away from high-risk pasture or sources of infection. However, the timing of peak risk of infection often depends on climate (or recent weather patterns) and farm management,[24] and the optimal timing of treatment or other interventions (such as grazing movements) depends on these factors as well as economic considerations. Since these factors are difficult for veterinarians and farmers to track, and it is difficult for a nonexpert to relate this to parasite risk because of the complexity of the host-parasite-environment system, models can play a key role in providing decision support (see **Table 1**).

Minimizing Selection for Anthelmintic Resistance

Along with decision support tools, models of anthelmintic resistance in gastrointestinal (GI) nematodes have been hailed as one of the 10 events defining anthelmintic research.[28] Models of anthelmintic resistance (**Table 2**) usually track GI nematode populations over time, dividing the population according to the genotype (eg, RR for homozygotic-resistant nematodes, RS for heterozygotic-resistant nematodes, and SS for homozygotic-susceptible nematodes). A different proportion of nematodes of each genotype are removed from the population when anthelmintic treatments are applied (eg, removing all or most of the susceptible nematodes, none or very few of the resistant nematodes, and an intermediate number of the heterozygotic nematodes). These models are valuable for comparing parasite control strategies and to identify methods that minimize selection for resistance[33] (**Fig. 4**).

Models of anthelmintic resistance have highlighted unsustainable parasite control practices, such as anthelmintic treatment of ewes at lambing[29] (see **Table 2**), which have later been confirmed by field data.[15] They have also demonstrated the considerable potential for sustainable parasite control guidelines[38] to slow the development of resistance.[35] High-risk practices identified by modeling studies (see plus signs in **Table 2**) could be avoided to minimize selection for resistance. If they cannot be avoided, practices that are predicted to slow the development of resistance could be implemented to help mitigate the impact of the high-risk practices (see minus signs in **Table 2**).

The responsible and strategic use of new anthelmintics (also known as "new actives") is of paramount importance. Just 1 year after the discovery of aminoacetonitrile derivatives (monepantel) was published, a modeling study provided evidence that a

---

60%–100% delay in AR; (A), depending on the treatments used (B) and regional weather/climatic conditions (C). Crucially, with the exception of MPL + COM combination treatment, which was always 96% to 100% effective, the optimal treatment strategy varied by region, highlighting the importance of considering environmental conditions in the development of sustainable parasite control strategies. –, treatments applied in rotation; +, treatments applied in combination; COM, combination treatment of benzimidazoles + imidazothiazoles + abamectin; MOX, moxidectin; MPL, monepantel.

single annual treatment with a novel anthelmintic could slow the development of resistance to other, older anthelmintics, especially when applied later in the grazing season.[11] The use of novel anthelmintics in lambs in the mid-to-late grazing season is now advocated.[38] Field trials to test this would have taken years to complete, at significant cost.

Two independent modeling studies subsequently simulated the development of resistance to novel anthelmintics such as monepantel and derquantel, predicting that over a period of 40 years the rate that anthelmintic resistance develops to a novel compound could be slowed when the novel anthelmintic is administered as a combination with another anthelmintic class.[32,35] These studies were notable because they were completed before the first report of detectable anthelmintic resistance to monepantel, at a time when field studies to track the development of resistance to novel anthelmintics would have been impossible.

Veterinarians and policymakers should also consider potential interactions that may or may not be included in modeling studies. For example, Le Jambre and colleagues[36] predicted that the use of persistent anthelmintics in lambs (controlled-release ivermectin or persistent moxidectin oral drench) would lead to rapidly developing anthelmintic resistance (compared with nonpersistent ivermectin oral drench). The investigators concluded that "treating sheep with a persistent ML [macrocyclic lactone] while grazing on a contaminated paddock should be seen as an emergency procedure when there are no alternatives." Similarly, other modeling studies predict that the magnitude of the impact of persistent anthelmintics on the development of resistance varies depending on grazing management.[31]

These examples highlight a central theme to managing and slowing the development of resistance: the size of the population of nematodes that are in *refugia*, having not been exposed to anthelmintic treatment. The impact of weather and climate on the abundance of parasites and seasonal dynamics of parasite populations (and thus the size of the *refugia* on pasture) is of increasing interest in the veterinary parasitology research community (eg, Verschave and colleagues[26]). Modeling studies exploring the interacting effects of climate and farm management on the development of anthelmintic resistance are limited to date. However, Dobson and colleagues[33] predicted that the optimum anthelmintic treatment strategy varied by Australian region and the resulting differences in the size of the *refugia* on pasture (see **Fig. 4**). Further model development is ongoing to evaluate the impact of climate and climate-management interactions on the development of anthelmintic resistance, and recent progress has been made with similar models evaluating the impacts of climate-based and *refugia*-based control strategies on the development of anthelmintic resistance in equine cyathostomins,[39,40] paving the way for similar developments in ruminant parasitology.

SUMMARY

Models of parasites, their transmission, and the evolution of anthelmintic resistance have made significant contributions to veterinary parasitology in recent decades. Most recently, models have provided evidence to guide the responsible use of novel anthelmintics at a time when field trials to optimize the timing and method of administration to minimize selection for resistance would have been impossible. In parallel with the threat of developing drug resistance, ruminant producers must contend with increasingly variable weather patterns and the threat of climate change, which affects parasite abundance and risk of infection. An array of decision support tools are now available to farmers and veterinarians to help plan and implement targeted parasite control strategies that are tailored to the prevailing weather conditions. The examples presented throughout this article highlight how modeling is an indispensable tool in veterinary parasitology.

ACKNOWLEDGMENTS

The author was funded by the BBSRC LoLa Consortium, "BUG: Building Upon the Genome" (Project reference: BB/M003949/1) and the University of Liverpool's Institute of Infection and Global Health. Thanks are extended to Brian Horton, Deborah Maxwell, Ludovica Beltrame, and Thorsten Wagener for providing additional information about their research.

DISCLOSURE

The author has nothing to disclose.

REFERENCES

1. Doherty E, Burgess S, Mitchell S, et al. First evidence of resistance to macrocyclic lactones in *Psoroptes ovis* sheep scab mites in the UK. Vet Rec 2018;182:106.
2. Kaplan RM. Anthelmintic resistance and strategies for sustainable control of parasites. Vet Clin North Am Food Anim Pract, in press.
3. Van Dijk J, David GP, Baird G, et al. Back to the future: developing hypotheses on the effects of climate change on ovine parasitic gastroenteritis from historical data. Vet Parasitol 2008;158:73–84.
4. Gethings OJ, Rose H, Mitchell S, et al. Asynchrony in host and parasite phenology may decrease disease risk in livestock under climate warming: *Nematodirus battus* in lambs as a case study. Parasitology 2015;142:1306–17.
5. Greer A. Refugia-based strategies for parasite control in livestock. Vet Clin North Am Food Anim Pract, in press.
6. Claerebout E, Geldhof P. Parasite vaccines. Vet Clin North Am Food Anim Pract, in press.
7. Burke J, Miller J. Novel approaches to parasite control in small ruminants. Vet Clin North Am Food Anim Pract, in press.
8. Bryan RP, Kerr JD. Factors affecting the survival and migration of the free-living stages of gastrointestinal nematode parasites of cattle in central Queensland. Vet Parasitol 1989;30:315–26.
9. Rose H, Wang T, van Dijk J, et al. GLOWORM-FL: a simulation model of the effects of climate and climate change on the free-living stages of gastrointestinal nematode parasites of ruminants. Ecol Model 2015;297:232–45.
10. Rose Vineer H, Baber P, White T, et al. Reduced egg shedding in nematode-resistant ewes and projected epidemiological benefits under climate change. Int J Parasitol 2019;49:901–10.
11. Leathwick DM, Hosking BC. Managing anthelmintic resistance: modelling strategic use of a new anthelmintic class to slow the development of resistance to existing classes. N Z Vet J 2009;57:203–7.
12. Turner J, Howell A, McCann C, et al. A model to assess the efficacy of vaccines for control of liver fluke infection. Sci Rep 2016;6:23345.
13. Box GEP. Science and statistics. J Am Stat Assoc 1976;71:791–9.
14. Leathwick DM, Waghorn TS, Miller CM, et al. Managing anthelmintic resistance—use of a combination anthelmintic and leaving some lambs untreated to slow the development of resistance to ivermectin. Vet Parasitol 2012;187:285–94.

15. Leathwick DM, Miller CM, Atkinson DS, et al. Drenching adult ewes: implications of anthelmintic treatments pre- and post-lambing on the development of anthelmintic resistance. N Z Vet J 2006;54:297–304.

16. Ollerenshaw CB, Rowlands WT. A method of forecasting the incidence of fascioliasis in anglesey. Vet Rec 1959;71:591–8.

17. Howell A, Williams DJ. Epidemiology and control of liver fluke. Vet Clin North Am Food Anim Pract, in press.

18. Beltrame L, Dunne T, Rose Vineer H, et al. A mechanistic hydro-epidemiological model of liver fluke risk. J R Soc Interface 2018;15:20180072.

19. Kahn LP, Johnson IR, Rowe JB, et al. ASKBILL as a web-based program to enhance sheep well-being and productivity. Anim Prod Sci 2017;57:2257–62.

20. Wang C, Torgerson PR, Höglund J, et al. Zero-inflated hierarchical models for faecal egg counts to assess anthelmintic efficacy. Vet Parasitol 2017;235:20–8.

21. Horton BJ, Hogan L. FlyBoss: a flystrike information and decision support system. Anim Prod Sci 2010;50:1069–76.

22. Lucas PG, Horton BJ. Guidelines for treatment of lice in sheep with long wool based on a model of the development of wool damage. Aust Vet J 2014;92:8–14.

23. Horton BJ, Evans DL, James PJ, et al. Development of a model based on Bayesian networks to estimate the probability of sheep lice presence at shearing. Anim Prod Sci 2009;49:48–55.

24. Wall R, French NP, Fenton A. Sheep blowfly strike: a model approach. Res Vet Sci 2000;69:1–9.

25. Charlier J, Van der Voort M, Hogeveen H, et al. Paracalc®—a novel tool to evaluate the economic importance of worm infection on the dairy farm. Vet Parasitol 2012;184:204–11.

26. Verschave SH, Charlier J, Rose H, et al. Cattle and nematodes under global change: transmission models as an ally. Trends Parasitol 2016;32:724–38.

27. Mahoney DF, Ross DR. Epizootological factors in the control of bovine babesiosis. Aust Vet J 1972;48:292–8.

28. Sangster NC, Cowling A, Woodgate RG. Ten events that defined anthelmintic resistance research. Trends Parasitol 2018;34:553–63.

29. Leathwick DM, Vlassoff A, Barlow ND. A model for nematodiasis in New Zealand lambs: the influence of drenching and grazing management on the development of anthelmintic resistance. Int J Parasitol 1995;25:1479–91.

30. Leathwick DM, Sutherland IA, Vlassoff A. Persistent drugs and anthelmintic resistance—part III. NZ J Zool 1997;24:298–9.

31. Barnes EH, Dobson RJ. Population dynamics of *Trichostrongylus colubriformis* in sheep: computer model to simulate grazing systems and the evolution of anthelmintic resistance. Int J Parasitol 1990;20:823–31.

32. Leathwick DM. Modelling the benefits of a new class of anthelmintic in combination. Vet Parasitol 2012;186:93–100.

33. Dobson RJ, Barnes EH, Tyrrell KL. A multi-species model to assess the effect of refugia on worm control and anthelmintic resistance in sheep grazing systems. Aust Vet J 2011;89:200–8.

34. Berk Z, Laurenson YCSM, Forbes AB, et al. Modelling the consequences of targeted selective treatment strategies on performance and emergence of anthelmintic resistance amongst grazing calves. Int J Parasitol Drugs Drug Resist 2016;3:258–71.

35. Learmount J, Taylor MA, Bartram DJ. A computer simulation study to evaluate resistance development with a derquantel-abamectin combination on UK sheep farms. Vet Parasitol 2012;187:244–53.

36. Le Jambre LF, Dobson RJ, Lenane IJ, et al. Selection for anthelmintic resistance by macrocyclic lactones in *Haemonchus contortus*. Int J Parasitol 1999;29: 1101–11.
37. Dobson RJ, Le Jambre L, Gill JH. Management of anthelmintic resistance: inheritance of resistance and selection with persistent drugs. Int J Parasitol 1996;26: 993–1000.
38. Abbott KA, Taylor M, Stubbings L. Sustainable worm control strategies for sheep. A technical manual for veterinary surgeons and advisers. 4th edition. SCOPS; 2012. Available at: https://www.scops.org.uk/workspace/pdfs/scops-technical-manual-4th-edition-updated-september-2013.pdf. Accessed May 31, 2019.
39. Nielsen MK, Sauermann CW, Leathwick DM. The effect of climate, season, and treatment intensity on anthelmintic resistance in cyathostomins: a modelling exercise. Vet Parasitol 2019;269:7–12.
40. Leathwick DM, Sauermann CW, Nielsen MK. Managing anthelmintic resistance in cyathostomin parasites: investigating the benefits of refugia-based strategies. Int J Parasitol Drugs Drug Resist 2019;10:118–24.

Helminth Vaccines in Ruminants

From Development to Application

Edwin Claerebout, DVM, PhD*, Peter Geldhof, PhD

KEYWORDS

- Gastrointestinal nematodes • Lungworm • Liver fluke • Vaccines

KEY POINTS

- Only a few vaccines against parasitic helminths of livestock are currently on the market; namely those against *Dictyocaulus viviparus* in cattle, *Haemonchus contortus* in sheep, and the tapeworm *Echinococcus granulosus* in sheep.
- Research is ongoing to develop vaccines based on purified or recombinantly expressed worm proteins for *Ostertagia ostertagi* and *Cooperia oncophora* in cattle, for *Teladorsagia circumcincta* and *H contortus* in sheep, and for *Fasciola hepatica* in ruminants.
- Recombinant expression of worm antigens with the correct conformation to induce protective immunity is still a major challenge in vaccine development.
- Vaccination is likely to be part of integrated worm control, together with other control measures, such as anthelmintic treatments, biological control, and grazing management.
- Interdisciplinary research, including social sciences, should investigate drivers of farmers' and veterinarians' decision making, to optimize uptake of vaccination by the end users.

INTRODUCTION

The major helminth infections in ruminants include gastrointestinal (GI) nematodes, liver fluke, and lungworms. At present, they are mainly controlled by regular treatments with anthelmintic drugs. However, decades of intensive use of anthelmintics have led to the development of anthelmintic resistance. High levels of resistance against all classes of anthelmintics are reported in GI nematodes of small ruminants worldwide. Resistance against macrocyclic lactones is also emerging in cattle parasites, mainly in *Cooperia* spp and, to a lesser extent, *Ostertagia ostertagi*. Resistance against flukicides has been reported in *Fasciola hepatica* in several countries.

Together with a more sustainable use of anthelmintics, potential alternative (or complementary) control methods include bioactive forages, selective breeding for host resistance or resilience, nematophagous fungi, and vaccines.[1] Vaccines are

Faculty of Veterinary Medicine, Laboratory of Parasitology, Ghent University, Salisburylaan 133, Merelbeke 9820, Belgium
* Corresponding author.
E-mail address: edwin.claerebout@ugent.be

Vet Clin Food Anim 36 (2020) 159–171
https://doi.org/10.1016/j.cvfa.2019.10.001
0749-0720/20/© 2019 Elsevier Inc. All rights reserved.

considered a favorable option, because of the durable protection they can provide and a lack of chemical residues in animal products and the environment.[2] The principle of vaccination is to induce immunologic protection in a host against a subsequent infection. For this, the immune system can be stimulated with either the weakened or killed pathogen or proteins/antigens from it, the so-called subunit vaccines (**Fig. 1**). Subunit vaccines can be based on a single antigen or a mixture of antigens, which can be purified from the parasites or produced through recombinant DNA technology. The approach of producing a commercial vaccine straight from worm material is not applicable for most parasite species because it is practically difficult or even impossible to obtain large enough quantities of parasite material. For this reason, recombinant vaccines have been evaluated against a range of helminths. However, maintaining the correct conformation of target antigens in recombinant form is a major challenge,[3] and only a few recombinant vaccine antigens have been shown to be protective. The challenge for further development lies in delivering these promising subunit vaccines in a manner feasible for large-scale commercial production, testing their efficacy in more extensive field trials, and in making them fit for purpose for commercial and end-user uptake.[2]

Despite strong efforts to develop antiparasitic vaccines, only 3 vaccines are currently on the market (**Table 1** for specifications): (1) a live attenuated vaccine for control of the bovine lungworm, *Dictyocaulus viviparus* (Bovilis Huskvac, MSD Animal Health); (2) a native gut antigen-based vaccine, recently launched for the control of haemonchosis in sheep in Australia (Barbervax, Wormvax Australia Pty Ltd) and South Africa (Wirevax, Afrivet Business Management Pty Ltd); and (3) a cestode vaccine

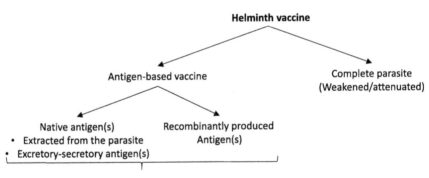

> ➤ **'Hidden' antigen:** antigen from the parasite that is typically not exposed to the immune system during the course of an infection, for example antigens from the gut of the worm.
> ➤ **'Conventional' antigen:** antigen that is typically exposed to the immune system of the host during an infection, for example the excretory-secretory proteins from a worm.
> ➤ **Excretory-secretory antigen:** antigen released in culture fluid by worms cultured *in vitro*
> ➤ **Somatic antigen:** antigen extracted from water-soluble or insoluble (fractions of) whole worm homogenate

Fig. 1. Different types of helminth vaccine antigens.

(Providean Hidatil EG95, Tecnovax) is available on the commercial market in parts of South America for the control of *Echinococcus granulosus* in sheep and goats.

This article summarizes the state of the art in vaccine research against sheep and cattle helminths, including the lungworm *D viviparus*, the GI nematodes *Haemonchus contortus*, *Teladorsagia circumcincta*, *O ostertagi*, and *Cooperia oncophora*, and the liver fluke *F hepatica*. Furthermore, safety and efficacy requirements for implementation of helminth vaccines in field conditions are discussed, as well as factors that may affect uptake of vaccines by the end users.

STATE OF THE ART IN VACCINE DEVELOPMENT
Dictyocaulus viviparus

A commercial lungworm vaccine (Bovilis Huskvac, MSD Animal Health), composed of live irradiated third-stage (L3) *D viviparus* larvae, was developed decades ago.[4] Two doses of 1000 viable irradiated larvae are delivered orally with an interval of approximately 4 weeks, and the full vaccination schedule should be completed at least 2 weeks before turnout of the vaccinated animals on pasture. Vaccinated cattle should not be treated with anthelmintics until at least 2 weeks after the second vaccination. The vaccine can be used in healthy cattle of 8 weeks of age or older, which includes grazing young stock and adult cows. Although vaccine-induced protection is generally good,[5] the vaccine has disadvantages associated with live vaccines, such as ethical issues (production of larvae in donor animals), batch heterogeneity, and a short shelf life. In an attempt to overcome these issues, several attempts were made to develop recombinant subunit vaccines, with limited success. Vaccination with recombinant acetylcholinesterase,[6] paramyosin,[7,8] or asparaginyl peptidase legumain-1[9] with different adjuvants did not result in significant and/or reproducible reduction in worm numbers or larval shedding.

Haemonchus contortus

An *H contortus* vaccine based on a worm gut membrane antigen mixture was recently commercialized for sheep (Barbervax, Wirevax) and has quickly become an invaluable tool to control haemonchosis in areas where anthelmintic resistance is rampant.[10] The vaccine is only registered in Australia and South Africa, but it can be used in the United Kingdom under Special Treatment Certificate and veterinary prescription. Vaccination with the vaccine also conferred protection against *Haemonchus placei* in grazing calves,[11] but the vaccine has not been registered for use in cattle. Vaccination of young goats did not sufficiently protect against *H contortus* infections on pasture.[12] For the production of this vaccine, the native antigens need to be extracted and purified locally from adult *H contortus* derived from infected sheep. A vaccine based on recombinantly expressed antigens would have advantages compared with a native antigen vaccine for reproducibility of product batches, biosafety, and global distribution. Many efforts have been made to identify and express a range of antigens from *H contortus*, but most recombinant proteins were unsuccessful in eliciting protective immunity.[2,10] Recently, a gene encoding an Hc23 somatic antigen was identified and expressed in *Escherichia coli*. Lambs vaccinated with the recombinant Hc23 antigen were significantly protected against an artificial challenge infection, with more than 80% reduction in fecal egg counts (FECs) and average abomasal parasite burdens, compared with challenge controls.[13] This work is a promising step toward a recombinant *Haemonchus* vaccine, but further experiments are needed to confirm these results and to test the vaccine in natural infection conditions.

Table 1
Commercialized vaccines against helminth parasites in ruminants

Brand Name	Parasite	Animal Species	Antigen	Adjuvant	Administration Route	Vaccination Schedule	Level of Protection	Withdrawal Period
Bovilis Huskvac	Dictyocaulus viviparus	Cattle	Live irradiated third-stage larvae	None	Oral	Basic scheme: 2 vaccinations with 4-wk interval before turnout. Revaccination: single dose before turnout	95%–98% (worm burden)	None
Barbervax, Wirevax	Haemonchus contortus	Sheep	Gut membrane proteins	Saponin	Subcutaneous	Basic scheme: 3 vaccinations with interval of 3–4 wk before Haemonchus season. Revaccination: 6-wk intervals	93%–95% (egg counts) 72%–94% (worm burden)	None
Providean Hidatil EG95	Echinococcus granulosus	Cattle, sheep, goats, camelids	EG95	Montanide and saponin	Subcutaneous or intramuscular	2 vaccinations with 1-mo interval	95%–100% (cysts)	None

Teladorsagia circumcincta

Similar to *H contortus*, over the years several antigens have been evaluated as vaccine candidates against the sheep abomasal parasite *T circumcincta*.[2] The most promising results have recently been obtained with an experimental vaccine that is based on a cocktail of 8 recombinant proteins. The native versions of these antigens were originally identified either as immunodominant excretory/secretory proteins or selected because of their potential immune modulatory role or as homologues of vaccine candidates in related nematode species.[2] All proteins were expressed in *E coli* or the yeast *Pichia pastoris*. Vaccination with this antigen cocktail with Quil A adjuvant protected 6- month-old to 7-month-old lambs and peripartturient ewes against a challenge infection, resulting in significantly reduced FECs (73%–92% reduction in lambs, 45% in ewes) and worm burdens (56%–75% reduction in lambs).[14,15] Work is ongoing to refine the protein cocktail by testing fewer recombinant protein combinations in vaccine trials.[16] Further, its protective capacity will be tested in newly weaned lambs and in field trials.

Ostertagia ostertagi

Over the last 40 years, several antigens and antigen mixtures have been evaluated against *O ostertagi* (reviewed in Rinaldi and Geldhof[17]). At present the most promising experimental vaccine against *O ostertagi* is based on activation-associated secreted proteins (ASPs).[2,18] Vaccination with a fraction of the adult excretory-secretory products containing ASP or with the purified protein has consistently resulted in a significantly reduced worm egg output (55%–62% reduction) after artificial trickle challenge infections.[18–21] Attempts to generate similar levels of protection with a recombinant ASP protein have been unsuccessful so far. Recombinant proteins, expressed in different expression systems, such as *E coli*, insect cells, and *P pastoris*, were either insoluble or did not protect vaccinated calves against challenge infection.[3,22] Current research focuses on eliciting differences in protein folding and glycosylation between the native and recombinant ASP proteins, to identify epitopes that are important to induce a protective immune response.[23,24]

Cooperia oncophora

Based on the promising results obtained with an ASP-based vaccine against *O ostertagi*, a double-domain ASP (ddASP) protein purified from the excretory-secretory material of adult *C oncophora* worms was recently successfully evaluated as a vaccine candidate.[25,26] Immunization with this antigen resulted in a significant reduction (91%) in cumulative FEC in an experimental challenge experiment. In a subsequent field trial, *C oncophora* cumulative FECs in vaccinates were reduced by 59%, resulting in 65% less infective *C oncophora* larvae on plots grazed by vaccinated calves and a significant reduction of 82% in worm counts in the vaccinates at housing.[26] Vaccination with the *C oncophora* ddASP also protected calves against a challenge infection with an Uruguayan isolate of mixed *C oncophora* and *Cooperia punctata*, suggesting that the protective epitopes are conserved between *Cooperia* species/isolates in different parts of the world. In contrast, the *C oncophora* ddASP vaccine did not protect sheep against *Cooperia curticei* (unpublished results). As with *O ostertagi*, the research is currently focused on the recombinant expression of the ASP in an immune-active form.

Fasciola Spp

An overview of individual antigens and combinations thereof that have been tested against the liver flukes *F hepatica* and *Fasciola gigantica* in cattle and sheep is given by Toet and colleagues.[27] Some antigens, such as cathepsin L1 and leucine amino-peptidase (LAP), induced significant protection levels in sheep and/or cattle, both as native, purified antigen and as recombinant protein. However, protection levels were highly variable, hence the need to test each vaccine in multiple vaccine trials to show consistent protection.[27] Combining different antigens, such as cathepsins, with LAP or hemoglobin, or vaccination with a chimeric protein composed of leucine aminopeptidase and cathepsin L1 has not substantially improved vaccine efficacy.[27,28] Despite multiple individual studies showing promising results for various DNA vaccine candidates against fascioliasis in animal models, a systematic review and meta-analysis did not show a significant pooled efficacy for all vaccine candidates against fasciola infection.[29]

VACCINE SAFETY, EFFICACY, AND USE OF VACCINES IN PARASITE CONTROL

The ideal parasitic vaccine should be safe, have a high efficacy, and ideally this activity should extent to a wide range of parasites.[30]

Vaccine Safety

Safety is an absolute requirement for any new vaccine. To avoid unwanted contamination with other proteins or pathogens and to ensure batch reproducibility, recombinant protein or DNA vaccines would be preferable to vaccines consisting of native proteins, purified from worms that are collected from animals. Vaccination with a (recombinant) protein (cocktail) in combination with a well-defined commercial adjuvant is not expected to raise important safety issues. Nevertheless, the development of a human hookworm vaccine based on ASPs caused allergic reactions in vaccinated preexposed individuals.[31] Several vaccines currently under experimental evaluation for livestock helminths also contain ASPs (*O ostertagi, C oncophora, T circumcincta*). No side effects were observed in calves that were vaccinated with a double-domain ASP from *C oncophora* before turnout on pasture,[26] but it has not been tested yet whether this vaccine is safe to use in regions with year-long grazing, where animals are likely to be infected before vaccination. However, Nisbet and colleagues[15] observed no adverse reactions in grazing ewes that were vaccinated with a recombinant *T circumcincta* vaccine containing ASP.

Vaccine Efficacy

The major aim in controlling helminth infections by vaccination is to reduce parasite transmission by decreasing the number of viable eggs that are excreted into the environment, because these determine the number of infective larvae on the pasture later in the grazing season. The fecundity of *Ostertagia* is highly regulated by host immunity,[32] and fecal egg output can be strongly reduced without a reduction in worm numbers.[33] In contrast, the fecundity of *Haemonchus* is not regulated by the intensity of the infection and there is a good correlation between total daily FECs and mature female worm burden.[34] Consequently, to prevent the buildup of a high pasture infection level, a *Haemonchus* vaccine needs to reduce the number of adult worms present in the animals early in the grazing season, either by reducing the establishment of infective larvae or by increasing the mortality of established worms.[30]

An advantage of vaccines based on hidden antigens (see **Fig. 1**) is that they can produce protective effects in situations in which natural immunity is either weak or ineffective, such as in young lambs or in periparturient ewes. A disadvantage is that vaccine-induced immunity is not boosted by a challenge infection, because the hidden antigens in the ingested worms are not exposed to the host's immune system. As a consequence, immunity induced by vaccination with hidden antigens is typically short lasting and animals need to be revaccinated regularly. This need is shown by the vaccination schedules for *H contortus* in sheep. When lambs first receive Barbervax, 3 doses of the vaccine with intervals of 3 to 4 weeks are required to reach an effective level of antibodies, whereas subsequent vaccinations are given each 6 weeks until *H contortus* infections are no longer a risk (www.wormboss.com.au).

Animals vaccinated with conventional antigens (see **Fig. 1**) benefit from restimulation of their immune systems by the corresponding antigens from the challenge infection. The level and duration of protection required depend on the local grazing management and climate conditions.[35]

In sheep, both lambs and their dams need to be vaccinated. The ewes contribute significantly to the pasture infection because of their periparturient increase in egg shedding, and the lambs are vulnerable because of a lack of acquired immunity. Therefore, experimental *T circumcincta* vaccines are tested in both these age categories,[14,15] and separate vaccine schedules were designed for lambs and ewes for the commercial *H contortus* vaccine (www.barbervax.com.au).

In dairy cattle, calves are typically separated from their dams at birth and the heifer calves are raised as a separate group of replacement stock. First grazing season calves are the most susceptible to infections with GI nematodes, and parasitic gastroenteritis is mainly seen in this age class when no appropriate preventive measures have been taken. In many parts of Europe, there is a well-defined grazing period, from spring to autumn. Helminth-naive calves should be vaccinated before turnout and the vaccine should protect them until natural immunity has sufficiently developed. Natural immunity against *C oncophora* develops within the first months of grazing, but immunity development against *O ostertagi* is slow,[36] and vaccination should protect calves during their entire first grazing season. Because the peak egg output occurs around 2 months after turnout,[37] it can be anticipated that reduction of worm egg shedding in the first 2 to 3 months after turnout may be sufficient to prevent accumulation of infective larvae on pasture and to protect vaccinated animals until housing in autumn.[35] The authors previously suggested that a vaccine that reduces the mean fecal egg output by around 60% during the first 2 months after turnout would sufficiently protect calves against GI nematodes during their first grazing season and allow them to develop a natural immunity without production loss.[30] For *C oncophora*, this has been shown to be an achievable goal,[26] but whether this assumption holds for *O ostertagi* in field conditions remains to be confirmed. Moreover, this expectation does not take into account individual variability of each calves' response to vaccination.

Required levels of vaccine efficacy and duration of protection depend on the host-parasite system and the grazing management, both of which are influenced by climate. Short-term protection may suffice for GI nematodes of cattle in regions with a restricted grazing season, such as in Europe.[26] In regions with continuous grazing throughout the year (eg, South America and New Zealand), the required duration of protection offered by vaccination may be similar for parasites that rapidly induce natural immunity, such as *Cooperia*, but longer protection by vaccination may be needed for parasites with a slower immune development, such as *Ostertagia* and *Fasciola*.

F hepatica infection levels greater than 30 to 40 flukes in cattle and 30 to 54 flukes in sheep have been associated with production losses.[38–40] In order to reduce fluke burdens below these threshold values, and taking into account reported fluke burdens in different countries, vaccine efficacy against *Fasciola* should reach 50% to 80% according to Toet and colleagues.[27] However, it was not specified whether this reduction in fluke burden should be obtained through a direct effect of vaccination on worm viability or indirectly by reducing worm egg output in vaccinated animals. Estimating an indirect effect of reduced egg shedding on adult fluke burdens is complicated by the role of the intermediate snail host in parasite transmission. Because a snail infected with a single miracidium can produce several hundred cercariae, the snail biology has a significant impact on the outcome of vaccination.

Vaccines Against Multiple Pathogens

In most regions, grazing ruminants are coinfected with several pathogenic worm species; for example, *H contortus*, *T circumcincta*, and *Trichostrongylus* spp in sheep, and in cattle *O ostertagi* and *Cooperia* spp, plus others at lower levels. Multivalent vaccines, protecting against multiple GI nematodes and/or lungworms and liver fluke, could have an obvious advantage compared with single-species vaccines.[2] However, monovalent vaccines may be useful in situations in which a single parasite species dominates (eg, *H contortus* in warmer regions), when other parasites are controlled by alternative measures, or in regions where the risk for other parasites is low (eg, in dry regions with a low risk for liver fluke infection).[2] Little or no research on multispecies helminth vaccines has been conducted, to our knowledge. No cross-protection was observed against *O ostertagi* when cattle were vaccinated against *C oncophora* with a ddASP vaccine[26] despite the similarity of the ASP antigens of both worm species.

Helminth vaccines could also be combined with vaccines against other pathogens. However, vaccines against multiple pathogens are particularly useful when they tackle a common disease complex, such as neonatal bovine diarrhea (a combined vaccine against *E coli*, rotavirus, and coronavirus) or bovine respiratory disease (eg, vaccine against bovine respiratory syncytial virus, parainfluenza virus, and *Mannheimia haemolytica*). Parasitic gastroenteritis and lungworm disease are well-defined disease entities in grazing ruminants, and combining a GI nematode or lungworm vaccine with bacterial or viral antigens may have little advantage.[1]

Vaccination and Other Worm Control Measures

In many cases, vaccination is not a stand-alone solution, especially if vaccines are targeted at single parasite species and/or confer only partial protection. However, vaccination, even if only partially effective, could become an important component of integrated worm control programs.[1] Anthelmintic treatment at particular time points during the vaccination schedule with the Barbervax vaccine is recommended in sheep, to cope with concurrent trichostrongylus infections or early haemonchus infections (www.barbervax.com.au). Because there is a large variability of immune responses to vaccination between individual animals,[14] animals that respond poorly to vaccination may need to be identified and either treated or removed from the group. Likewise, herd immunity leads to reduced levels of pasture contamination that then helps protect those few animals that respond poorly. It would be an impossible task to test the huge number of possible scenarios arising from the combination of (multispecies) vaccines with other worm control measures in different management systems and climatic conditions in field vaccine trials. In contrast, helminth transmission models can be a useful tool for evaluating different scenarios in silico, and to select the most promising (combinations of) control methods for field testing.[41,42] Barnes and colleagues[43] modeled the population dynamics of *Trichostrongylus colubriformis* in sheep to predict the effect of different vaccines on worm population dynamics in grazing lambs. They concluded that, with vaccines based on conventional antigens, substantial benefits can be obtained with a decrease of 60% in larval establishment in 80% of the flock. These simulations have been referred to in several articles to argue that it is not essential for a vaccine against GI nematodes in ruminants to obtain 100% efficacy (or even >90%) in all animals. However, these results cannot be readily extrapolated to other host-parasite systems; for example, when suppressed egg production is the main effect of vaccine-induced immunity rather than decreased larval establishment.[35] Turner and colleagues[44] developed a mathematical model to simulate the effectiveness of liver fluke vaccines under field conditions. The model output suggests that current vaccine candidates have the potential to reduce the mean total fluke burden by 43% and mean daily egg output by as much as 99% under field conditions. However, to be effective, a vaccine should protect at least 90% of the animals during the whole grazing season. It seems unlikely that this level and duration of protection can be achieved with vaccination alone, but vaccines could contribute substantially toward fasciolosis control, reducing usage of anthelmintics and thus delaying the spread of anthelmintic resistance.[44]

POTENTIAL UPTAKE OF VACCINES BY END USERS

It is unlikely that the use of helminth vaccines will be imposed by policy makers, because helminth infections in livestock are considered as production diseases, without importance for public health or international trade.[45] Consequently, the decision to vaccinate will be the farmer's responsibility and among other things will depend on the vaccine's performance and cost-effectiveness in comparison with alternative control measures, as shown by the success of the Barbervax vaccine. Despite the need to vaccinate sheep on a regular basis and to combine vaccination with anthelmintic treatments, farmers are willing to use the vaccine because anthelmintics alone have become insufficient to control haemonchus infections in regions with high levels of anthelmintic resistance. In contrast, the lungworm vaccine is not used extensively in many countries, despite good vaccine efficacy. Practical concerns, such as a short shelf life, and the availability of anthelmintics with a persistent efficacy against *Dictyocaulus*, apparently have made the vaccine a less attractive control option.

Although ultimately it may be the farmer's decision to vaccinate, veterinarians have an important role to implement and improve vaccination strategies.[46] More sociopsychological studies to identify drivers of farmers' and veterinarians' decision making will be crucial to optimize uptake of novel parasite control tools, such as vaccines.[47]

FUTURE PROSPECTS AND SUMMARY

Expressing recombinant vaccine antigens in the right conformation to induce a protective immune response remains an issue for many nematode vaccines. Studies on allelic variability of the target genes and on the protein conformation and secondary modifications of the antigens should help to steer the recombinant expression work and ultimately lead to the development of protective recombinant antigens. In addition, increasing knowledge on vaccine-induced immune responses will lead to optimized antigen-adjuvant combinations and improved vaccine delivery.[2] The sustainability of vaccines, like anthelmintics, will depend on parasite evolution, and the ability of helminths to develop resistance to vaccine-induced host responses remains an open question.[41] Vaccines containing multiple antigens of a single parasite species could slow down adaptation of the parasites to the vaccine, such as an experimental *Teladorsagia* vaccine in sheep that comprises multiple recombinant proteins.[14,16]

The effect of the level and duration of vaccine efficacy on parasite transmission and animal productivity and the combined use of vaccines and other control methods in different management systems and climate regions should be simulated using mathematical models to inform vaccine developers and regulatory authorities about possible outcome scenarios.

In parallel, consumer expectations about helminth vaccines should be investigated and drivers and inhibitors of farmers' and veterinarians' uptake of parasite vaccines should be identified to ensure that vaccines, once they are ready for commercialization, will be effectively used and incorporated into routine farm management and disease control.

ACKNOWLEDGMENTS

This article is based on work funded by the European Union's Horizon 2020 Research and Innovation Programme under grant agreement no. 635408EU (PARAGONE) and COST Action COMBAR CA16230, supported by COST (European Cooperation in Science and Technology).

DISCLOSURE

The research on vaccine development against *O ostertagi* and *C oncophora* described in this article is financially supported by Zoetis.

REFERENCES

1. Vercruysse J, Charlier J, van Dijk J, et al. Control of helminth ruminant infections by 2030. Parasitology 2018;45(13):1655–64.
2. Matthews JB, Geldhof P, Tzelos T, et al. Progress in the development of subunit vaccines for gastrointestinal nematodes of ruminants. Parasite Immunol 2016;38: 744–53.
3. Geldhof P, De Maere V, Vercruysse J, et al. Recombinant expression systems: the obstacle to helminth vaccines? Trends Parasitol 2007;23:527–32.
4. Jarrett WF, Jennings FW, McIntyre WI, et al. Immunological studies on Dictyocaulus viviparus infection: active immunization with whole worm vaccine. Immunology 1960;3:135–44.
5. Benitez-Usher C, Armour J, Urquhart GM. Studies on immunisation of suckling calves with dictol. Vet Parasitol 1976;2:209–22.
6. Matthews JB, Davidson AJ, Freeman KL, et al. Immunisation of cattle with recombinant acetylcholinesterase from Dictyocaulus viviparus and with adult worm ES products. Int J Parasitol 2001;31:307–17.
7. Joekel D, Hinse P, Raulf MK, et al. Vaccination of calves with yeast- and bacterial-expressed paramyosin from the bovine lungworm Dictyocaulus viviparus. Parasite Immunol 2015;37:614–23.
8. Strube C, Haake C, Sager H, et al. Vaccination with recombinant paramyosin against the bovine lungworm Dictyocaulus viviparus considerably reduces worm burden and larvae shedding. Parasit Vectors 2015;8:119.
9. Holzhausen J, Haake C, Schicht S, et al. Biological function of Dictyocaulus viviparus asparaginyl peptidase legumain-1 and its suitability as a vaccine target. Parasitology 2018;145:387–92.
10. Nisbet AJ, Meeusen EN, Gonzalez JF, et al. Immunity to Haemonchus contortus and vaccine development. Adv Parasitol 2016;93:353–96.

11. Bassetto CC, Silva MRL, Newlands GFJ, et al. Vaccination of grazing calves with antigens from the intestinal membranes of Haemonchus contortus: effects against natural challenge with Haemonchus placei and Haemonchus similis. Int J Parasitol 2014;44:697–702.

12. Meier L, Torgerson PR, Hertzberg H. Vaccination of goats against Haemonchus contortus with the gut membrane proteins H11/H-gal-GP. Vet Parasitol 2016; 229:15–21.

13. Fawzi EM, González-Sánchez ME, Corral MJ, et al. Vaccination of lambs with the recombinant protein rHc23 elicits significant protection against Haemonchus contortus challenge. Vet Parasitol 2015;211:54–9.

14. Nisbet AJ, McNeilly TN, Wildblood LA, et al. Successful immunization against a parasitic nematode by vaccination with recombinant proteins. Vaccine 2013; 31(37):4017–23, 23.

15. Nisbet AJ, McNeilly TN, Greer AW, et al. Protection of ewes against Teladorsagia circumcincta infection in the periparturient period by vaccination with recombinant antigens. Vet Parasitol 2016;228:130–6.

16. Nisbet AJ, McNeilly TN, Price DRG, et al. The rational simplification of a recombinant cocktail vaccine to control the parasitic nematode Teladorsagia circumcincta. Int J Parasitol 2019;49:257–65.

17. Rinaldi M, Geldhof P. Immunologically based control strategies for ostertagiosis in cattle: where do we stand? Parasite Immunol 2012;34:254–64.

18. Geldhof P, Vercauteren I, Gevaert K, et al. Activation-associated secreted proteins are the most abundant proteins in a host protective fraction of *Ostertagia ostertagi*. Mol Biochem Parasitol 2003;128:111–4.

19. Geldhof P, Claerebout E, Knox DP, et al. Vaccination of calves against *Ostertagia ostertagi* with cysteine proteinase enriched protein fractions. Parasite Immunol 2002;24:263–70.

20. Geldhof P, Vercauteren I, Vercruysse J, et al. Validation of the protective capacity of the *Ostertagia ostertagi* ES-thiol antigens with different adjuvantia. Parasite Immunol 2004;26:37–43.

21. Meyvis Y, Geldhof P, Gevaert K, et al. Vaccination against Ostertagia ostertagi with subfractions of the protective ES-thiol fraction. Vet Parasitol 2007;149: 239–45.

22. Geldhof P, Meyvis Y, Vercruysse J, et al. Vaccine testing of a recombinant activation-associated secreted protein (ASP1) from Ostertagia ostertagi. Parasite Immunol 2008;30:57–60.

23. Borloo J, Geldhof P, Peelaers I, et al. Structure of Ostertagia ostertagi ASP-1: insights into disulfide mediated cyclization and dimerization. Acta Crystallogr D Biol Crystallogr 2013;69:493–503.

24. Meyvis Y, Callewaert N, Gevaert K, et al. Hybrid N-glycans on the host protective activation-associated secreted proteins of Ostertagia ostertagi and their importance in immunogenicity. Mol Biochem Parasitol 2008;161:67–71.

25. Borloo J, Claerebout E, De Graef J, et al. In-depth proteomic and glycomic analysis of the adult-stage Cooperia oncophora excretome/secretome. J Proteome Res 2013;12(9):3900–11.

26. Vlaminck J, Borloo J, Vercruysse J, et al. Vaccination of calves against Cooperia oncophora with a double-domain activation-associated secreted protein reduces parasite egg output and pasture contamination. Int J Parasitol 2015; 45:209–13.

27. Toet H, Piedrafita DM, Spithill TW. Liver fluke vaccines in ruminants: strategies, progress and future opportunities. Int J Parasitol 2014;44:915–27.

28. Ortega-Vargas S, Espitia C, Sahagún-Ruiz A, et al. Moderate protection is induced by a chimeric protein composed of leucine aminopeptidase and cathepsin L1 against Fasciola hepatica challenge in sheep. Vaccine 2019;37:3234–40.

29. Jayaraj R, Kumarasamy C, Norbury L, et al. Protective efficacy of liver fluke DNA vaccines: a systematic review and meta-analysis: Guiding novel vaccine development. Vet Parasitol 2019;267:90–8.

30. Claerebout E, Knox DP, Vercruysse J. Current research and future prospects in the development of vaccines against gastrointestinal nematodes in cattle. Expert Rev Vaccines 2003;2:147–57.

31. Diemert DJ, Pinto AG, Freire J, et al. Generalized urticaria induced by the Na-ASP-2 hookworm vaccine: implications for the development of vaccines against helminths. J Allergy Clin Immunol 2012;130:169–76.

32. Smith G, Grenfell BT, Anderson RM. The regulation of Ostertagia ostertagi populations in calves: density-dependent control of fecundity. Parasitology 1987;95:373–88.

33. Gasbarre LC. Effects of gastrointestinal nematode infection on the ruminant immune system. Vet Parasitol 1997;72:327–43.

34. Coyne MJ, Smith G. Trichostrongylid parasites of domestic ruminants. In: Scott ME, Smith G, editors. Parasitic and infectious diseases: epidemiology and ecology. San Diego (CA): Academic Press; 1994. p. 235–56.

35. Vercruysse J, Claerebout E. Assessment of the efficacy of helminth vaccines. J Parasitol 2003;89(Suppl):S202–9.

36. Claerebout E, Vercruysse J. The immune response and the evaluation of acquired immunity against gastrointestinal nematodes in cattle: a review. Parasitology 2000;120:S25–42.

37. Shaw DJ, Vercruysse J, Claerebout E, et al. Gastrointestinal nematode infections of first-season grazing calves in Western Europe: general patterns and the effect of chemoprophylaxis. Vet Parasitol 1998;75:115–31.

38. Dargie JD. The impact on production and mechanisms of pathogenesis of trematode infections in cattle and sheep. Int J Parasitol 1987;17:453–63.

39. Hawkins CD, Morris RS. Depression of productivity in sheep infected with Fasciola hepatica. Vet Parasitol 1978;4:341–51.

40. Hope Cawdery MJ, Strickland KL, Conway A, et al. Production effects of liver fluke in cattle. I. The effects of infection on liveweight gain, feed intake and food conversion efficiency in beef cattle. Br Vet J 1977;133:145–59.

41. Morgan ER, Aziz N-AA, Blanchard A, et al. 100 important research questions in livestock helminthology. Trends Parasitol 2018;35(1):52–71.

42. Verschave SH, Charlier J, Rose H, et al. Cattle and nematodes under global change: transmission models as an ally. Trends Parasitol 2016;32(9):724–38.

43. Barnes EH, Dobson RJ, Barger IA. Worm control and anthelmintic resistance: adventures with a model. Parasitol Today 1995;11:56–63.

44. Turner J, Howell A, McCann C, et al. A model to assess the efficacy of vaccines for control of liver fluke infection. Sci Rep 2016;6:23345.

45. Charlier J, Vande Velde F, van der Voort M, et al. ECONOHEALTH: placing helminth infections of livestock in an economic and social context. Vet Parasitol 2015;212:62–7.

46. Cresswell E, Brennan ML, Barkema HW, et al. A questionnaire-based survey on the uptake and use of cattle vaccines in the UK. Vet Rec Open 2014;1: e000042.
47. Vande Velde F, Charlier J, Claerebout E. Farmer behaviour and gastrointestinal nematodes in ruminant livestock–uptake of sustainable control approaches. Front Vet Sci 2018;5:255.

Ectoparasites of Cattle

Adalberto A. Pérez de León, DVM, MS, PhD[a],*,
Robert D. Mitchell III, MS, PhD[a], David W. Watson, MS, PhD[b]

KEYWORDS

- Cattle • Ectoparasites • Flies • Myiasis • Lice • Mites • Ticks
- Integrated management

KEY POINTS

- Most of the approximately 1.49 billion head of cattle worldwide are susceptible to infestation with ectoparasites, several of which are also vectors of bovine pathogens.
- Diseases listed by the World Organization for Animal Health include some caused directly by ectoparasites and by ectoparasite-borne pathogens affecting cattle.
- Some ectoparasites of cattle are of One Health importance because they can be invasive and of high socioeconomic consequence, and several zoonotic ectoparasite-borne pathogens can affect public health.
- Arthropods, mainly insects, mites, and ticks, represent the most economically important group of cattle ectoparasites because of the direct effect associated with heavy infestations on health and food production.
- Integrated approaches are required to manage cattle ectoparasites in a sustainable manner.

Most of the approximately 1.49 billion head of cattle worldwide are susceptible to infestation with diverse ectoparasitic fauna. Arthropods, mainly insects, mites, and ticks, represent the most economically important group of cattle ectoparasites because of the direct effect associated with heavy infestations on health and food production.[1] Multiple species of arthropod ectoparasites are also vectors of pathogens causing bovine diseases, some of which are zoonotic.[2] Moreover, several diseases caused directly by ectoparasites or the pathogens they transmit to cattle are listed as notifiable by the World Organization for Animal Health.[3] An overview of common ectoparasites and current practices to treat or prevent ectoparasitoses in cattle is presented here.

The biology and ecology of ectoparasites are unique. Interactions between characteristics of the farming system under consideration and complex epidemiologic aspects influence the prevalence and incidence of ectoparasitoses and arthropod

[a] United States Department of Agriculture – Agricultural Research Service, Knipling-Bushland U.S. Livestock Insects Research Laboratory and Veterinary Pest Genomics Center, 2700 Fredericksburg Road, Kerrville, TX 78028, USA; [b] Entomology and Plant Pathology Department, North Carolina State University, Campus Box 7616, 1575 Varsity Drive, Raleigh, NC 27695-7616, USA
* Corresponding author.
E-mail address: beto.perezdeleon@usda.gov

Vet Clin Food Anim 36 (2020) 173–185
https://doi.org/10.1016/j.cvfa.2019.12.004
vetfood.theclinics.com
0749-0720/20/Published by Elsevier Inc. This is an open access article under the CC BY-NC-ND license (http://creativecommons.org/licenses/by-nc-nd/4.0/).

vector-borne diseases in cattle. Permutations of conventional and nonconventional beef or dairy cattle farming systems across world regions can range from extensive subsistence farming involving one resource-poor farmer to intense commercial production under ownership of multinational corporations where the latest technologies are used to manage ectoparasites.[4,5] Thus, the veterinary practitioner must consider husbandry practices to treat infestations effectively in cattle herds.[6,7] For example, grazing beef cattle, including cows and their calves, in the United States can be infested with horn flies and face flies. During the dry season or winter, hay wagons or round bale feeders used to supplement feeding operations can become stable fly-breeding sites unless hay residues are managed. Cattle-wildlife interactions in extensive farming systems can provide the medium for tick infestations and the transmission of tick-borne diseases. Biosecurity is another critical practice used to avoid the introduction of ectoparasites into a cattle herd and prevent their spread within and between farms. Practitioners must observe best veterinary drug-use practices to treat infestations, caused, for example, by latent lice or mite populations, in cattle that must be transported for managing or marketing purposes. Breeding conditions tend to be unfavorable for horn flies and face flies in properly managed cattle-feeding operations, feedlots, and feed yards. Cattle shipped from remote rangelands may be infested with cattle grubs and should be examined for warbles where these ectoparasites are endemic.

Veterinary drugs and mechanical/environmental, biological, and genetic methods have been used alone or in combination to control or eradicate ectoparasites. Veterinary products containing ectoparasiticides are used commonly by practitioners and producers to treat or prevent ectoparasitoses and mitigate exposure to vector-borne pathogens.[8] However, the intense use of ectoparasiticides in several parts of the world has selected for resistance in ectoparasite populations exposed to them continuously. Strategies combining other methods for sustainable cattle ectoparasite management are needed to address societal concerns with the massive application of ectoparasiticides in the context of food safety, global change, animal welfare, and environmental health.

Injurious ectoparasite infestations impair the productivity of cattle and, in extreme cases, result in mortality. This inflicts significant economic loss on cattle producers around the world. For example, estimates indicate that ectoparasitic flies and ticks infesting cattle in Brazil cause US$6.86 billion in economic losses annually.[9] Adopting the principles of integrated pest management to practice integrated ectoparasite management mitigates the risk for the development of resistance to ectoparasiticides while maximizing their longevity as useful tools used rationally with decreased impact on nontarget species.[10] Best ectoparasiticide use practices contribute to achieving One Health by safeguarding animal, public, and environmental health.[11]

COMMON CATTLE ECTOPARASITES
Ectoparasitic Flies

Many species of Diptera (two-winged insects, or true flies) are ectoparasites because they bite to feed on blood, that is, hematophagous, or cause nuisance to the animals during the adult stage, cause myiasis at the immature stages or larvae, invade living soft tissue, or transmit pathogens to cattle as biological or mechanical vectors.[12] Examples of common ectoparasitic flies affecting cattle health and production causing economic damage are briefly reviewed.

Horn and buffalo flies
Haematobia irritans, commonly known as the horn fly, is a cosmopolitan hematophagous ectoparasite closely associated with cattle grazing in open pastures and

rangeland. Adults spend most of their life on the host and tend to congregate on the back and shoulders of cattle or on their underbelly during the heat of the day. Persistent blood feeding irritates cattle and can cause significant production losses. Larvae breed in undisturbed dung pats, and adult populations build up during the warmer months of the year. Treatment is warranted when adult horn fly counts per animal exceed 200.[13] In northern Australia and Southeast Asia, the buffalo fly, *Haematobia exigua*, is an economically important biting fly closely related to the horn fly.

Horn flies are mechanical vectors of bacteria causing bovine mastitis.[14] Buffalo and horn flies are intermediate hosts of spirurid nematodes causing bleeding sores from stephanofilariasis in cattle.[15] Several classes of ectoparasiticides and formulations are used to treat infestations.[16] Insecticide resistance is a problem among these biting flies in several parts of their geographic range. Cattle-feed additives containing larvacides and insect growth regulators excreted in the dung that prevent the adult stage are used to control *Haematobia* spp. populations.[17]

Stable fly

With a worldwide distribution, unique breeding habits, strong flying ability, and transient host association to acquire a blood meal through a painful bite, the stable fly, *Stomoxys calcitrans*, is a pestiferous ectoparasite of cattle. Larvae breeding in moist decaying organic material from multiple sources including crop residues, lawn clippings, silage, and animal bedding can result in stable fly outbreaks. Stable flies tend to blood feed on the lower parts of cattle. The threshold for treatment is 5 flies per front leg.[18]

The stable fly can be a pest in open pastures or in confined cattle production facilities. Although considered a poor vector, viruses, bacteria, and protozoans pathogenic to cattle have been recovered from the stable fly. Sanitation in and around cattle-raising areas prevents fly population growth locally.[19] Ectoparasiticide treatment helps control adult flies. Biological control methods augment the effect of other stable fly interventions.

Face fly

Cattle in Europe, central Asia, and parts of Africa, the United States, and Canada are hosts for the face fly, *Musca autumnalis*. Ectoparasitism by face flies is associated with pastured cattle where, as with the horn fly, fresh cattle dung provides the immature stages the nourishment to develop.[20] Adult flies consume secretions from the eyes and nostrils, and sanguineous fluid from wounds around the host face. When face flies attempt to feed, the abrasive action of their mouthparts can create superficial skin lesions and ocular irritation and damage. The threshold of greater than 15 flies per face is generally accepted, and cattle with infestations of 20 or more flies on the face spend less time grazing and exhibit avoidance behavior.[21,22]

The face fly is the mechanical vector of *Moraxella bovis*, causing infectious bovine keratoconjunctivitis (IBK) or pinkeye. As fly feeding increases and cattle exhibit more defensive behaviors, the spread of IBK is augmented. The face fly serves as the intermediate host of *Thelazia* eyeworms, the causative agent of thelaziasis. Ectoparasiticides to aid in the control of the adults are often used in feed additives and are an effective means of preventing heavy infestations.

Mosquitoes

The adult females of several mosquito species in the insect family Culicidae blood feed on cattle. Mosquito larvae develop in many aquatic environments including ditches, ponds, open containers, tree holes, and flood-irrigated pastures. Blood feeding by female mosquitoes decreases milk production and weight gains.[23] Massive mosquito attacks can suffocate cattle and result in death.

Mosquito biting activity is mostly crepuscular or nocturnal, but some species will blood feed during the day.[24] Mosquitoes are vectors of pathogens that affect cattle, some of which are zoonotic, including Rift Valley fever virus, which has caused outbreaks in several African countries and in the Arabian Peninsula. Breeding-site management and the use of products targeting larvae prevent the local buildup of large mosquito populations. Ectoparasiticides, including those with repellent activity, can be used to protect cattle from mosquito bites.

Black flies

The distribution around the world of black fly species of the family Simuliidae is determined by the presence of flowing water where the larvae develop. Herd health and productivity are affected when cattle are attacked by swarms of adult female black flies. Significant blood loss and exposure of the host, including cattle, to considerable amounts of bioactive salivary factors at feeding sites associated with persistent biting by swarms of black flies results in a syndrome called simuliotoxicosis. Cattle can die in large numbers from severe blood loss in areas where population explosions of black flies occur.[25]

Black flies are vectors of vesicular stomatitis virus–New Jersey in North America, and filarial nematodes causing bovine onchocerciasis in various parts of the world. The microfilaria of *Onchocerca lienalis* infect the umbilical region of cattle, where feeding black flies acquire the nematode for transmission to other susceptible hosts. This parasitic nematode is suspected to cause zoonotic ocular onchocerciasis.

In large geographic areas where black flies are problematic, engineered manipulation of stream flow is an effective management tool. Treating the larval habitat with *Bacillus thuriengiensis israelensis* is an effective means of controlling local populations. Additional protection can be afforded by treating cattle with ectoparasiticides, which have repellent activity. In the presence of black fly swarms, ruminants should be provided shelter in stables or barns to relieve cattle from heavy black fly attack, and in extreme cases thorough coverage spraying with an ectoparasiticide can prevent mortality caused by simuliotoxicosis.

Tabanids

Tabanidae is the family of flies that includes several species in the genera *Tabanus* and *Hybomitra* commonly known as horse flies, and deer fly species in the genus *Chrysops*. The vermiform larvae develop in aquatic or semiaquatic environments where they prey on other insects or feed on decaying organic matter depending on the species. Adults are most abundant in open areas along the edge of woods and only the females are hematophagous, which results in persistent attacks on cattle.[26] Horse flies inflict painful bites to take a blood meal, in part caused by the action of their cutting-lapping mouthparts.

Blood-feeding activity by tabanids can alter daily cattle movement patterns and influence herd structure. As strong fliers and painful biters that are frequently interrupted during blood feeding, tabanids are efficient mechanical vectors of pathogens given their tendency to return to the same host or attempt to feed on another host nearby.[27] Traps and repellent ectoparasiticides can be used for tabanid control. However, local conditions and seasonal phenology can make it challenging to manage large tabanid populations.

Biting midges

In contrast to their tiny size, biting midge species in the *Culicoides* genus of the Ceratopogonidae family are of considerable economic impact on cattle health and production worldwide. The adult females are hematophagous, feeding from blood in a pool formed by the scissor-like action of their mouthparts that lacerates the skin. Larvae hatching from the eggs laid by the females in semiaquatic or aquatic environments rich in organic matter feed on the environmental microbiota to develop and continue the life cycle. Adults are minute, measuring ∼2 mm in body length and difficult to detect until they inflict their painful bite.

Bluetongue and epizootic hemorrhagic disease viruses are economically important groups of arboviruses transmitted by *Culicoides* spp. that affect cattle in several parts of the world.[28] Some parasitic nematode and protozoan species are suspected to be transmitted to cattle by biting midges. *Culicoides* spp. are among the group of biting flies incriminated as vectors of vesicular stomatitis viruses in the Americas. Vector control remains the primary approach to attempt the interruption of transmission of *Culicoides*-borne bluetongue and epizootic hemorrhagic disease viruses to cattle in the absence of commercial vaccines against these arboviruses. Although challenging, environmental management to prevent breeding sites is an effective way to prevent large biting midge populations. Ectoparasiticide treatment aids in the control of biting midges.

Sand flies

Several species of Old World sand flies in the genus *Phlebotomus* and New World sand flies in the genus *Lutzomyia* of the family Psychodidae are ectoparasites of cattle in tropical and subtropical regions of the world. Adult flies are characteristically small insects <5 mm in length and brown to yellow in color, with hairy wings and bodies. Gravid female sand flies lay their eggs in humid terrestrial habitats with highly organic soils including leaf litter, animal burrows, barns, livestock pens, and shelters where decomposing cattle manure may accumulate. The recently emerged adults rest near the larval site until old enough to seek food. Being weak fliers, adult females disperse through a series of short hopping flights to find a host.[29]

Females will take blood meals from a variety of vertebrate hosts including cattle. Feeding activity can distress cattle, resulting in avoidance behaviors leading to decreased productivity. In addition to skin irritation from their bite, some *Lutzomyia* species are vectors of vesiculoviruses in the Rhabdoviridae family, including vesicular stomatitis viruses.[30] Protection of cattle from nuisance and hematophagy by sand flies must be practiced because breeding-source reduction for population control is challenging. Repellent ectoparasiticides can be used to control adult sand flies attacking cattle.

Tsetse flies

Tsetse fly species in the genus *Glossina* are of great economic importance as ectoparasites and vectors of pathogens that affect cattle health in a significant portion of sub-Saharan Africa spanning savanna, forest, and riverine ecosystems. Tsetse flies transmit *Trypanosoma* spp. causing African animal trypanosomiasis, or nagana, in cattle and other domestic animals. Some of these fly ectoparasites are of One Health relevance because they are also cyclical vectors of trypanosomes causing human African trypanosomiasis or sleeping sickness. African animal trypanosomiasis is a major impediment to the development of cattle production in Africa, where the disease is endemic.[31] Male and female tsetse flies are obligate blood feeders. Adenotrophic viviparity is a unique reproductive mode evolved by tsetse flies whereby maternal nourishment of the progeny is provided by glandular secretions within viviparous females, which is followed by live birth.

Tsetse flies can detect moving cattle 180 m away, attracted to host odors from 100 m, and disperse approximately 1 km per day.[4] These ecologic characteristics have influenced the development of control methods targeting the adult stage. Area-wide integrated pest management has been adapted, taking a phase-conditional approach to control tsetse flies in Africa.

Myiasis-causing flies

Myiasis is an infestation with the immature stages, generally referred to as maggots, of several fly species that feed on living or necrotic tissue of a live animal to develop and complete their life cycle. Most myiasis-producing fly species make up the superfamilies Muscoidea and Oestroidea. Members of the Calliphoridae (blow flies) and Sarcophagidae (flesh flies) are generally some of the most damaging to cattle. The winged adult females do not bite but are opportunistic and generally exploit open wounds in cattle produced by common farm practices, including branding, dehorning, and castration, to lay their eggs from which the maggots emerge. They are also a nuisance and can induce cattle to injure themselves.

The list of notifiable diseases by the World Organization for Animal Health includes infestation with the invasive New World screwworm (*Cochliomyia hominivorax*) and Old World screwworm (*Chrysomya bezziana*).[3] These myiases are of One Health importance because they can affect warm-blooded animals including humans, cattle, and other domesticated animal and wildlife species. When a myiasis is left untreated it generally results in host mortality. New World and Old World screwworms cause millions of dollars in loss annually for cattle producers wherever these pests remain endemic. Experiences eradicating the New World screwworm from North and Central America applying the sterile insect technique, followed by elimination of outbreaks first in Libya starting in the late 1980s and then one occurring in Florida in 2016, are testament to the scientific and technical complexities of area-wide efforts to protect cattle from high-consequence foreign livestock pests requiring national and international multiagency coordination through public-private partnerships.[32] In endemic areas, ectoparasiticides can be applied in several ways to treat myiasis in cattle and other domestic animals.

Economically important fly species in the family Oestridae causing myiasis in cattle include *Hypoderma lineatum*, also known as the common cattle grub, *Hypoderma bovis* or the northern cattle grub, and *Dermatobia hominis*, commonly called the torsalo or human bot fly. The cutaneous ulcer caused by the developing oestrid larva, or bot, appears as an open cyst termed a warble—hence the name warble flies. Cattle bots are also called grubs. Adult flies have a bumblebee-like appearance and are commonly known as heel flies or gadflies. Cattle grubs are found on all continents of the northern hemisphere, whereas *D hominis* affects cattle in tropical and subtropical regions of the Americas.

Frantic behavior by cattle to avoid hovering female grub flies attempting to lay their eggs on them, known as gadding, is observed generally in response to *H bovis*. This can result in reduced weight gains, lowered weaning weights, and reduced milk production. After burrowing into the skin, larvae then translocate to development sites in the host and migrate to superficial tissue, where the warble is formed to eventually drop off through the exit pore. Dropped larvae pupate in the ground to complete the life cycle. In addition to tissue damage, warbles diminish the value of hides from infested cattle. Macrocyclic lactones can be used to control cattle grubs by treating in autumn and spring.[33] However, ensure treatment is avoided when *H lineatum* and *H bovis* grubs cluster along the esophagus and the spinal column, respectively. Otherwise components leaking from dead grubs can trigger respiratory distress, paralysis, and shock in treated cattle.

Lice

Lice, representing the insect order Phthiraptera, are relatively small ($\leq$2.5–3.0 mm) with a dorsoventrally flattened body, and are morphologically divided into sucking and chewing groups. *Bovicola bovis*, commonly known as the cattle biting louse, is the chewing louse associated with cattle. The main species of cattle sucking lice are: *Haematopinus eurysternus*, or short-nosed cattle louse; *Haematopinus quadripertusus*, or cattle tail louse; *Linognathus vituli*, or long-nosed cattle louse; and *Solenopotes capillatus*, or little blue cattle louse. Lice complete all the stages of their life cycle on the host. Sucking lice are hematophagous and typically have a narrow, pointed head, whereas biting lice feed on skin and hair and have a broad head. Unlike the cattle tail louse that can be more abundant in the summer, burdens are low on cattle with other louse species during the summer months but typically increase during the winter and early spring.[10]

Heavy lice infestation is associated with signs of pruritus, can cause severe anemia, and may also be an indicator of other underlying conditions in affected cattle. Infested animals will scratch and rub the skin, trying to relieve themselves of the irritation.[34] Dip or spray ectoparasiticide treatment of cattle can control lice infestations. Macrocyclic lactones are also used but are more effective against sucking lice than chewing lice. However, they are inactive against lice eggs, or nits, so additional treatments may be required to ensure that newly hatched nymphs are killed. Ectoparasiticide application can be part of the schedule to treat lice and other parasites when cattle are prepared for the winter months.

Mites

Mites are arachnids in the subclass Acari and are approximately 1 mm long. Acariasis describes an infestation with mites that complete their life cycle on the host by feeding on the skin and its secretions or by ingesting fluids oozing from lesions inflicted with their mouthparts.[35] Severe dermatitis caused by cutaneous acariasis is called mange. Cattle can be affected by 5 types of mange according to the mite species causing it. Ectoparasite biology and ecology influence the clinical picture of mange—for example, whether the mite burrows into the skin or whether it inhabits the hair follicles or sebaceous glands.

Sarcoptic mange, or scabies, caused by *Sarcoptes scabiei* var. *bovis*, a skin-burrowing mite, is highly contagious and zoonotic, causing intense pruritus and papules. If left untreated the skin thickens, forming large folds, and the entire outer body surface can be affected in a few weeks. *Psoroptes ovis* is a nonburrowing mite causing psoroptic mange that pierces the skin to imbibe the fluids emanating from the wound, which can form a thick crust. Exudative dermatitis, alopecia, and intense pruritus characterize psoroptic mange that can kill untreated calves.[36] *Chorioptes bovis*, the chorioptic mange mite, typically inhabits the skin surface of the tail and lower legs and therefore the condition may be called tail, foot, or leg mange. Although *C bovis* can survive off the host for up to 3 weeks, chorioptic mange is relatively less pathogenic to cattle than sarcoptic or psoroptic mange. *Demodex bovis* is the most common of 3 *Demodex* species that can infest the hair follicles and sebaceous glands of cattle where they feed on sebum, oozing plasma, and epidermal debris. Cases of demodectic mange occur frequently during late winter and early spring; lesions are susceptible to secondary bacterial infection. Young cattle appear to be more susceptible to heavy infestations, which can also result in hide damage. The cattle itch mite, *Psorobia bos*, can cause psorergatic mange of limited pathogenicity. Cases involve slight skin thickening and some scaling where low-grade pruritus can occur. Cattle are also susceptible to infestation by the ear mites *Raillietia auris* and *Raillietia flechtmanni*. In addition to subclinical otitis, ear mite cases include the accumulation of wax and the involvement of neurologic symptoms. Early detection and diagnosis using the proper sampling method are important for the control of infestations and prevention of mite transmission to the herd.

Ticks

Ticks are larger and close relatives of the mites in the arachnid subclass Acari. Their obligate blood-feeding habit requires that ticks subvert innate and acquired host immune responses through bioactive factors secreted in their saliva to remain attached at the bite site for days at a time, sometimes on multiple occasions parasitizing the same host.[37] Besides having direct effects on their hosts, ticks are also the most important parasitic arthropod group as vectors of pathogens affecting domestic animals and wildlife. Ticks are remarkable in their vector ability to transmit diverse pathogens including protozoa, bacteria, and viruses. Tick-borne pathogens are the cause of transboundary cattle diseases. Bovine babesiosis, anaplasmosis, theileriosis, and heartwater are among the diseases listed as notifiable by the World Organization for Animal Health caused by tick-borne pathogens that affect cattle.[3]

Ticks of veterinary relevance belong to the family Ixodidae, also known as hard ticks, and the family Argasidae, which are known as soft ticks. Ixodid tick species in the genera *Ixodes*, *Dermacentor*, *Amblyomma*, *Haemophysalis*, *Hyalomma*, and *Rhipicephalus* affect cattle health and production around the world. Depending on the species, ixodid ticks will parasitize 1, 2, or 3 hosts to complete the larval, nymphal, and adult stages. Mated adult females drop off the host to lay their eggs on the ground. Compared with ixodid ticks, argasid ticks are faster feeders and nidicolous, living in or near shelters used by their hosts. Argasid genera with species that are ectoparasites of cattle include *Ornithodoros* and *Otobius*.

The importance of ticks in animal agriculture is reflected in efforts by different countries spanning more than a century trying to control or eradicate ticks and tick-borne diseases. The southern cattle fever tick, *Rhipicephalus microplus*, is considered to be the most economically important ectoparasite of livestock worldwide.[5] This invasive tick species is the vector of *B bovis* and *Bovicola bigemina*, causing babesiosis in cattle in tropical and subtropical parts of the world. Estimates place bovine babesiosis at the top of arthropod-borne diseases causing financial losses for cattle producers.[37] As a result of the intense use of ectoparasiticides against it, *R microplus* is ranked sixth among the most resistant arthropods globally. The detection of *Haemaphysalis longicornis* in several states of the United States by 2019 is an emerging disease threat for cattle, other domesticated animals, wildlife, and humans in North America, which highlights the One Health importance of invasive ticks and associated tick-borne diseases.[38] Several research groups are investigating alternative technologies that could ease the dependence on ectoparasiticide treatments to deal with the problem of ticks and tick-borne diseases of cattle.

ADVANCING INTEGRATED ECTOPARASITE MANAGEMENT

Compounds from several chemical classes with insecticidal and acaricidal activities are marketed as cattle ectoparasiticides.[39] The macrocyclic lactones represent another important group of chemicals that because of their mode of action also have activity against endoparasites and thus are defined as endectocidal. Their administration requires attention because of the relative susceptibility of endoparasites and ectoparasites. This, for example, can result in the exposure of ticks infesting treated cattle to a sublethal dose when the macrocyclic lactone product is applied as indicated on the label for an endoparasite infection, which in this scenario will select for resistance in that tick population.[40] In addition, it is unlawful to use an ectoparasiticide product in a manner inconsistent with the label instructions. Farmers should consult a veterinarian, extension agent, or local veterinary entomologist to obtain information on products authorized for use in their area to ensure they are handled safely. Overuse and misuse of ectoparasiticides selects for resistance to the veterinary drug in the product and can be hazardous to animals, food, and the environment.

The combined use of emerging technologies is being tested. However, habitat reduction and sanitation must remain key management goals. Where commercially available, the integrated use of antitick vaccines can reduce the frequency of ectoparasiticide applications and diminish the total amount of product used.[41] Research on vaccines against other cattle ectoparasites such as the horn fly must be resumed now that its genome is sequenced and bioinformatic tools that can accelerate the development process are available.[42] Botanic ectoparasiticides that could be used to treat cattle continue to be commercialized. The combined use of biopesticides, such as acaropathogenic fungi, with ectoparasiticides can result in synergistic effects to control cattle tick populations resistant to the widely applied pyrethroid ectoparasiticides. Additional research in this area is facilitated by testing samples available at entomopathogenic fungal collections. An example is the US Department of Agriculture Agricultural Research Service collection, which maintains more than 130,000 isolates and provides information and taxonomic services on the characterization and identification of fungi.[43] This collection contains 188 records of fungi pathogenic to mosquitoes, 91 records for muscoid flies, and 47 records for black flies. Continued research is needed to assess the integrated use of traps to manage biting and nuisance fly populations.[44,45] The strategic use of barriers impregnated with ectoparasiticides for fly control and foot baths to manage tick infestations enhances integrated strategies.[46]

Organic cattle farming continues to grow in some parts of the world. Methods to control cattle ectoparasites in organic farms have been developed.[47] Preventive practices are also paramount for the management of ectoparasites in organic operations.[48] These practices include selecting species and types of cattle suitable for local conditions and resistant to endemic parasites, providing adequate nutrition, establishing housing with proper pasture conditions, observing sanitation practices to minimize predisposing conditions for ectoparasitoses, and keeping stress low.[49] Natural enemies serve as a focal point for the biological control of pests. Naturally occurring populations of parasitoids are amenable to augmentative releases, which significantly enhance the biological control effort for cattle production. Parasitoids prey on fly pupa wherein their offspring develop.

Research on livestock genomics is being applied to advance the breeding of cattle resistant to ectoparasites, especially ticks. Likewise, biotechnology-enhanced sterile insect technique approaches are being enabled by advances in ectoparasite genomic science.[50] These include progress with genetic pest management for ectoparasites of cattle. For example, RNA interference (RNAi) affords protection by silencing mRNA, resulting in the suppression of critical gene functions. RNAi technology is being developed for the control of bluetongue viruses in *C sonorensis*.[51] Lethal gene and gene drive technology could be developed for cattle ectoparasite management.[52] Lethal gene technology demonstrated yellow fever mosquito control in small studies and on islands without the use of insecticides. Gene editing using CRISPR (clustered regularly interspaced short palindromic repeats)/Cas9 relies on the insertion of another sequence into the genome of the male. Once introduced into the population all offspring inherit the altered gene sequence, and within a few generations the population becomes dominated by the transgene constructs, eliminating or neutralizing the population.[53]

SUMMARY

Diverse groups of ectoparasitic arthropods cause significant morbidity and mortality in cattle globally. Ectoparasites affect cattle health and production through the different ways that they infest their hosts to obtain nutrients and complete their life cycle, and as vectors of pathogens. Some ectoparasites and ectoparasite-borne pathogens affecting cattle are listed by the World Organization for Animal Health as notifiable. Hematophagous flies, myiasis-causing flies, lice, mites, and ticks are the most important groups of cattle ectoparasites. Several of these ectoparasitic species are of One Health relevance because of their impact on public health. The intense use of ectoparasiticides to treat infestations in cattle has selected for ectoparasite populations that are resistant to this treatment method. Although ectoparasiticide resistance is prevalent in most of the important arthropods infesting cattle, the alternatives currently available for cattle producers are limited. This limitation of cost-effective control measures should be evaluated in relation to current cattle-management systems. Approaches integrating the use of different technologies are required to manage cattle ectoparasites effectively while addressing societal expectations regarding food safety and environmental health.[54] Assessing the status of coparasitism with ectoparasites and endoparasites in cattle across agroecosystems is critical for the advancement of integrated parasite management.

DISCLOSURE

The research of Drs. Pérez de Leónand Mitchell is supported by appropriated funds for projects 3094-32000-041-00D and 3094-32000-042-00D. Research by Dr. Watson was supported in part by Multistate Research Project S-1076: Fly Management in Animal Agriculture Systems and Impacts on Animal Health and Food Safety. USDA is an equal opportunity provider and employer.

REFERENCES

1. Wall RL, Shearer D. Veterinary ectoparasites: biology, pathology and control. 2nd edition. Malden (MA): Blackwell Science Ltd.; 2001.
2. Garros C, Bouyer J, Takken W, et al. Pests and vector-borne diseases in the livestock industry. Wageningen (the Netherlands): Wageningen Academic Publishers; 2018.
3. World Animal Health Organization. OIE-Listed diseases. In: OIE-Listed diseases, infections and infestations in force in 2019. 2019. Available at: https://www.oie.int/en/animal-health-in-the-world/oie-listed-diseases-2019/. Accessed November 29, 2019.
4. Endres MI, Schwartzkopf-Genswein K. Overview of cattle production systems. In: Tucker CB, editor. Advances in cattle welfare. Kidlington (United Kingdom): Woodhead Publishing; 2018. p. 1–26.
5. Henrioud AN. Towards sustainable parasite control practices in livestock production with emphasis in Latin America. Vet Parasitol 2011;180:2–11.
6. Wileman BW, Thomson DU, Reinhardt CD, et al. Analysis of modern technologies commonly used in beef cattle production: conventional beef production versus nonconventional production using meta-analysis. J Anim Sci 2009;87:3418–26.

7. Narladkar BW. Projected economic losses due to vector and vector-borne parasitic diseases in livestock of India and its significance in implementing the concept of integrated practices for vector management. Vet World 2018;11: 151–60.

8. Meng CQ, Sluder AE, Selzer PM. Ectoparasites: drug discovery against moving targets. Weinheim (Germany): Wiley-VCH; 2018.

9. Grisi L, Leite RC, Martins JRDS, et al. Reassessment of the potential economic impact of cattle parasites in Brazil. Rev Bras Parasitol Vet 2014;23:150–6.

10. Scasta JD. Livestock parasite management on high-elevation rangelands: ecological interactions of climate, habitat, and wildlife. J Integr Pest Manag 2015;6:8–17.

11. Laing G, Aragrande M, Canali M, et al. Control of cattle ticks and tick-borne diseases by acaricide in southern province of Zambia: a retrospective evaluation of animal health measures according to current One Health concepts. Front Public Health 2018;6:45.

12. Mullen GR, Durden LA. Medical and veterinary entomology. 3rd edition. San Diego (CA): Academic Press; 2019.

13. Schreiber ET, Campbell JB, Kunz SE, et al. Effects of horn fly (Diptera: Muscidae) control on cows and gastrointestinal worm (Nematode: Trichostrongylidae) treatment for calves on cow and calf weight gains. J Econ Entomol 1987;80:451–4.

14. Owens WE, Oliver SP, Gillespie BE, et al. Role of horn flies (*Haematobia irritans*) in *Staphylococcus aureus*-induced mastitis in dairy heifers. Am J Vet Res 1998; 59:1122–4.

15. Shaw SA, Sutherland IA. The prevalence of *Stephanofilaria* sp. in buffalo fly, *Haematobia irritans exigua*, in Central Queensland. Aust J Entomol 2006;45:198–201.

16. Swiger SL, Payne RD. Selected insecticide delivery devices for management of horn flies (*Haematobia irritans*) (Diptera: Muscidae) on beef cattle. J Med Entomol 2017;54:173–7.

17. Meat and Livestock Australia. Recommendations for integrated buffalo fly control 2011. North Sydney (Australia); Available at: https://www.mla.com.au/CustomControls/PaymentGateway/ViewFile.aspx?co4Y6oDDU7HwRLRFUnQltcN/p+2lSe3gz2BcevceelqHyRBj3V47auHcoqsAMbBA3EYMKKAfsht7d1Tnt3BqiA==. Accessed November 1, 2019.

18. Campbell JB, Berry IL. Economic threshold for stable flies on confined livestock. In: Petersen J, Greene GL, editors. Current status of stable fly (Diptera: Muscidae) research, vol. 74. Lanham (MD): Entomological Society of America; 1989. p. 18–22.

19. Patra G, Behera P, Das SK, et al. *Stomoxys calcitrans* and its importance in livestock: a review. Int J Adv Agric Res 2018;6:30–7.

20. Fowler FE, Chirico J, Sandelin BA, et al. Seasonality and Diapause of *Musca autumnalis* (Diptera: Muscidae) at its southern limits in North America, with observations on *Haematobia irritans* (Diptera: Muscidae). J Med Entomol 2015;52: 1213–24.

21. Krafsur ES, Moon RD. Bionomics of the face fly, *Musca autumnalis*. Annu Rev Entomol 1997;42:503–23.

22. Schmidtmann ET, Valla ME, Chase LE. Effect of face flies on grazing time and weight gain in dairy heifers. J Econ Entomol 1981;74:33–9.

23. Steelman CD, White TW, Schilling PE. Effects of mosquitoes on the average daily gain of feedlot steers in southern Louisiana. J Econ Entomol 1972;65:462–6.

24. Hartman DA, Rice LM, DeMaria J, et al. Entomological risk factors for potential transmission of Rift Valley fever virus around concentrations of livestock in Colorado. Transbound Emerg Dis 2019;66:1709–17.

25. Adler PH, Kúdelová T, Kúdela M, et al. Cryptic biodiversity and the origins of pest status revealed in the macrogenome of *Simulium colombaschense* (Diptera: Simuliidae), history's most destructive black fly. PLoS One 2016;11:e0147673.

26. Baldacchino F, Porciani A, Bernard C, et al. Spatial and temporal distribution of Tabanidae in the Pyrenees Mountains: the influence of altitude and landscape structure. Bull Entomol Res 2014;104:1–11.

27. Baldacchino F, Desquesnes M, Mihok S, et al. Tabanids: neglected subjects of research, but important vectors of disease agents! Infect Genet Evol 2014;28: 596–615.

28. Harrup L, Miranda M, Carpenter S. Advances in control techniques for *Culicoides* and future prospects. Vet Ital 2016;52:247–64.

29. Faiman R, Kirstein O, Moncaz A, et al. Studies on the flight patterns of foraging sand flies. Acta Trop 2011;120:110–4.

30. Ayhan N, Charrel RN. Sandfly-borne viruses of demonstrated/relevant medical importance. In: Savić S, editor. Vectors and vector-borne zoonotic diseases. London: IntechOpen; 2018. p. 1–22. https://doi.org/10.5772/intechopen.81023. Available at: https://www.intechopen.com/books/vectors-and-vector-borne-zoonotic-diseases/sandfly-borne-viruses-of-demonstrated-relevant-medical-importance. Accessed November 1, 2019.

31. Harris KM. Agricultural and veterinary significance of Diptera. In: Kirk-Spriggs AH, Sinclair BJ, editors. Manual of Afrotropical Diptera, vol. 1. Pretoria (South Africa): South African National Biodiversity Institute; 2017. p. 153–62.

32. Hennessey MJ, Hsi DJ, Davis JS, et al. Use of a multiagency approach to eradicate New World screwworm flies from Big Pine Key, Florida, following an outbreak of screwworm infestation (September 2016-March 2017). J Am Vet Med Assoc 2019;255:908–14.

33. Lia RP, Rehbein S, Giannelli A. LONGRANGE® (eprinomectin 5% w/v extended-release injection) efficacy against *Hypoderma lineatum* in an endemic area in southern Italy. Parasit Vectors 2019;12:231.

34. Egri B. Louse infestation of ruminants. In: Sadashiv SO, Patil SJ, editors. Bovine science—a key to sustainable development. London: IntechOpen; 2018. p. 79–88. Available at: https://www.intechopen.com/books/bovine-science-a-key-to-sustainable-development/louse-infestation-of-ruminants. Accessed November 1, 2019.

35. Control of ectoparasites and insect pests of cattle. 2014. In: Control of worms sustainably (COWS). Available at: https://www.cattleparasites.org.uk/app/uploads/2018/04/Control-of-ectoparasites-and-insect-pests-of-cattle.pdf. Accessed November 1, 2019.

36. Mauldin EA, Peters-Kennedy J. Integumentary system. In: Maxie MG, editor. Jubb, Kennedy, and Palmer's pathology of domestic animals:, vol. 1, 6th edition. St Louis (MO): WB Saunders; 2016. p. 509–736.

37. Sonenshine DE, Roe RM. 2nd edition. Biology of ticks, vols. 1 and 2. New York: Oxford University Press; 2014.

38. Beard CB, Occi J, Bonilla DL, et al. Multistate infestation with the exotic disease-vector tick *Haemaphysalis longicornis*—United States, August 2017-September 2018. Morb Mortal Wkly Rep 2018;67:1310–3.

39. Shaurub E. Arthropod ectoparasites of domestic animals: biology, pathology, dermatology, diagnosis, and control. Saarbrüken (Germany): Lambert Academic Publishing; 2012.

40. Rodriguez-Vivas RI, Jonsson NN, Bhushan C. Strategies for the control of *Rhipicephalus microplus* ticks in a world of conventional acaricide and macrocyclic lactone resistance. Parasitol Res 2018;117:3–29.

41. Suarez M, Rubi J, Pérez D, et al. High impact and effectiveness of Gavac™ vaccine in the national program for control of bovine ticks *Rhipicephalus microplus* in Venezuela. Livest Sci 2016;187:48–52.

42. Konganti K, Guerrero FD, Schilkey F, et al. A whole genome assembly of the horn fly, *Haematobia irritans*, and prediction of genes with roles in metabolism and sex determination. G3 (Bethesda) 2018;8:1675–86.

43. U.S. Department of Agriculture—Agricultural Research Service. ARS collection of entomopathogenic fungal cultures. 2019. Available at: https://data.nal.usda.gov/dataset/ars-collection-entomopathogenic-fungal-cultures-arsef. Accessed November 1, 2019.

44. Denning SS, Washburn SP, Watson DW. Development of a novel walk-through fly trap for the control of horn flies and other pests on pastured dairy cows. J Dairy Sci 2014;97:4624–31.

45. Hogsette JA, Foil LD. Blue and black cloth targets: effects of size, shape, and color on stable fly (Diptera: Muscidae) attraction. J Econ Entomol 2018;111:974–9.

46. Garros C, Bouyer J, Takken W, et al. Control of vector-borne diseases in the livestock industry: new opportunities and challenges. In: Garros C, Bouyer J, Takken W, et al, editors. Pests and vector-borne diseases in the livestock industry. Wageningen (the Netherlands): Wageningen Academic Publishers; 2018. p. 575–80.

47. Sorge US, Moon RD, Stromberg BE, et al. Parasites and parasite management practices of organic and conventional dairy herds in Minnesota. J Dairy Sci 2015;98:3143–51.

48. Rutz DA, Waldron JK. 2016 Integrated pest management (IPM) guide for organic dairies. New York State IPM Program. Ithaca (NY): Cornell University; 2016. NYS IPM Publication number 323 version 3.

49. Coffey L. Tipsheet: organic management of internal and external livestock parasites. Butte (MT): National Center for Appropriate Technology; 2015. Available at: https://www.ams.usda.gov/sites/default/files/media/Organic%20Management%20of%20Internal%20and%20External%20Livestock%20Parasites_FINAL.pdf. Accessed November 1, 2019.

50. Bourtzis K, Lees RS, Hendrichs J, et al. More than one rabbit out of the hat: radiation, transgenic and symbiont-based approaches for sustainable management of mosquito and tsetse fly populations. Acta Trop 2016;157:115–30.

51. Schnettler E, Ratinier M, Watson M, et al. RNA interference targets arbovirus replication in *Culicoides* cells. J Virol 2013;87:2441–54.

52. Paulo DF, Williamson ME, Arp AP, et al. Specific gene disruption in the major livestock pests *Cochliomyia hominivorax* and *Lucilia cuprina* using CRISPR/Cas9. G3 (Bethesda) 2019;9:3045–55.

53. Gould F, Dhole S, Lloyd AL. Pest management by genetic addiction. Proc Natl Acad Sci U S A 2019;116:5849–51.

54. Integrated parasite control on cattle farms. In: Control of worms sustainably (COWS). 2014. Available at: https://www.cattleparasites.org.uk/app/uploads/2018/04/Integrated-parasite-control-on-cattle-farms.pdf. Accessed November 1, 2019.

Ruminant Coccidiosis

Berit Bangoura, DVM, PhD*, Katherine D. Bardsley, MS

KEYWORDS

- *Eimeria* • Intestinal • Diarrhea • Anticoccidial • Pathogenicity • Prepatent
- Patent period • Management

KEY POINTS

- Coccidiosis is a common disease in ruminants worldwide and causes significant economic losses in livestock; it is caused by highly host-specific *Eimeria* species.
- Coccidiosis is identified by observing clinical diarrhea and by detecting *Eimeria* species oocysts in fecal samples. Not all *Eimeria* species are equally pathogenic, thus proper diagnosis requires species differentiation.
- Effective coccidiosis control relies heavily on both management measures and chemical control by anticoccidial drugs. Drug resistance should be considered a significant potential threat in coccidiosis treatment.
- The life cycle of *Eimeria* species is self-limiting, that is, young animals stop excreting high numbers at about 1 week after onset of clinical signs.
- *Eimeria* species infections induce protective immunity but no cross-protection. Initial exposure of young animals to only low infection pressure and timing of anticoccidial treatment, are crucial.

INTRODUCTION

Taxonomically, ruminant coccidia are a group of unicellular parasites comprising representatives of several different genera. *Toxoplasma gondii*, *Neospora caninum*, *Sarcocystis* species, and *Eimeria* species are summarized under the wide term of coccidia. However, in ruminants the genus *Eimeria* is commonly referred to by the term coccidia. This genus contains a diversity of species. In ruminants, *Eimeria* species are generally gastrointestinal parasites, and most species of *Eimeria* are exclusively located in the intestine. In contrast to other genera of related coccidia species, they feature a one-host (homoxenous) life cycle and are highly host specific. They are not transmissible between different domestic ruminant species; cattle, sheep, and goats have several specific *Eimeria* species infecting each. *Eimeria* are a group of economically important parasites and a common cause of diarrhea in young ruminants. Thus, coccidia-related disease, also known as eimeriosis or coccidiosis, represents one of the major challenges in raising cattle, sheep, and goats. Coccidiosis produces both acute and chronic damage, and may predispose to secondary

Department of Veterinary Sciences, Wyoming State Veterinary Laboratory, University of Wyoming, 1174 Snowy Range Road, Laramie, WY 82070, USA
* Corresponding author.
E-mail address: bbangour@uwyo.edu

Vet Clin Food Anim 36 (2020) 187–203
https://doi.org/10.1016/j.cvfa.2019.12.006
0749-0720/20/© 2019 Elsevier Inc. All rights reserved.

diseases. Of importance, not all *Eimeria* species in ruminants are problematic. Some of them can parasitize the host without causing considerable damage to the intestinal mucosa and are not regarded as significant pathogens.

EIMERIA SPECIES IN RUMINANT HOSTS

A vast number of *Eimeria* species have been described in ruminant hosts. This article focuses on the 3 major livestock species cattle (*Bos taurus*), sheep (*Ovis aries*), and goats (*Capra hircus*). For cattle, 13 intestinal *Eimeria* species are recognized as valid, although many more were originally described.[1,2] Decades ago it was assumed that sheep and goats share *Eimeria* species. Only later was it discovered that each of the small ruminant species harbors its own panel of *Eimeria* species, which leads to some confusion in the literature. Some species names were revised and some publications still confound sheep and goat *Eimeria* species. However, recently 12 intestinal and 1 abomasal *Eimeria* species have been observed in sheep,[3,4] with the abomasal *Eimeria gilruthi* being assumed to be a stage of another intestinal *Eimeria* species rather than an individual species. Ten different intestinal species have been recently found in goats.[5,6] Older literature sources may list higher numbers for both sheep and goat and are partially still referred to. Moreover, species names of small ruminant *Eimeria* have changed several times over the decades, leading to even more confusion when comparing different literature. The history of species identification and denomination has been reviewed in detail elsewhere.[7] The valid ruminant *Eimeria* species responsible for clinical coccidiosis are listed by host in **Table 1** along with the species of lesser clinical relevance. In cattle, the highest pathogenicity is observed with *Eimeria bovis* and *Eimeria zuernii*; in sheep, *Eimeria ovinoidalis*, *Eimeria ahsata*, *Eimeria bakuensis*, and *Eimeria crandallis* are the most relevant pathogens; and in goats, *Eimeria ninakohlyakimovae* and *Eimeria caprina* are the major pathogens.

Table 1
Valid *Eimeria* species of domestic ruminants by host

Pathogenicity	Cattle	Sheep	Goat
+++	E bovis E zuernii	E ovinoidalis	E ninakohlyakimovae E caprina
++	E alabamensis	E ahsata E bakuensis (syn. E ovina) E crandallis E gilruthi[a]	
+	E auburnensis E ellipsoidalis	E faurei	E alijevi E arloingi E apsheronica
−	E brasiliensis E bukidnonensis E canadensis E cylindrica E illinoisensis E pellita E subspherica E wyomingensis	E granulosa E intricata E marsica E pallida E parva E punctata E weybridgensis	E caprovina E christenseni E hirci E jolchijevi E kocharli

Pathogenicity is given as +++, high; ++, moderate, +, low; −, not present.
[a] Parasite meronts observed in the sheep abomasum; this species is suspected to be invalid and represent the developmental stage of one of the other listed *Eimeria* spp. (although the species has not been identified).

PARASITE LIFE CYCLE AND TRANSMISSION

The life cycle of *Eimeria* species is shown in **Fig. 1** and contains 3 major phases; the first 2 phases are internal (asexual and sexual replication), followed by environmental sporogony (sporulation). The internal development of the parasite takes about 1 to 3 weeks, with variations that are *Eimeria* species specific. The life cycle is homoxenous; thus, one host suffices to complete the development of the parasite, starting with infection by the sporulated oocyst, which is the environmental and infective stage. Sporulated oocysts are ingested from a contaminated environment and are then swallowed and transported to the intestine. Owing to the influence of pepsin, bile, trypsin, temperature, and pH, the oocysts rupture and set free the infectious contents, the sporozoites.[8,9] Each sporulated oocyst contains a total of 8 infective sporozoites. Each single sporozoite invades one enterocyte and stays within the cell inside a parasitophorous vacuole (PV). The parasite is able to gain nutrients from its host cell through the PV wall.[10] Inside the PV, the parasite replication starts by several asexual replication cycles, also known as schizogony or merogony. The schizogony is a multiple fission, leading to a varying number of daughter parasite cells derived from one initial stage. Most *Eimeria* species feature 2 subsequent schizogony cycles, and a few have 3 merogonies.[11,12] During each schizogony, hundreds to thousands of new stages (merozoites) are formed in each host cell. After completion of one schizogony cycle, the merozoites leave the host cell by rupturing it and each of them is able to infect a new enterocyte. After undergoing all predetermined merogonies, the parasite enters the sexual replication phase, the gamogony. Within host cells, the parasites form either a microgamont, which is the male stage, or a macrogamont, the

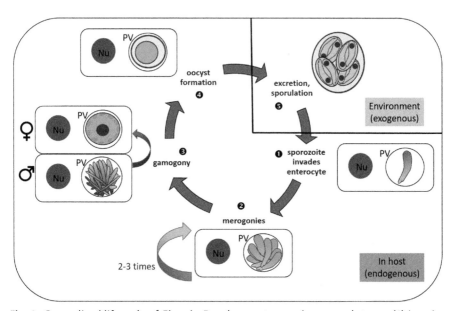

Fig. 1. Generalized life cycle of *Eimeria*. Development comprises several stages: (1) invasion of host cells; (2) asexual replication (schizogony): the number of merogonies is species-dependent and most common are 2 merogonic cycles; (3) sexual replication step (gamogony) with formation of macrogamonts (♀) and microgamonts (♂) and fertilization; (4) oocyst formation and release into gut lumen; (5) environmental sporulation that renders oocyst infective. Nu, host cell nucleus; PV, parasitophorous vacuole.

female parasite stage. On maturation, the microgamont releases many microgametes, motile stages that fertilize the macrogamont. This leads to the formation of a zygote that matures into the oocyst. The oocyst leaves the host cell and is excreted by the host by defecation. The time period from infection until the start of fecal oocyst excretion (prepatent period) varies greatly by *Eimeria* species. The same is true for the duration of oocyst excretion (patent period) until the infection is cleared by the host. The prepatent and patent periods of ruminant *Eimeria* species, as far as is known, are summarized in **Table 2**. Of importance is that *Eimeria* oocysts are not infective on excretion but need a period in the environment to gain infectivity.[11] This process is called sporulation and is expedited by warm and moist conditions. Under optimal conditions, sporulation can take place within as few as 2 to 3 days.[13] The final infective oocyst contains 2 inner membrane-covered vesicles, the sporocysts, each of them containing 4 sporozoites, so that each sporulated oocyst contains 8 infective sporozoites. The environmental oocysts are transmitted directly by fecal-oral infection route, the susceptible hosts ingesting contaminated feed, drinking from contaminated water sources, licking on surfaces contaminated with fecal material, and so forth. According to the parasites' life cycle, coccidiosis is a self-limiting infection because there are no stages left inside the gut after the life cycle is completed and the oocysts are excreted.

EPIDEMIOLOGY AND IMMUNOLOGY

Coccidiosis should always be regarded as herd disease rather than as a problem in individual animals. Once *Eimeria* species are present in an operation, they spread

Table 2
Internal development of *Eimeria* developmental stages in ruminants: major locations and prepatent and patent periods

	Meronts	Gamonts	Prepatent Period (days)	Patent Period (days)
E bovis	Small intestine	Distal ileum, cecum, colon	15–23	5–26
E zuernii	Small intestine	Distal ileum, cecum, colon, rectum	15–22	2–11
E alabamensis	Distal ileum	Distal ileum, massive infections; also cecum and proximal colon[a]	6–11	1–13
E auburnensis	Middle and distal third of small intestine	Middle and distal third of small intestine	18–20	2–8
E ellipsoidalis	Small intestine	Small intestine, mainly distal ileum	8–13	12
E bukidnonensis	Small intestine	Ileum	10–25	2–12
E cylindrica	ND	ND	11–20	ND
E subspherica	Jejunum[a]	Jejunum[a]	7–18	4–15
E wyomingensis	ND	Distal 5 m of small intestine	13–15	1–7

No data available on *E brasiliensis*, *E canadensis*, *E illinoisensis*, *E pellita*.
Abbreviation: ND, not described.
[a] Intranuclear parasite stages.
Data from Vieira LS, Lima JD, Rosa JS. Development of *Eimeria ninakohlyakimovae* Yakimoff & Rastegaieff, 1930 emend. Levine, 1961 in experimentally infected goats (*Capra hircus*). J Parasitol 1997 Dec;83(6):1015–8.

widely in the herd within a few life cycles of the parasite. Older animals develop a partial immunity to the infection, so they excrete only a small number of oocysts on reinfection. Younger animals are naïve up to their first infection, leading to a considerable multiplication of the parasite and excretion of high numbers of oocysts, further contaminating the environment for the next naïve animals. During primary infections, ruminants can shed more than a million oocysts per each gram of feces.[14] It is widely assumed that adult animals play a minor role in the epidemiology of the disease, and the major problem on commercial farms is the transmission within the young animal population.[1] However, nursing calves, lambs, and kids can acquire a primary infection from their mothers.[15] Transmission is most efficient on farms with high stocking densities and a concentration of young animals. It occurs by the fecal-oral route within a group, and can also be introduced into a susceptible herd by contaminated boots, tools, tires, or feed. Most clinical cases of coccidiosis are observed in animals younger than 12 months of age. Although all farm types may be affected by coccidia infections, operations such as feedlots and other intensive production settings are at highest risk to struggle with coccidiosis owing to the facilitated transmission. *Eimeria* oocysts have a high survival potential in the environment. They can remain viable and infectious for at least 1 year[16] and withstand many adverse environmental influences because of their thick oocyst wall. Few chemical and physical stressors are capable of inactivating *Eimeria* oocysts. They are resistant to freezing, extreme pH changes, and low oxygen availability. However, direct exposure to ultraviolet light over several hours or extreme dryness is detrimental to the oocysts.[17] Therefore, good environmental hygiene and exposure of the premises to direct sunlight can be of great benefit in minimizing problems with coccidiosis. By contrast, covered areas that are wet and contaminated by feces provide optimal conditions for transmission. High temperatures (about 39°C) over longer time periods are able to prevent oocyst sporulation[18] but only if applied uninterrupted. Regarding natural conditions whereby oocysts are commonly covered in feces and nights in many regions are much cooler than 39°C, this leaves many environmental oocysts unaffected long enough to infect another host animal.

The global prevalence of coccidia is high; infections are common in all ruminants and most infections involve multiple species. A study from England indicated a prevalence of 98% in goats, with pathogenic species being most common in the examined goat kids.[7] In cattle, a study from the United States (Georgia) indicated 86% prevalence of *Eimeria* oocysts in young calves,[19] with a high percentage of highly pathogenic *E bovis*. In sheep, 86% of ewes in a Louisiana flock were positive for a variety of *Eimeria* species.[20] Thus, *Eimeria* are considered ubiquitous pathogens.

Although *Eimeria* species are highly host specific and not transmissible between different livestock species, they may be transmitted between defined wildlife and domestic animals, each serving as a potential reservoir to infect each other. According to the current knowledge, cattle *Eimeria* are assumed to be transmissible to bison (*Bison bison*, *Bison bonasus*)[21,22] and other bovines, and domestic sheep share *Eimeria* species with ovines such as Bighorn sheep (*Ovis canadensis*).[23]

Immunity occurs after primary infection. The immunity is strictly *Eimeria* species specific, that is, infections with one *Eimeria* species do not cross-protect against later infections with another species. This implies that animals can be prone to coccidiosis several times in their life, mostly during their young ages. The acquired immunity is largely based on a Th1 (T helper cell 1) cellular immune response. A detectable humoral response with formation of specific antibodies also occurs but contributes little to immunoprotection.[24] The immunity is partial; it is protective against clinical coccidiosis but does not completely suppress parasite replication on reinfection. Thus, animals may be reinfected and shed oocysts transiently throughout their life, although excreted parasite numbers are much lower because the immune system controls the parasite infection to a major extent.[1] In chickens, a relation between breed and coccidia replication and intestinal damage is established. However, regarding ruminants, a study in sheep did not demonstrate significant breed-dependent effects for the degree of clinical coccidiosis in young lambs.[25]

PATHOGENESIS AND PATHOLOGY

Owing to the intracellular localization of all internal developmental stages, significant damage to the intestinal mucosa occurs. Several factors influence the pathologic and clinical outcome, such as the *Eimeria* species present, infection dose, its replication potential, inflammatory immune response, and concurrent infections with other pathogens, as well as management practices and related stress. Accordingly, the outcome of *Eimeria* infections can vary greatly by parasite species as well as by individual host animal and farm. The initial invasion site for the sporozoites is generally the small intestine except for *E gilruthi*, an early developmental stage of an intestinal sheep *Eimeria* species that is able to parasitize the abomasum. In the pathogenesis of intestinal lesions during infections with pathogenic *Eimeria* species, 2 major elements are involved. On the one hand, the parasite causes direct damage arising from mucosal host cell destruction during its multiplication steps. In *E bovis*, destruction of deeper submucosal layers also occurs, including invasion of lymphatic vessels[26] and even mesenterial lymph nodes.[27] On the other hand, the immune system contributes largely to the local damage and dysfunction by a severe inflammatory response with attraction of immune cell populations.[28] After completion of parasitic development, prolonged tissue repair is seen before normal intestinal function is largely restored; in other words, pathologic changes often persist longer than the duration of the patent period and detectable parasite excretion.

The direct damage caused by the parasite infection and replication is generally greatest during the late schizogony and even more during the gamogony.[29] This is due to the high level of multiplication the parasite undergoes during its first schizogony, leading to infection of an exponentially increasing number of intestinal cells during later multiplication rounds. Thus, most of the damage occurs shortly before oocyst excretion starts in affected animals. Interestingly, also in *Eimeria* species that feature macroschizonts during their first asexual generation, for example, *E bovis* and *E zuernii*, damage during the first schizogony is less pronounced than during the subsequent stages.[29]

To date it is not completely clear why some *Eimeria* species cause significant damage, inflammation, and clinical disease while others are much less pathogenic or even lack a detectable pathogenicity. It is highly likely that invasion of deeper layers of the intestinal wall, such as seen in *E bovis*, as well as a high replication potential, are factors that increase pathogenicity. Furthermore, it is assumed that species-specific virulence factors are involved in the pathogenesis of coccidiosis; however, in contrast to chickens, not a lot of research has been performed in this area in ruminants so far. Virulence factor candidates are proteins involved in host cell invasion, remodeling, and modulation of host cell metabolism such as the rhoptry proteins and cathepsins. Their presence, structure, and function may be essential for the induced damage similar to other coccidian genera,[30] although little is known regarding this issue.

Regarding the different pathologic effects of coccidia, intestinal hemorrhagic lesions can be observed in most severe cases in cattle, sheep, and goats. The exact intestinal location of the developmental stages and the extent of damage depend on the *Eimeria* species (see **Table 2**; **Tables 3** and **4**).

Table 3
Sheep *Eimeria*

	Meronts	Gamonts	Prepatent Period (days)	Patent Period (days)
E ovinoidalis (based on description of E ninakohlyakimovae in sheep)	Small intestine	Ileum, cecum, proximal colon	11–15 and more	8–30
E ahsata	Small intestine	Small intestine	9–28	10–12
E bakuensis (syn. E ovina)	Small intestine	Small intestine	9–23	10
E crandallis	Small intestine	Small intestine	15–20	ND
E gilruthi*	Abomasum	ND	ND	ND
E faurei	Small intestine	Small intestine	12–14	9–10
E intricata	Distal small intestine	Distal half of small intestine, colon, rectum	20–27	3–11
E parva	Small intestine	Small intestine, cecum, colon	11–15	6–8
E weybridgensis	ND	ND	23–29	9–18

No data available on *E granulosa, E marsica, E pallida, E punctata.*
Abbreviation: ND, not described.
  * Parasite meronts observed in the sheep abomasum; this species is suspected to be invalid and represent the developmental stage of one of the other listed Eimeria spp (although the species has not been identified).

Cattle

The highly pathogenic species *E bovis* and *E zuernii* cause the most pronounced lesions. The first generation of meronts (macromeronts) might be visible by the naked eye on necropsy; they often are much bigger than the following replication stages and may contain more than 100,000 merozoites.[26,31–33] Severe coccidiosis in cattle is marked by extensive epithelial destruction in the distal small intestine and throughout the large intestine, leading to hemorrhagic and diphtheritic enteritis in these sections.[29,34,35] With the less pathogenic *Eimeria alabamensis*, the pathologic

Table 4
Goat *Eimeria*

	Meronts	Gamonts	Prepatent Period	Patent Period
E ninakohlyakimovae	Ileum, cecum, proximal colon	Ileum, cecum, proximal colon	10–17	4–10
E caprina	ND	Colon, cecum, rectum	21	7
E arloingi	Jejunum, mesenteric lymph nodes	Small intestine, proximal third of colon	21	ND
E christenseni	Small intestine	ND	21–24	ND

No data available on *E alijevi, E apsheronica, E caprovina, E hirci, E jolchijevi, E kocharli.*
Abbreviation: ND, not described.

profile greatly relies on the infection dose, and only high-dose infections lead to hyperemia and destruction of villi in the distal half of the small intestine.[36]

Sheep

Lambs aged 4 to 5 weeks are the most susceptible to intestinal injuries.[37] *E ovinoidalis* infections induce severe and potentially lethal enteritis. First-generation meronts may be macromeronts that are detectable during necropsy[38] and are accompanied by diphtheroid to hemorrhagic jejunitis. Late developmental stages cause hemorrhagic typhlitis in massive infections. Other ovine *Eimeria* species with pathogenic effects include *E crandallis* and *E bakuensis*. *E crandallis* infection leads to a similar but lesser infection in lambs with pathology similar to *E ovinoidalis* but mostly milder, with cecum and colon being most affected.[39] *E bakuensis* may lead to formation of polyps in the small intestine owing to localized replication of late parasitic stages.[40]

Of importance, coinfections of different *Eimeria* species in sheep have been shown to result in increased oocyst production,[41] which may lead to increased disorder resulting from more enterocytes being destroyed. Because multispecies infections are far more common than single-species infections in the field, an aggravated pathologic status may also be seen in animals with moderate infection doses.

Goats

Early infections with *E ninakohlyakimovae* or *E caprina*, respectively, in goat kids are characterized by hemorrhagic enteritis.[40] *Eimeria arloingi* infections may produce polyps in the small intestine,[42] and *Eimeria apsheronica* stages induce formation of white nodules in the mucosa that are visible from the serosal surface.[43]

It has been shown in cattle and sheep that coinfections with other intestinal pathogens exacerbate the disorder and the clinical outcome. In cattle, hemorrhagic enteritis during *E zuernii* infections seems to be associated with massive intestinal *Clostridium perfringens* colonization.[44] Also, coinfection with bovine parvovirus leads to much more pronounced disease than infection with each pathogen.[45] In sheep, *Nematodirus* (thread-necked strongyle) infections have been shown to severely aggravate *Eimeria*-induced enteritis and vice versa.[46]

CLINICAL SIGNS

The lead symptom of clinical coccidiosis is diarrhea. The diarrheal quality can vary greatly from softened fecal consistency, to watery diarrhea, to hemorrhagic character.[14,47,48] The highly pathogenic pathogens often lead to bloody diarrhea in a proportion of the infected animals (**Fig. 2**), and transient fever may occur.[49] In severely affected animals, dehydration, anorexia, electrolyte imbalances, weight loss, and impaired nitrogen balance have been described in domestic ruminants.[47,50–52] Significant long-term losses including mortality, reduced final body weight, and delayed fertility have been extrapolated for cattle.[53]

Cattle

Hemorrhagic diarrhea and severe systemic disease is seen only in infections with *E bovis* and *E zuernii*. *E alabamensis* can lead to watery diarrhea,[54,55] whereas infections with all other species generally do not cause disease,[1] with no adverse long-term effect on animal performance. The same seems to apply to farmed bison.

Bovine winter coccidiosis

In North American cattle, the term "winter coccidiosis" has been coined for herd issues arising during the winter months. Winter coccidiosis is associated with higher

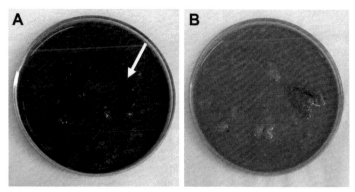

Fig. 2. Diarrhea samples from calves infected with *E bovis*. (*A*) Hemorrhagic quality 23 days after infection at the end of oocyst excretion (*arrow*: fibrin strands, mucosa parts, and blood clots). (*B*) Liquid diarrhea with mucosa parts still discharged 26 days after infection, which was after clearance of the infection.

mortality and, on a herd-level basis, a generally increased incidence and severity of coccidiosis caused by *E bovis* and/or *E zuernii*. Mostly 6- to 12-month-old animals are affected, and up to 20% to 50% of animals from this age group may show diarrhea.[56,57] Rather than reflecting higher infection doses, winter coccidiosis is attributed to generally increased susceptibility to diseases during cold weather conditions.[56]

Bovine nervous coccidiosis

A special form of coccidiosis in cattle is the phenomenon of "nervous coccidiosis." Both *E bovis* and *E zuernii* infections may cause neurologic symptoms,[58] such as epileptiform seizures with opisthotonus and nystagmus. Only a small proportion of infected calves develop nervous symptoms, and feedlot cattle seem most prone to this aggravated syndrome. In North America, nervous coccidiosis is mostly observed during winter,[57] and high mortality rates up to 75% are possible.[59] The pathogenesis is not known; however, it has been hypothesized that *Eimeria*-related neurotoxins, electrolyte imbalances, or vitamin A deficiency may be underlying factors.[59,60] Diagnosis of nervous coccidiosis proves difficult because there are no gross lesions in the central nervous system specifically related to the observed clinical signs.[59]

Sheep

E ovinoidalis can lead to hemorrhagic diarrhea.[40] Less often, similar symptoms develop naturally in animals infected with *E crandallis*. *E bakuensis* and *E ahsata* infections mostly remain subclinical unless massive infection doses are ingested. Naturally infected lambs often show prolonged disease and excrete more oocysts of each species if several *Eimeria* species are present.[41]

Goats

E ninakohlyakimovae and *E caprina* are highly pathogenic pathogens capable of inducing watery to bloody diarrhea.[61] *E arloingi* infections can also lead to watery diarrhea.[52]

In older animals after reinfection or after primary infection with low infection doses, acute symptoms may not be present at all or only in a small proportion of the affected animals. Nonetheless, subacute to chronic adverse effects on growth, feed conversion ratio, and long-term performance can be expected from subclinical coccidiosis after infection with pathogenic species.[62]

ECONOMIC IMPACT

The economic impact of coccidiosis is estimated to be high. Current estimates, however, are not available regarding bovine coccidiosis only. Fitzgerald[63] calculated annual losses of up to US$723 million worldwide. For sheep and goats, he estimated global losses up to $140 million. Losses occur from mortality, costs for targeted treatment (eg, feed additives) of animal groups, symptomatic treatment of diarrheic animals, enhanced susceptibility of affected animals to secondary infections, and lowered animal productivity. Besides the acute effects, a long-term impact in terms of a lower feed conversion ratio, a lower final body weight gain, and a lower life-time fertility potential have been proposed,[53] although long-term studies are largely missing for ruminants. It is assumed, interestingly, that subclinical coccidiosis may lead to higher production losses than clinical coccidiosis because more animals are affected and the long-term effects caused by reduced intestinal integrity are considerable.[1] Winter coccidiosis in cattle causes significant economic losses particularly in first-year cattle.

DIAGNOSIS

Diagnosis of coccidiosis is mostly based on clinical observations—for example, diarrhea in young animals. Fecal samples are collected and analyzed for the presence of *Eimeria* oocysts (**Figs. 3** and **4A**). Although high oocyst densities may be demonstrated by simple wet-mount techniques, the method of choice is fecal flotation allowing oocysts to be concentrated, which significantly increases the sensitivity. It is important that not only the presence of oocysts should be assessed; it is also imperative to perform a species-level identification as far as possible (see **Fig. 3**). Because many *Eimeria* species are not or mildly pathogenic, *Eimeria* species determination allows for evaluation to ascertain whether the detected *Eimeria* oocysts are linked to clinical disease or just an incidental finding and whether the cause of disease needs to be further investigated. A semiquantitative result is sufficient to judge current severity of infection, primarily if several samples from an affected herd or flock are tested. However, the oocyst excretion level varies greatly over time in infected animals, and detection of low numbers does not exclude a prior or subsequent shedding of high oocyst numbers. As a rule of thumb, the mere presence of highly pathogenic *Eimeria* species in a group of young animals is considered a potential threat to herd health. The situation in affected groups may be monitored by repeated sampling of the same animals and over several years to check the herd situation, prevent sudden outbreaks, and assure efficacy of any applied preventive or treatment measures. For monitoring purposes pooled fecal samples may be used, while clinically ill individuals

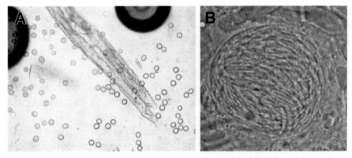

Fig. 3. Diagnostic stages. (*A*) High concentration of oocysts after fecal flotation (*E zuernii*, 200× magnification, from a calf with clinical coccidiosis). (*B*) Meront (with numerous merozoites inside) in intestinal mucosa scraping in deceased animal.

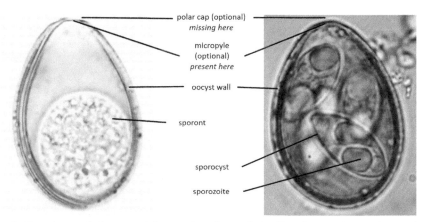

polar cap (optional)
missing here

micropyle
(optional)
present here

oocyst wall

sporont

sporocyst

sporozoite

Fig. 4. Oocyst morphology used for species diagnosis in *Eimeria* oocysts, naming major oocyst structures (exemplary here: *E pellita* from cattle).

should be sampled separately so that the excreted amount of pathogenic *Eimeria* oocysts can be easily estimated.

Notably for the latter purpose, an exact quantification of oocyst excretion in individual samples from animals in the focus groups can be helpful. There are several quantitative flotation methods available, the most common method being the McMaster counting technique. In cattle, 500 or more oocysts per gram of feces of pathogenic *Eimeria* species are considered significant findings for the individual's health,[64] whereas lower numbers justify further herd monitoring. In sheep and goats, no exact numbers for relevant excretion have been established thus far.

Serologic detection methods have been established for *E bovis* in cattle[65] but are not available for routine use. Herd monitoring might potentially be simplified by using serologic methods; however, for disease diagnosis in individual animals the use is highly limited because antibodies may persist long after the self-limiting infection has ended. Molecular biological tools such as the polymerase chain reaction have been described but are much more expensive than fecal flotation and are thus currently not used routinely. In postmortem analyses, native mucosal scrapings from different parts of the intestine may be examined by light microscopy for developmental *Eimeria* stages (see **Fig. 4**).

CONTROL

In general, effective coccidiosis control is not based on complete elimination of *Eimeria* from affected premises. It is considered neither possible nor useful to avoid contact of naïve hosts with *Eimeria* on operations dealing with this parasite. Uptake of low infection doses is generally not linked to disease, and low-dose infections are beneficial to the host because they permits them to develop a protective, nonsterile immunity and protect against future challenge infections. Therefore, the focus of ruminant coccidiosis control lies in the reduction of infection pressure to uncritical levels and endemic stability,[1] rather than pathogen eradication.

Prevention

Prevention is largely based on herd management including hygienic measures because, as there is no vaccine available. Coccidiosis outbreaks are a herd-level problem and are fostered by stress. Infected animals need a responsive immune system to avoid a severe disease outcome. Thus, minimizing or alleviating stressors such as diet changes, harsh climate conditions, crowding, repeated shipment, regrouping of animals, and exposure to other disease agents is a crucial part of disease prevention. Furthermore, oocysts persist for a long time in the environment, especially under moist conditions. Accordingly, good overall management that ensures low infection pressure by timely manure removal, deep litter usage, or a noncrowded pasture is beneficial. Furthermore, facilities designed to allow direct natural sunlight can be beneficial in reducing the levels of oocysts in the environment. The lower the infection dose, the less is the impact of coccidia infections on gut health. It must be stressed that complete elimination of the pathogen from the premises is neither possible nor desirable because contact with low-dose infections ensures development of immunity in host animals. Disinfection, for example with bleach, cresols, or chlorocresols (the latter 2 being unavailable in the United States), helps reduce infection pressure in indoor facilities. Most other disinfectants display a highly limited activity against coccidia stages. Separation of different age groups (ie, naïve from previously infected animals) will help minimize transmission. Pasture rotation, where possible, is a useful tool to avoid buildup of high concentrations of coccidia oocysts in areas dedicated for use by susceptible animals. Colostrum uptake is important for newborn ruminants; even if the protection against *Eimeria* is not efficient, the protection against other pathogens will support the animals' immune system and prevent complications.

On operations with reported coccidiosis problems, specific drugs for anticoccidial prophylaxis are commonly applied. The available drugs are administered as feed additives over a prolonged period of several weeks. In general, coccidiostatic and coccidiocidal drugs are available. Coccidiostats inhibit the development of internal coccidia stages, whereas coccidiocidal drugs kill the parasites. At present, drugs of both modes of action are available on the market. Coccidiostats are represented by amprolium, decoquinate, and sulfonamide drugs,[66] although the exact mode of action for the sulfonamide drugs is still unknown.[67] By contrast, polyether ionophores such as monensin, lasalocid, and salinomycin as well as symmetric triazines such as toltrazuril and diclazuril are coccidiocides.[68,69] Although diclazuril is not available in the United States and Canada, toltrazuril is licensed in Canada for cattle and sheep. In contrast to the other available drugs, toltrazuril is intended for a single-dose oral application; it is highly effective against all internal stages of *Eimeria*[69] and can be used for suckling calves or lambs.

Regarding the other available anticoccidials, they are commonly supplied as feed additives, in drinking water, or in feed supplements such as salt. Thus, their use often is most feasible in weaned animals. However, depending on the operation, anticoccidial prevention may need to be started as early as within the first weeks of life.

The optimal time point for prophylactic treatment would allow for the susceptible animals to be infected and establish an immune response but not for full parasite development and related intestinal damage. This effective timing of treatment after infection and before the start of oocyst excretion and clinical disease is also called metaphylaxis. Thus, optimally, anticoccidial treatment would be applied after infection but before the late developmental stages of the parasites have formed; this is roughly within 14 days after infection for the most relevant ruminant *Eimeria* species, when first and second merogonies take place. The important advantage of metaphylaxis over prophylaxis is the development of immunity and protection against reinfection, making later anticoccidial treatments unlikely to be necessary. In general, prophylactic and metaphylactic treatment need to be applied on a herd or animal group basis because the infected animals cannot be determined and all animals residing in the same contaminated environment will be exposed to *Eimeria* infections.

Several coccidiostats are currently available in the United States and Canada. All of them should be used optimally for at least 28 days (even though some are labeled for shorter usage) to ensure that the treated animals are under protection, because these drugs do not kill the parasite stages immediately but rather inhibit their further development. An early withdrawal of a coccidiostat will lead to a delayed internal development of the parasite and accordingly may still result in coccidiosis later on. Decoquinate (Deccox) should be fed at a daily dose of 0.5 mg/kg body weight in cattle, sheep, or goats. Amprolium is available as a feed additive (Corid crumbles) or as additive for drinking water (Ampromed; Corid also as drench) for cattle at a daily dose of 5 mg/kg body weight.

Regarding coccidiocidal drugs, lasalocid and monensin are available for prevention of coccidiosis in cattle, and prolonged feeding (28 days) is also recommended because the exact time point of infection is largely unknown for the individual animals in the group. Lasalocid (Bovatec) is available as feed additive (also for early use in milk replacer powder) or in salt blocks (mineral licks) to be used at a dose of 1 mg/kg body weight in cattle. Lasalocid is also licensed as a feed additive for sheep in confinement (15–70 mg/head/day). For monensin (Rumensin), available for cattle only, a level of 0.3 to 1.0 mg/kg body weight per day is recommended.

There are no known significant differences in the efficacy of the currently available products containing monensin, amprolium, lasalocid, or decoquinate if administered according to the manufacturer's recommendations. As in other pathogens controlled with anti-infectives (eg, bacteria and antibiotics), there is a general potential for development of drug resistance in coccidia. In the poultry industry, anticoccidial resistances are seen in many *Eimeria* field strains, resulting from widespread long-term use of the available drugs.[70] Recent studies from Norway that describe toltrazuril resistance in sheep *Eimeria* substantiate the ability of ruminant *Eimeria* to develop resistance against commonly used anticoccidials in the field.[71] Therefore, cautious use of anticoccidials based on thorough diagnostics and combined with management measures is highly recommended to avoid a similar scenario in ruminants. This includes consideration of anticoccidial drug rotation, limiting the total amount of anticoccidial drugs used on operations, and choosing a reliable administration option that allows for most secure uptake of the necessary drug amounts, such as drenching or checking for proper feed intake by individual animals.

Therapeutic Treatment

With coccidiosis, a therapeutic treatment approach is not the method of choice. Once the oocysts are detected in the feces and coccidiosis is diagnosed, the majority of the internal parasite population has already fulfilled its life cycle and the intestinal damage is set. With and without treatment, animals with patent coccidiosis will need time to recover and will suffer from prolonged dysentery. However, treatment may still have a limited beneficial effect, mainly at the herd level. The total number of excreted oocysts may still be reduced by stopping the development in the remaining proportion of the internal parasites: this helps in keeping the infection pressure down. Nonetheless, rather than treating therapeutically, a metaphylactic treatment approach is clearly preferred.

In cattle, amprolium (Corid) is also licensed for therapeutic treatment (for 5 days, double dose of 10 mg/kg body weight). Sulfonamides can be applied to control clinical coccidiosis in cattle. In addition, symptomatic therapy (fluids, electrolytes) and control of secondary intestinal bacterial infections are recommended.

DISCLOSURE

The authors have nothing to disclose.

REFERENCES

1. Daugschies A, Najdrowski M. Eimeriosis in cattle: current understanding [review]. J Vet Med B Infect Dis Vet Public Health 2005;52(10):417–27.
2. Duszynski DW, Lee C, Upton SJ. Coccidia (Eimeriidae) of Bovidae (excluding Caprinae). 2001. Available at: http://www.k-state.edu/parasitology/worldcoccidia/BOVIDAE. Accessed December 19, 2019.
3. Ammar SI, Watson AM, Craig LE, et al. *Eimeria gilruthi*-associated abomasitis in a group of ewes. J Vet Diagn Invest 2019;31(1):128–32.
4. Dittmar K, Mundt HC, Grzonka E, et al. Ovine coccidiosis in housed lambs in Saxony-Anhalt (central Germany). Berl Munch Tierarztl Wochenschr 2010; 123(1–2):49–57.
5. da Silva LMR, Vila-Viçosa MJM, Nunes T, et al. Eimeria infections in goats in Southern Portugal. Braz J Vet Parasitol. Jaboticabal 2014;23(2):280–6.
6. Das M, Laha R, Goswami A. Gastrointestinal parasitism of goats in hilly region of Meghalaya, India. Vet World 2017;10(1):81–5.
7. Norton CC. Coccidia of the domestic goat *Capra hircus*, with notes on *Eimeria ovinoidalis* and *E. bakuensis* (syn. *E. ovina*) from the sheep *Ovis aries*. Parasitology 1986;92(Pt 2):279–89.
8. Chapman HD. Studies on the excystation of different species of *Eimeria in vitro*. Z Parasitenkd 1978;56(2):115–21.
9. Kowalik S, Zahner H. *Eimeria separata*: method for the excystation of sporozoites. Parasitol Res 1999;85(6):496–9.
10. Saliba KJ, Kirk K. Nutrient acquisition by intracellular apicomplexan parasites: staying in for dinner [review]. Int J Parasitol 2001;31(12):1321–30.
11. Bangoura B, Daugschies A. Eimeria. In: Florin-Christensen M, Schnittger L, editors. Parasitic protozoa of farm animals and pets. Cham (Switzerland): Springer Nature; 2018. p. 55–101. ISBN 978-3-319-70131-8.
12. Hammond DM, Andersen FL, Miner ML. The occurrence of a second asexual generation in the life cycle of *Eimeria bovis* in calves. J Parasitol 1963;49:428–34.
13. Levine N. Protozoan parasites of animals and man. 2nd edition. Minneapolis (MN): Burgess Publishing Company; 1973. p. 164–86.
14. Bangoura B, Daugschies A. Parasitological and clinical parameters of experimental *Eimeria zuernii* infection in calves and influence on weight gain and haemogram. Parasitol Res 2007;100(6):1331–40.
15. Carrau T, Silva LMR, Pérez D, et al. Associated risk factors influencing ovine *Eimeria* infections in southern Spain. Vet Parasitol 2018;263:54–8.
16. Roesicke E, Greuel E. The survival ability of salmonella, coccidia oocysts and ascarid eggs in laying hen feces from different housing systems. Dtsch Tierarztl Wochenschr 1992;99(12):492–4.
17. Marquardt WC, Senger CM, Seghetti L. The effect of physical and chemical agents on the oocyst of *Eimeria zurnii* (protozoa, coccidia). J Protozool 1960; 7(2):186–9.
18. Marquardt WC. Effect of high temperature on sporulation of *Eimeria zurnii*. Exp Parasitol 1960;10:58–65.
19. Ernst JV, Stewart TB, Witlock DR. Quantitative determination of coccidian oocysts in beef calves from the coastal plain area of Georgia (U.S.A.). Vet Parasitol 1987; 23(1–2):1–10.
20. da Silva NR, Miller JE. Survey of *Eimeria* spp. oocysts in feces from Louisiana State University ewes. Vet Parasitol 1991;40(1–2):147–50.

21. Penzhorn BL, Knapp SE, Speer CA. Enteric coccidia in free-ranging American bison (*Bison bison*) in Montana. J Wildl Dis 1994;30(2):267–9.

22. Pyziel AM, Demiaszkiewicz AW, Klich D, et al. A morphological and molecular comparison of *Eimeria bovis*-like oocysts (Apicomplexa: Eimeriidae) from European bison, *Bison bonasus* L., and cattle, *Bos taurus* L., and the development of two multiplex PCR assays for their identification. Vet Parasitol 2019;275 [pii: S0304-4017(19)30193-1].

23. Duszynski DW, Samuel WM, Gray DR. Three new *Eimeria* spp. (Protozoa, Eimeriidae) from muskoxen, *Ovibos moschattus*, with redescriptions of *E. faurei*, *E. granulosa*, and *E. ovina* from muskoxen and from a Rocky Mountain bighorn sheep, *Ovis canadensis*. Can J Zool 1977;55(6):990–9.

24. Rose ME, Wakelin D. Immunity to coccidiosis. In: Long PL, editor. Coccidiosis of man and domestic animals. Boca Raton (FL): CRC Press; 1990. p. 191. ISBN 0-8493-6269-5.

25. Reeg KJ, Gauly M, Bauer C, et al. Coccidial infections in housed lambs: oocyst excretion, antibody levels and genetic influences on the infection. Vet Parasitol 2005;127(3–4):209–19.

26. Hammond DM, Bowman GW, Davis LR, et al. The endogenous phase of the life cycle of *Eimeria bovis*. J Parasitol 1946;32(4):409–27.

27. Lindsay DS, Dubey JP, Fayer R. Extraintestinal stages of *Eimeria bovis* in calves and attempts to induce relapse of clinical disease. Vet Parasitol 1990; 36(1–2):1–9.

28. Gregory MW. Pathology of coccidial infections. In: Long PL, editor. Coccidiosis of man and domestic animals. Boca Raton (FL): CRC Press; 1990. p. 240. ISBN 0-8493-6269-5.

29. Friend SC, Stockdale PH. Experimental *Eimeria bovis* infection in calves: a histopathological study. Can J Comp Med 1980;44(2):129–40.

30. Weilhammer DR, Rasley A. Genetic approaches for understanding virulence in *Toxoplasma gondii*. Brief Funct Genomics 2011;10(6):365–73.

31. Davis LR, Bowman GW. The endogenous development of *Eimeria zurnii*, a pathogenic coccidium of cattle. Am J Vet Res 1957;18(68):569–74.

32. Hamid PH, Hirzmann J, Kerner K, et al. *Eimeria bovis* infection modulates endothelial host cell cholesterol metabolism for successful replication. Vet Res 2015; 46:100.

33. Stockdale PHG. Proposed life cycle of *Eimeria zuernii*. Br Vet J 1977;133:471–3.

34. Mundt HC, Bangoura B, Rinke M, et al. Pathology and treatment of *Eimeria zuernii* coccidiosis in calves: investigations in an infection model. Parasitol Int 2005;54: 223–30.

35. Stockdale PHG. The pathogenesis of the lesions produced by *Eimeria zuernii* in calves. Can J Comp Med 1977;41:338–44.

36. Davis LR, Bowman GW, Boughton DC. The endogenous development of *Eimeria alabamensis* Christensen, 1941, an intranuclear coccidium of cattle. J Protozool 1957;4:219–25.

37. Foreyt WJ. Coccidiosis and cryptosporidiosis in sheep and goats [review]. Vet Clin North Am Food Anim Pract 1990;6(3):655–70.

38. Gregory MW, Catchpole J. Ovine coccidiosis: pathology of *Eimeria ovinoidalis* infection. Int J Parasitol 1987;17(6):1099–111.

39. Gregory MW, Catchpole J. Ovine coccidiosis: the pathology of Eimeria crandallis infection. Int J Parasitol 1990;20(7):849–60.

40. Taylor MA, Catchpole J. Review article: coccidiosis of domestic ruminants [review]. Appl Parasitol 1994;35(2):73–86.

41. Catchpole J, Norton CC, Joyner LP. Experiments with defined multispecific coccidial infections in lambs. Parasitology 1976;72(2):137–47.

42. Gregory MW, Norton CC. Caprine coccidiosis. Goat Vet J 1986;7:32–4.

43. Kanyari PW. *Eimeria apsheronica* in the goat: endogenous development and host cellular response. Int J Parasitol 1990;20(5):625–30.

44. Kirino Y, Tanida M, Hasunuma H, et al. Increase of *Clostridium perfringens* in association with *Eimeria* in haemorrhagic enteritis in Japanese beef cattle. Vet Rec 2015;177(8):202.

45. Durham PJ, Johnson RH, Parker RJ. Exacerbation of experimental parvoviral enteritis in calves by coccidia and weaning stress. Res Vet Sci 1985;39(1):16–23.

46. Catchpole J, Harris TJ. Interaction between coccidia and *Nematodirus battus* in lambs on pasture. Vet Rec 1989;124(23):603–5.

47. Bangoura B, Daugschies A. Influence of experimental *Eimeria zuernii* infection in calves on electrolyte concentrations, acid-base balance and blood gases. Parasitol Res 2007;101(6):1637–45.

48. Leek RG, Lotze JC. Experimental infection of newborn lambs with *Eimeria ninakohlyakimovae* and *E. ovina*. J Parasitol 1972;58(6):1205–6.

49. Heath HL, Blagburn BL, Elsasser TH, et al. Hormonal modulation of the physiologic responses of calves infected with *Eimeria bovis*. Am J Vet Res 1997;58(8):891–6.

50. Aleksandersen M, Landsverk T, Gjerde B, et al. Scarcity of gamma delta T cells in intestinal epithelia containing coccidia despite general increase of epithelial lymphocytes. Vet Pathol 1995;32(5):504–12.

51. Daugschies A, Bürger HJ, Akimaru M. Apparent digestibility of nutrients and nitrogen balance during experimental infection of calves with *Eimeria bovis*. Vet Parasitol 1998;77(2–3):93–102.

52. Koudela B, Boková A. Coccidiosis in goats in the Czech Republic. Vet Parasitol 1998;76(4):261–7.

53. Lassen B, Ostergaard S. Estimation of the economical effects of *Eimeria* infections in Estonian dairy herds using a stochastic model. Prev Vet Med 2012;106(3–4):258–65.

54. Hooshmand-Rad P, Svensson C, Uggla A. Experimental *Eimeria alabamensis* infection in calves. Vet Parasitol 1994;53(1–2):23–32.

55. Svensson C, Uggla A, Pehrson B. *Eimeria alabamensis* infection as a cause of diarrhoea in calves at pasture. Vet Parasitol 1994;53(1–2):33–43.

56. Niilo L. Experimental winter coccidiosis in sheltered and unsheltered calves. Can J Comp Med 1970;34(1):20–5.

57. Radostits OM, Stockdale PH. A brief review of bovine coccidiosis in Western Canada. Can Vet J 1980;21(8):227–30.

58. Julian RJ. Nervous signs in bovine coccidiosis. Mod Vet Pract 1976;711–8.

59. Reppert JF, Kemp R. Nervous coccidiosis. Iowa State Univ Veterinarian 1972;34:9–12.

60. Isler CM, Bellamy JEC, Wobeser GA. Pathogenesis of neurological signs associated with bovine enteric coccidiosis: a prospective study and review. Can J Vet Res 1987;51:261–70.

61. Matos L, Muñoz MC, Molina JM, et al. Protective immune responses during prepatency in goat kids experimentally infected with *Eimeria ninakohlyakimovae*. Vet Parasitol 2017;242:1–9.

62. Khodakaram-Tafti A, Hashemnia M. An overview of intestinal coccidiosis in sheep and goats. Revue Méd Vét 2017;167(1–2):9–20.

63. Fitzgerald PR. The economic impact of coccidiosis in domestic animals. Adv Vet Sci Comp Med 1980;24:121–43.
64. Joachim A, Altreuther G, Bangoura B, et al. WAAVP guideline for evaluating the efficacy of anticoccidials in mammals (pigs, dogs, cattle, sheep). Vet Parasitol 2018;253:102–19.
65. Fiege N, Klatte D, Kollmann D, et al. *Eimeria bovis* in cattle: colostral transfer of antibodies and immune response to experimental infections. Parasitol Res 1992; 78(1):32–8.
66. Rogers EF, Clark RL, Pessolano AA, et al. Antiparastitic drugs. III. Thiamine-reversible Coccidiostats. J Am Chem Soc 1960;82:2974–5.
67. Keeton STN, Navarre CB. Coccidiosis in large and small ruminants. Vet Clin North Am Food Anim Pract 2018;34(1):201–8.
68. Mehlhorn H, Pooch H, Raether W. The action of polyether ionophorous antibiotics (monensin, salinomycin, lasalocid) on developmental stages of *Eimeria tenella* (Coccidia, Sporozoa) *in vivo* and *in vitro*: study by light and electron microscopy. Z Parasitenkd 1983;69(4):457–71.
69. Mehlhorn H, Ortmann-Falkenstein G, Haberkorn A. The effects of sym. Triazinones on developmental stages of *Eimeria tenella*, *E. maxima* and *E. acervulina*: a light and electron microscopical study. Z Parasitenkd 1984;70(2):173–82.
70. Blake DP, Tomley FM. Securing poultry production from the ever-present *Eimeria* challenge. Trends Parasitol 2014;30(1):12–9.
71. Odden A, Enemark HL, Ruiz A, et al. Controlled efficacy trial confirming toltrazuril resistance in a field isolate of ovine *Eimeria* spp. Parasit Vectors 2018;11(1):394.

Neosporosis, Toxoplasmosis, and Sarcocystosis in Ruminants: An Update

David S. Lindsay, PhD[a],*, J.P. Dubey, MVSc, PhD[b]

KEYWORDS

- *Neospora caninum* • *T gondii* • *Sarcocystis* spp. • Cattle • Sheep • Goats
- Water buffalo • White-tailed deer

KEY POINTS

- Neosporosis, toxoplasmosis, sarcocystosis are parasitic diseases that are transmitted to ruminants by oocysts shed in the feces of a carnivore or omnivore definitive hosts.
- Neosporosis causes of abortion in cattle, dogs are definitive hosts; it is transmitted transplacentally, and this is the major way it is transmitted in cattle.
- Toxoplasmosis is a cause of abortion in sheep and goats; cats are the definitive hosts.
- Sarcocystosis can cause abortion and carcass condemnation in ruminants. Dogs, cats, and wild predators are definitive hosts.
- No effective preventative chemotherapeutics or vaccines are available for these parasites in ruminants in North America.

NEOSPOROSIS
Etiology

Neosporosis is a disease caused by the *Toxoplasmosis gondii*-like parasite, *Neospora caninum*. Until 1988, *N caninum* was confused with the structurally similar coccidian *T gondii*.[1] The disease was recognized and the features of the clinical disease it causes in congenitally infected dogs was reported in dogs from Norway in 1984.[2] This report prompted a retrospective study that provided a scientific description of the parasite and the name *N caninum*.[3] The parasite was isolated in cell cultures from congenitally infected Labrador retriever pups.[4] This process provided a source of antigen for immunologic[4] and immunohistochemical[5] studies. Researchers used these tools and within a few years it became apparent that neosporosis was an important cause

---

[a] Department of Biomedical Sciences and Pathobiology, Center for One Health Research, Virginia Maryland College of Veterinary Medicine, Virginia Tech, 1410 Prices Fork Road, Blacksburg, VA 24061-0342, USA; [b] United States Department of Agriculture, Agricultural Research Service, Beltsville Agricultural Research Center, Building 1001, Beltsville, MD 20705-2350, USA
* Corresponding author.
E-mail address: lindsayd@vt.edu

Vet Clin Food Anim 36 (2020) 205–222
https://doi.org/10.1016/j.cvfa.2019.11.004
0749-0720/20/© 2019 Elsevier Inc. All rights reserved.
vetfood.theclinics.com

of abortion and neonatal mortality in cattle-rearing regions worldwide.[1] In 1998, domestic dogs were found to be the definitive host and also excrete oocysts.[6,7] Coyotes and wolves[8,9] are also definitive hosts and maintain the parasite in a sylvatic cycle with white-tailed deer (*Odocoileus virginianus*) where they are present.[10] Viable *N caninum* has been isolated from dogs, cattle, white-tailed deer, water buffaloes, and sheep.[1] *N caninum* is not known to naturally infect primates or humans, but experimental infections in rhesus macaque tachyzoite crossed the placenta and infected the fetus.[1]

The life cycle is typified by 3 infectious stages: tachyzoites, tissue cysts, and oocysts (**Fig. 1**). Tachyzoites disseminate the infection extracellularly by moving between host cells or via the blood. Tissue cysts are latent stages found in the intermediate hosts and both occur intracellularly in vacuoles derived from the host cell plasma membrane.[1,3,4] Tachyzoites are approximately 6 × 2 μm. They are rapidly dividing stages that cause tissue damage, disseminate the infection in the intermediate host and are transplacentally transmitted to the fetus. Tachyzoites divide asexually into 2 organisms by a type of longitudinal binary fission called endodyogeny. The tachyzoites eventually produce bradyzoites by endodyogeny after receiving a cue from the host to undergo stage conversion to produce the dormant thick-walled tissue cyst stage.

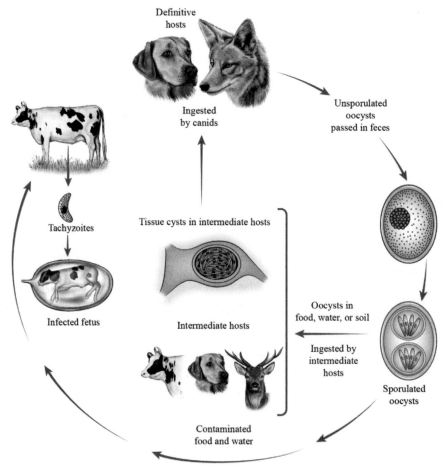

Fig. 1. Life cycle of *Neospora caninum*. (*Courtesy of* J. P. Dubey, MVSc, PhD, Beltsville, MD.)

Tissue cysts are seen detected in the central nervous system.[11] These tissue cysts are round or oval in shape, up to 107 μm long, and contain up to 100 slow-growing bradyzoites. The tissue cyst wall is up to 4 μm thick and the enclosed bradyzoites are 7 to 8 × 2 μm. Bradyzoites are believed to produce asexual and sexual stages in the intestines of canines that results in oocysts in their feces.

N caninum oocysts are excreted unsporulated in the feces and measure 10 to 12 μm in diameter and sporulation occurs outside the host.[6] Presently, little is known regarding the frequency of shedding of *N caninum* oocysts, the survival of the oocysts in the environment, and how many different canines can serve as definitive hosts.[1] Oocysts are most likely susceptible to environmental conditions that inhibit oocysts of *T gondii*. The parasite can be transmitted transplacentally in several hosts and the vertical route is the major mode of its transmission in domestic dairy antibody cattle.[11] There is no adult cow to adult cow transmission of *N caninum*. Although most *N caninum* infections in cattle are transmitted transplacentally, reports of postnatal rates have been variable depending on the region of the country, the type of test used, and the antibody cut-off values used.[1,11] Although *N caninum* has been found in bovine semen,[12] it is unlikely that *N caninum* is transmitted in semen or by embryo transfer from the donor cows. Embryo transfer has been recommended as a method of control to prevent vertical transmission.[13] However, it is prudent to test all recipients, and embryos should not be transferred to seropositive cows. Lactogenic transmission of *N caninum* is considered unlikely.[14–16] Canids can acquire infection by ingestion of infected tissues.

Neosporosis in Cattle

Clinical signs
N caninum is responsible for inducing abortion both dairy and beef cattle.[1,17–20] Cows of any age may abort from 3-month gestation to near full term. Most neosporosis-induced abortions occur at 5 to 6 months of gestation. Fetuses may die in utero, be resorbed, mummified, autolyzed, stillborn, born alive with clinical signs, or born clinically normal but chronically infected. Neosporosis-induced abortions occur year round. Cows with *N caninum* antibodies (seropositive) are more likely to abort than seronegative cows and this applies to both dairy and beef cattle. However, up to 95% of calves born congenitally infected from seropositive dams remain clinically normal. The age of dam, lactation number, and history of abortion generally do not affect rate of congenital infection, but there are reports indicating that in persistently infected cattle vertical transmission is more efficient in younger than older cows. If replacement heifers are infected, they may either abort or transplacentally infect their offspring.

Clinical signs have only been reported in cattle younger than 2 month of age.[1,11] *N caninum*-infected calves may have neurologic signs, be underweight, unable to rise, or be born without clinical signs of disease. Hind limbs or forelimbs or both may be flexed or hyperextended. Neurologic examination may reveal ataxia, decreased patellar reflexes, and loss of conscious proprioception. Calves may have exophthalmia or asymmetrical appearance in the eyes. *N caninum* occasionally causes birth defects including hydrocephalus and narrowing of the spinal cord.[1]

Abortions may be epidemic or endemic.[17–20] Up to 33% of dairy cow abortions owing to *N caninum* occur within a few months of pregnancy. Abortions are considered epidemic if more than 10% of cows at risk have aborted within 6 to 8 weeks. A small proportion (<5%) of cows are reported to have repeated abortions owing to neosporosis.[21] Cows with *N caninum* antibodies (seropositive) are more likely to abort than seronegative cows. There is an increase in antibody titers 4 to 5 months before parturition. These observations strongly suggest reactivation of latent infection; however, little is known regarding the mechanism of reactivation. It is likely that there is parasitemia during pregnancy leading to fetal infection. However, N caninum has never been identified in histologic sections of adult cows and viable N caninum has been isolated from the brains of only 2 cows.[22,23] Although it is reasonable to speculate that pregnancy-induced immunosuppression or hormonal imbalance may reactivate latent tissue cysts of N caninum, such a mechanism has not been demonstrated experimentally or in natural infections. N caninum DNA has been found in blood of naturally infected cattle indicating parasitemia.[24] N caninum is one of the most efficiently transplacentally transmitted organisms in cattle. In some herds, up to 90% of cattle are infected, and most calves born congenitally infected with N caninum remain healthy.

Prevalence

N caninum infections have been reported from most parts of the world. Serologic prevalence in cattle varies, depending on the country, region, type of serologic test used, and antibody titer cut-off level used to determine exposure. In some dairies up to 87% of cows are seropositive[1] and studies involving a large number of fetuses in many countries indicate that 12% to 42% of aborted fetuses from dairy cattle are infected with N caninum.[1] Less is known of the causes of abortion in beef cattle than in dairy cattle owing to the difficulty of finding small aborted fetuses expelled in the field during the first trimester. There is no evidence of N caninum-associated morbidity in beef cattle more than 2 months of age.[1]

Diagnosis

Examination of the serum from an aborting cow is only indicative of exposure to N caninum and histologic examination of the fetus is necessary for a definitive diagnosis of abortion owing to neosporosis.[25] The brain, heart, liver, placenta, and body fluids or blood serum are the best specimens for diagnosis and diagnostic rates are higher if multiple tissues are examined.[25] Although lesions of neosporosis are found in several organs, fetal brain is the most consistently affected organ.[25] Because most aborted fetuses are likely to be autolyzed, even semiliquid brain tissue should be fixed in 10% buffered neutral formalin for histologic examination of hematoxylin and eosin–stained sections. Immunohistochemistry is necessary because there are generally only a few N caninum present in autolyzed tissues and these are often not visible in hematoxylin and eosin–stained sections. The most characteristic lesion of neosporosis is focal encephalitis characterized by necrosis and nonsuppurative inflammation.[25] Hepatitis is more common in epizootic than sporadic abortions.[26] Lesions are also present in the placenta, but protozoa are difficult to find.

The efficiency of the diagnosis by polymerase chain reaction (PCR) depends on the laboratory, stage of the autolysis of the fetus, and sampling procedures.[25,27,28] Fresh or frozen tissues are superior to formalin-fixed tissues. N caninum DNA can be detected by PCR in formalin-fixed, paraffin-embedded bovine tissue, but it is less sensitive than PCR on fresh/frozen tissue.

Serologic tests can be used to detect N caninum antibodies including various enzyme-linked immunosorbent assays (ELISAs), the indirect fluorescent antibody test, and the Neospora agglutination test.[1,29,30] There are several modifications of the ELISA test to detect antibodies to N caninum in sera or milk using whole parasite, whole parasite lysate, purified proteins, recombinant proteins, tachyzoite proteins absorbed on immunostimulating complex adjuvant particles and some of these teats were compared recently in a multicentered study in various laboratories in Europe.[31]

Avidity ELISAs designed to distinguish acute and chronic infections in cattle seem to be promising to distinguish endemic and epidemic abortion.[32] In the avidity ELISA sera are treated with urea to release low-avidity (low-affinity) antibodies and differences in values obtained before and after treatment with urea are used to evaluate recency of infection. In recently acquired infection, avidity values are low.[32] Another modification of ELISA is antigen capture. This test detects (captures) a 65-kD antigen in sera of infected cattle using a specific monoclonal antibody and this test is commercially available.[33] Immunoblots are useful in detecting N caninum-specific antibodies.[25]

Finding N caninum antibody in serum from the fetus can establish N caninum infection, but a negative result is not informative because antibody synthesis in the fetus depends on the stage of gestation, level of exposure, and the time between infection and abortion. Although blood, serum, or other body fluids from the fetus may be used for serologic diagnosis, peritoneal fluid is better than other body fluids. In calves, presuckling serum can be submitted for diagnosis of congenital infection.

The definitive antibody level that should be considered diagnostic for neosporosis has not been established for bovines because of the uncertainty of serologic diagnosis in chronically infected animals and the availability of sera from noninfected cattle. In serologic assays, titer and absorbance values depend on antigen composition, secondary antibodies, and other reagents.[25] Further, antibody titer cut-off levels can be arbitrarily selected to provide sensitivity and specificity requested for a particular application. The age and class of an animal may also affect selection of an antibody titer cut-off level. Although N caninum is closely related to T gondii, cut-off titers in general are higher in cattle that have aborted owing to neosporosis than those with normal pregnancy; however, titers in individual cows cannot determine the etiology of abortions.

Control

N caninum is efficiently transmitted vertically in cattle, perhaps for several generations. Culling is 1 way at present to prevent this transmission from cow to heifer.[34] However, culling is impractical if the prevalence of N caninum in a herd is very high. Before making the decision to cull, it is advisable to estimate the prevalence of N caninum in the herd. Bulk milk testing can provide preliminary data about the prevalence of N caninum infection. If a bulk milk test is positive, antibody prevalence in dam-heifer samples and cattle of different ages can provide insight to the transmission of N caninum in a given herd. In herds with a high transplacental transmission, the prevalence of N caninum in cattle of different ages is about the same and there is high correlation between infection in dams and daughters. To decrease vertical transmission of N caninum, culling of seropositive dams and/or heifer calves from seropositive cows, and embryo transfer from seropositive cows to seronegative cows are some management strategies that can be adapted. There are no drugs that kill N caninum bradyzoites within tissue cysts.

To prevent horizontal (from outside sources) transmission, it is important to prevent exposure of the cows to feed and water contaminated with oocysts.[35,36] Domestic dogs and other canids should not be allowed to defecate in cattle feed, barns, or pasture, although this is not easy to achieve. How dogs become infected with N caninum is not well-understood. Consumption of aborted bovine fetuses does not seem to be an important source of N caninum infection in dogs. The consumption of placental membranes may be a source of N caninum infection in dogs because the parasite has been found in naturally infected placentas and dogs fed placentas shed N caninum oocysts.[16] Little is known at present regarding the frequency of shedding of *N caninum* oocysts by canids in nature, the resistance of the oocysts, or whether dogs shed oocysts more than once. Domestic and wild canines should not be allowed to eat aborted fetuses, fetal membranes, or dead calves. Other factors such as farm location can be a risk factor.[36] There is evidence that cattle can develop protective immunity to subsequent neosporosis abortion.[37,38] This protective immunity seems to be more effective in cows that are subsequently infected with an exogenous source (oocysts) than in cows in which there is a recrudescence of a persistent infection.[38] Inducing protective immunity through vaccination against abortion in cows that already harbor a latent infection is problematic.

The only commercial *N caninum* vaccine (Neo Guard) has been removed from the market because of lack of convincing data about the efficiency of the vaccine to prevent *N caninum* associated abortions in cattle.[39,40]

NEOSPOROSIS IN OTHER ANIMALS

Neosporosis is a primary disease of dogs. In addition to dogs and cattle, sporadic cases of clinical neosporosis have been reported in other animals including adult horses, in a 16 day-old rhinoceros (*Ceratotherium simum*), in a juvenile raccoon (*Procyon lotor*), in a 2-month-old black-tailed deer (*Odocoileus hemionus columbianus*), in neonatal alpacas (*Vicugna pacos*) and llamas (*Lama glama*), goats, sheep, Eld's deer (*Cervus eldi siamensis*), Fallow deer (*Dama dama*), and an antelope (*Tragelaphus imberbis*).[1] A new species, *Neospora hughesi*, has been described in horses.[41] It is molecularly different from *N caninum*[42,43] and tissue cysts of *N hughesi* were not infectious for dogs.[44] It is presently not known if *N caninum* infects horses or *N hughesi* infects ruminants or other animals.

TOXOPLASMOSIS
Etiology

Toxoplasmosis is caused by the infection with the protozoan *T gondii*.[45] It is among the most common of parasites of animals and *T gondii* is the only known species. Felids are the definitive hosts, and warm-blooded animals are intermediate hosts.[45] There are 3 infectious stages of *T gondii* for all hosts: tachyzoites (individually and in groups), bradyzoites (in tissue cysts), and sporozoites (in sporocysts within sporulated oocysts) (**Fig. 2**).[46]

The tachyzoite and bradyzoite stages of *T gondii* are morphologically and biologically nearly identical to those of *N caninum*.[1,45,46] The tachyzoites are metabolically active and are susceptible to agents used to treat coccidia infections. The slow-growing bradyzoites in tissue cysts are not as metabolically active and are not affected by drugs used to treat coccidia. Tissue cysts grow and remain intracellular. They vary in size from 5 to 70 μm and contain a few to several hundred bradyzoites.[46,47] Although tissue cysts may develop in visceral organs, including lungs, liver, and kidneys, they are more prevalent in muscular and neural tissues, including the brain, eye, skeletal, and cardiac muscle. Intact tissue cysts of *T gondii* are probably harmless and can persist for the life of the host.[45]

The tissue cyst wall is elastic, thin (<0.5 μm), and may enclose hundreds of crescent-shaped slender bradyzoites each measuring 7.0×1.5 μm. Bradyzoites differ only slightly structurally from tachyzoites in having a nucleus situated toward the posterior end whereas the nucleus in tachyzoites is more central. Bradyzoites are more slender than are tachyzoites and less susceptible to destruction by acid conditions and proteolytic enzymes in the stomach than tachyzoites. Tissue cysts are believed to periodically release bradyzoites and quickly destroyed by the hosts immune system contributing to life-long exposure and ongoing immunity to the parasite.

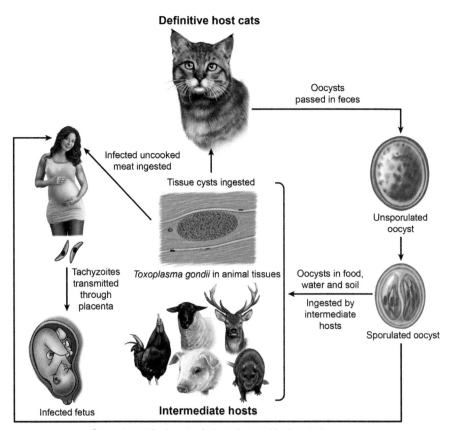

Fig. 2. Life cycle of *Toxoplasma gondii*. (*Courtesy of* J. P. Dubey, MVSc, PhD, Beltsville, MD.)

Upon ingestion by cats, the wall of the tissue cyst is digested and bradyzoites are released. Some penetrate the lamina propria of the intestine and multiple as tachyzoites.[47] Within a few hours, *T gondii* may disseminate to extraintestinal tissues. Other bradyzoites penetrate epithelial cells of the cat small intestine and initiate 5 cycles (types A to E schizonts) of schizonts[47,48] and then become sexual stages. Some become male stages (microgamonts) and produce microgametes (sperm) but most become female stages that will be fertilized by the microgametes and will form a zygote. The zygote produces an oocyst wall around the sporont. When oocysts are mature, they are discharged into the intestinal lumen by the rupture of intestinal epithelial cells.

Oocysts of *T gondii* are formed only in cats, including both domestic and wild felids. Domestic cats shed oocysts after ingesting tachyzoites,[49] bradyzoites,[47] or sporozoites.[50] However, less than 50% of cats shed oocysts after ingesting tachyzoites or oocysts, whereas nearly all shed oocysts after ingesting tissue cysts.[47,49,50]

Oocysts in freshly passed feces are unsporulated (noninfective) and subspherical or spherical in shape and 10 to 12 × 10 to 12 μm in diameter. Sporulation occurs outside the cat and within 1 to 5 days, depending on humidity, oxygen, and temperature. Sporulated oocysts contain 2 ellipsoidal sporocysts. Each sporocyst contains 4 sporozoites. The sporozoites are 6 to 8 × 2 μm in size.

Hosts, including felids can acquire *T gondii* by ingesting either tissue cysts in tissues of infected animals or sporulated oocysts in food or drink, or by transplacental transmission of tachyzoites from mother to fetus. After ingestion, bradyzoites released from tissue cysts or sporozoites from oocysts penetrate intestinal tissues, transform to tachyzoites, multiply locally as tachyzoites, and are disseminated in the body via blood or lymph as tachyzoites to leukocytes that contain viable tachyzoites. After a few multiplication cycles, tachyzoites give rise to bradyzoites in a variety of tissues and undergo stage transformation to produce tissue cysts. *T gondii* infection during pregnancy can lead to infection of the fetus. Congenital toxoplasmosis in sheep and goats can kill the fetus. Oocysts are more pathogenic than tissue cysts for hosts during a primary infection and edema, necrosis of the lamina propria, and sloughing of the intestinal mucosa can produce severe enteritis.

Host–Parasite Relationship

T gondii can multiply in most nucleated cell types in the body. How *T gondii* stages are destroyed by immune cells is not completely known. All extracellular forms of the parasite are directly affected by antibodies, but intracellular forms are not. Cellular factors, including lymphocytes and lymphokines, are thought to be more important than humoral factors (antibodies) in the immune-mediated destruction of *T gondii* stages in hosts.

Acquired immunity does not eliminate an established infection, but tachyzoites stages convert to bradyzoites in response to a host stimulus and develop into tissue cysts. During early stage conversion and production of tissue cysts, tachyzoites and bradyzoites can be seen in the same developing tissue cyst. As the tissue cyst matures, the numbers of tachyzoites-like stages become less and eventually only bradyzoites are present in the tissue cyst. *T gondii* tissue cysts persist for several years after acute infection. The fate of tissue cysts residing in an immunocompetent host is not fully known. Some tissue cysts may rupture during the life of the host and the released bradyzoites are destroyed by the host's immune responses locally. However, in immunosuppressed individuals, infection can be reactivated and bradyzoites stages convert to tachyzoites, which leads to dissemination of infection in the host.

The pathogenicity of *T gondii* is determined by many factors, including the innate susceptibility of the host species, virulence of the parasitic (its genotype), and the stage that is acquired by the host.[45] Oocyst-induced infections are the most severe clinically in intermediate hosts, and this is not dose dependent.[45] *T gondii* genotypes differ remarkably in their virulence to outbred mice. However, the virulence of *T gondii* in mice does not always equate to virulence in domestic animals.

T gondii has also adapted to an oocyst–oral cycle in herbivores (intermediate hosts) because these animals do not consume tissue cysts. The tissue cyst–oral cycle in carnivores and omnivores is efficient and a means to be maintained the life cycle when cat populations are low. Epidemiologic evidence indicates that cats are essential in perpetuation of the life cycle as *T gondii* infection is rare or absent in areas devoid of cats.[51–53] *T gondii* oocysts are less infective and less pathogenic for cats than for mice.[45]

Epidemiology

Domestic cats are the major source of contamination of the environment with oocysts, as they are more common than wild fields (bobcats) and produce large numbers of *T gondii* oocysts.[45] Sporulated oocysts survive for long periods under moderate environmental conditions and can be spread by erosion of topsoil, and mechanically by flies, cockroaches, dung beetles, and earthworms.

Although only a few cats may be shedding *T gondii* oocysts at any given time the millions produced by each infected cat and their resistance to destruction assure widespread environmental contamination.[54] Seroprevalence in cats is largely determined by the prevalence of infection in the local avian and rodent populations, which serve as prey. For epidemiologic surveys, seroprevalence data for cats are more useful than results of fecal examination because cats with antibodies have likely shed oocysts and are an indicator of environmental contamination.[45]

Clinical Toxoplasmosis

T gondii is capable of causing severe disease in small ruminants and is responsible for great losses to the livestock industry.[45] In sheep and goats, primary maternal infections may cause embryonic death and resorption, fetal death and mummification, abortion, stillbirth, and neonatal death. The disease is more severe in goats than in sheep. Cattle and water buffaloes are more resistant to acute clinical toxoplasmosis than are other species of livestock and there are no confirmed reports of clinical toxoplasmosis in these animals.

T gondii infection is widespread in humans and prevalence varies with geography and increases as a population ages. In the United States and the UK it is estimated that 16% to 40% of people become infected, whereas in Central and South America and continental Europe infection estimates reach 50% to 80%.[45,55] Infections in healthy adults are usually asymptomatic; however, severe disease can occur in immunocompromised individuals and newborns. Congenital infection may occur following maternal infection during pregnancy.[56,57] The severity of the disease depends on the immune status of the mother, parasite genotype,[58] and stage of pregnancy at the time of infection.[56–58] A wide spectrum of clinical disease occurs in congenitally infected children.

Diagnosis

Diagnosis can be made by biological, serologic, molecular, or histologic methods or by a combination of these methods.[45] Clinical signs are nonspecific and insufficiently characteristic for a definite diagnosis because toxoplasmosis mimics several other infectious diseases.

Numerous serologic procedures are available for use in diagnostic laboratories for the detection of humoral antibodies, including indirect hemagglutination assays, indirect fluorescent antibody assays, direct agglutination tests, latex agglutination tests, ELISA, and the immunosorbent agglutination assay test.[45,57] The indirect fluorescent antibody assays, immunosorbent agglutination assay test, and ELISA have been modified to detect IgM antibodies, which appear sooner after infection than IgG and disappear faster than IgG after recovery. The finding of antibodies to *T gondii* in 1 serum sample merely establishes that the host has been infected at some time in the past, so it is best to collect 2 samples from the same individual, the second 2 to 4 weeks after the first.[45] A 4- to 16-fold increase in antibody titer in the second sample indicates an acute infection. A high antibody titer sometimes persists for months after infection. Tissues samples submitted to diagnostic laboratories can be examined by immunohistochemical staining for *T gondii* or for PCR detection of parasite DNA.

Chemotherapy

Sulfadiazine and pyrimethamine are widely used for therapy of human and animal toxoplasmosis.[45,57] These drugs act synergistically by blocking the metabolic pathway involving *p*-aminobenzoic acid and the folic–folinic acid cycle, respectively. The drugs are usually well-tolerated; sometimes thrombocytopenia or leukopenia may develop, but these effects can be overcome by administering folinic acid and yeast without interfering with treatment, because the vertebrate host can transport presynthesized folinic acid into its cells, whereas *T gondii* cannot. Although these drugs have a beneficial action when given in the acute stage of the disease, when there is active multiplication of the parasite, they will not usually eradicate infection. Spiramycin, clindamycin, atovaquone, azithromycin, roxithromycin, clarithromycin, dapsone, and ponazuril and several other less commonly used drugs are available for treatment of toxoplasmosis, but none are approved for this purpose and restrictions on their use in food animals may limit their usage. Clindamycin is absorbed quickly and diffuses well into the central nervous system and therefore, has been used as alternative to sulfadiazine.[45,57]

Prevention and Control

It is difficult to prevent cats from being on farms that have grazing stock. In the farm environment, young cats that have recently been weaned are more likely to be passing *T gondii* oocysts than are older cats that have been on the farm for several months to years. The producer should take measures to control rodents and wild birds to help decrease the source of potentially infected prey. Cats should be prevented from entering feed storage areas.

Vaccination

There is no commercial vaccine to prevent *T gondii* infection in ruminants in North America. One live vaccine that contains a genotype (S48) of *T gondii* that does not persist in the tissues of sheep is available in Europe and New Zealand, where it is used to decrease fetal losses attributable to toxoplasmosis.[59] Ewes vaccinated with the S48 strain vaccine retain immunity for at least 18 months.[59] The S48b is not for use in pregnant ewes.

SARCOCYSTOSIS
Etiology

Unlike *N caninum* and *T gondii,* the genus *Sarcocystis* is much more diverse in the types of animals that can serve as definitive hosts (and excrete oocysts) and the types of animals that can serve as intermediate hosts (and contain the sarcocyst) and be eaten by the definitive host.[60] The genus *Sarcocystis* contains more than 100 named species that cycle between mammals, marsupials, birds, and reptiles as either the definitive host or the intermediate host. *Sarcocystis* has an obligatory prey–predator (2-host) life cycle (**Fig. 3**). Oocysts are passed fully sporulated by the definitive host and can be confused with the sporulated oocysts of *N caninum, T gondii,* and *Cystoisospora* spp. because they have 2 ellipsoidal sporocysts that enclose 4 sporozoites. Asexual stages develop only in the intermediate host, which in nature is often an herbivore (prey animal), and sexual stages develop only in the definitive host, which is a carnivore or omnivore. There are different intermediate and definitive hosts for each species of *Sarcocystis;* for example, there are 5 named species of *Sarcocystis* in cattle: *Sarcocystis cruzi, Sarcocystis heydorni, Sarcocystis hirsuta, S hominis,* and *Sarcocystis rommeli,* the definitive hosts for these species being canines (*S cruzi*), felines (*S hirsuta, S rommeli*), and primates (*S heydorni, S hominis*), respectively. Species of *Sarcocystis* parasites are generally more specific for their intermediate hosts than for their definitive hosts; for *S cruzi,* for example, ox and bison are the only intermediate hosts whereas dogs, wolves, coyotes, raccoons, jackals, and foxes can act as definitive hosts. In the following description of the life cycle and structure, *S cruzi* will serve as the example because its complete life cycle is known from experimental infections of intermediate and definitive hosts.

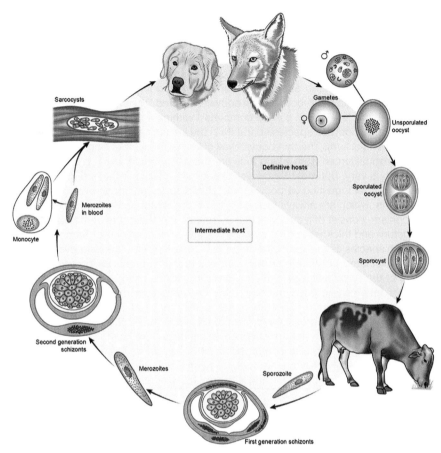

Fig. 3. Life cycle of *Sarcocystis cruzi*. (*Courtesy of* J. P. Dubey, MVSc, PhD, Beltsville, MD.)

The intermediate host becomes infected by ingesting sporocysts in food or water. Sporozoites excyst from sporocysts in the small intestine and the first generation of schizonts are formed in endothelial cells of arteries 7 to 15 days after inoculation while the second generation of schizonts occur 19 to 46 days after inoculation in capillaries throughout the body. Some merozoites are can also be found in mononuclear blood cells 24 to 46 days after inoculation. Both generations of schizonts develop asexually by a type of schizogony (asexual division) called endopolygeny, wherein the nucleus becomes lobulated and divides into several nuclei. Merozoites form at the periphery of the schizont. Both generation schizonts are located within the host cytoplasm and are not surrounded by a parasitophorous vacuole. Merozoites liberated from the last generation of schizonts initiate sarcocyst formation after penetration of appropriate host cells (striated and cardiac muscle, and occasionally the central nervous system). The intracellular merozoites are surrounded by a parasitophorous vacuole, unlike developing schizonts. The merozoite becomes a round to ovoid metrocyte and undergoes repeated division producing many metrocytes that eventually produce bradyzoites. As the sarcocyst matures, the numbers of bradyzoites increase and the numbers of metrocytes decrease. Eventually the sarcocyst is filled with bradyzoites. Sarcocysts generally become infectious about 75 days after infection, but there is considerable variation among species of *Sarcocystis*. Immature sarcocysts containing only metrocytes are not infectious for the definitive host.

The definitive host becomes infected by ingesting tissues containing mature sarcocysts. Bradyzoites liberated from the sarcocyst by digestion in the stomach and intestine penetrate the mucosa of the small intestine and transform into male (micro) and female (macro) stages and after fertilization of a macrogamete by a microgamete a wall develops around the zygote and an oocyst is formed. The entire process of sexual development and fertilization can be completed within 24 hours.

Oocysts of *Sarcocystis* species sporulate in the lamina propria. Sporulated oocysts are thin walled (<1 μm). The thin oocyst wall often ruptures, releasing the sporocysts into the intestinal lumen from which they are passed in the feces. The prepatent and patent periods vary, but most *Sarcocystis* species oocysts are first shed in the feces 7 to 14 days after ingesting sarcocysts and shedding occurs for weeks to months.

Sarcocysts, which are always located within a parasitophorous vacuole in the host cell cytoplasm, consist of a cyst wall that surrounds the metrocyte or the bradyzoites. The structure and thickness of the cyst wall differs among species of *Sarcocystis* and within each species as the sarcocyst matures.[60] Histologically, the sarcocyst wall may be smooth, striated or hirsute, or may possess complex branched protrusions. The structure of the sarcocyst wall is of taxonomic importance and used in species identification.[60] Internally, groups of zoites may be segregated into compartments by septa that originate from the sarcocyst wall or they may not be compartmentalized. Transmission electron microscopy of sarcocysts and PCR are often needed to identify sarcocysts to species.[60] Immunohistochemical tests are useful in experimental studies and are more helpful in locating schizonts in capillaries that sarcocysts in muscles. The presence of schizonts and only immature sarcocysts with metrocytes indicates acute or early infection and the presence of only mature sarcocysts indicates chronic infection.

Clinical Sarcocystosis in Ruminants

Sarcocystis are generally nonpathogenic for the definitive host, and some species of *Sarcocystis* are also nonpathogenic for intermediate hosts (**Table 1**). Generally, species transmitted by canids are pathogenic, whereas those transmitted by felids are nonpathogenic. *S cruzi*, *Sarcocystis capracanis*, and *S tenella* are the most pathogenic species for cattle, goats, and sheep, respectively. Clinical signs are generally seen during the time that second generation schizonts are developing in blood vessels (acute phase). Three to 4 weeks after infection with a large dose of sporocysts (≥50,000), fever, anorexia, anemia, emaciation, and hair loss (particularly on the rump and tail in cattle) develop, and some animals may die. Pregnant animals may abort, and growth is slowed or arrested. Animals recover as sarcocysts begin to mature.

Dramatic gross lesions are seen in animals that die during the acute phase. Edema, hemorrhage, and atrophy of fat are commonly seen. The hemorrhages are most evident on the serosa of viscera, in cardiac and skeletal muscles, and in the sclera of the eyes. Hemorrhages vary from petechiae to ecchymoses several centimeters in diameter. Microscopic lesions may be seen in many organs and consist of necrosis, edema, and infiltrations of mononuclear cells. During the chronic phase, lesions are restricted to muscles and consist of nonsuppurative myositis and degeneration of sarcocysts.

Zoonotic Sarcocystosis

Humans serve as the definitive host for *S hominis* and *S heydorni* of cattle and also serve as accidental intermediate hosts for several unidentified species of *Sarcocystis*.

Table 1				
Common species of *Sarcocystis* in ruminants				
Intermediate Hosts	*Sarcocystis* Species	Sarcocyst Grossly Visible	Pathogenicity[a]	Definitive Hosts
Cattle (*Bos taurus*)	*S cruzi*	No, <1 mm	++	Dog, coyote, raccoon, red fox, wolf
	S heydorni	No, <1 mm	+	Human
	S hirsuta	Yes, ≤7 mm	+	Cat
	S hominis	Yes, ≤7 mm	+	Human, other primates
	S rommeli	No, <1 mm	ND	Cat
Sheep (*Ovis aries*)	*S arieticanis*	No, <1 mm	+	Dog
	S gigantea	Yes, ≤10 mm	-	Cat
	S medusiformis	Yes, ≤8 mm	-	Cat
	S tenella	No, <1 mm	++	Dog, coyote, red fox
Goat (*Capra hircus*)	*S capracanis*	No, <1 mm	++	Dog, coyote, red fox
	S hircicanis	Yes, ≤2.5 mm	++	Dog
	S moule	Yes, ≤7.5 mm	ND	Cat
Water Buffalo (*Bubalus bubalis*)	*S buffalonis*	Yes, ≤3 mm	ND	ND
	S dubeyi	No, <1 mm	ND	ND
	S fusiformis	Yes, ≤3 mm	-	Cat
	S levinei	No, <1 mm	-	Dog

[a] ++ = Pathogenic, + = moderately pathogenic, - = not pathogenic, ND = not determined.

Intestinal sarcocystosis is acquired by ingesting uncooked beef containing sarcocysts of *S hominis* symptoms include nausea, stomachache and abdominal pain. Sporocysts are shed 11 to 13 days after ingesting the infected beef.[60]

Eosinophilic Myositis

Eosinophilic myositis (EM) is a specific inflammatory condition of striated muscles, mainly owing to accumulations of eosinophils.[60,61] It has been found mainly in cattle and occasionally in sheep. The affected animals are usually clinically normal and EM lesions are discovered at meat inspection after slaughter. Gross lesions consist of green to pale yellow areas that may be up to 15 cm long. The pathogenesis of EM is not clear and EM lesions have never been found in livestock species experimentally infected with *Sarcocystis* species.[60] Degenerating sarcocysts have been found in sections of lesions of EM,[61] but the high prevalence of *Sarcocystis* spp. infection in naturally infected cattle with no EM makes it difficult to designate *Sarcocystis* as the cause of EM in cattle.

Condemnation of beef containing lesions of EM or grossly visible sarcocysts (*S hirsuta*) can be a serious economic problem.[62,63] In a study, 974 of 1,622,402 cattle (0.06%) slaughtered in 1965 to 1966 in the United States were condemned because of EM.[63] In another report 18 bovine carcasses from 1 slaughter plant in the United States were condemned because of grossly visible *S hirsuta* sarcocysts.[62]

Diagnosis

The antemortem diagnosis of muscular sarcocystosis can only be made by histologic examination of muscle collected by biopsy or at necropsy.[60] The finding of immature sarcocysts with metrocytes suggests recently acquired infection but if only mature sarcocysts are present then the infection is chronic.[60]

An inflammatory response associated with sarcocysts may help to distinguish an active disease process from incidental finding of sarcocysts. There are several serologic tests and PCR techniques developed experimentally to distinguish *Sarcocystis* species in ruminants but there are pitfalls to serologic and molecular diagnosis of sarcocystosis in animals and none are commercially available.[63]

The diagnosis of intestinal *Sarcocystis* infection in a definitive host can be made by is by fecal examination. As has been mentioned, sporocysts or oocysts of *Sarcocystis* are shed fully sporulated in feces whereas those of *N caninum*, *T gondii*, and *Cystoisospora spp.* are shed unsporulated. It is not possible to distinguish one species of *Sarcocystis* from another by the structure of sporocysts in the feces. PCR on sporocysts can be used to determine the species present in definitive hosts.

Epidemiology and Control

Sarcocystis infection is common in ruminants worldwide.[60] Several factors contribute to the high prevalence in muscular infections in ruminants. Several species may infect a particular host and there maybe abundant definitive hosts for each species infecting that host. Each infected definitive host can shed millions of infectious sporocysts over several months contaminating the environment. *Sarcocystis* sporocysts and oocysts remain viable for many months in the environment, are resistant to freezing, and can overwinter on pasture. Oocysts and sporocysts are spread by invertebrate transport hosts to other areas. The definitive host develops little or no immunity, and repeat shedding of sporocysts occurs each time a meal of infected meat is consumed. *Sarcocystis* oocysts, unlike those of many other species of coccidia, are passed in feces in the infective form freeing them from dependence on warm moist weather conditions for maturation to infectivity.[60]

There is no vaccine to protect ruminants against sarcocystosis. Shedding of *Sarcocystis* oocysts and sporocysts in feces of the definitive hosts is the key factor in the spread of *Sarcocystis* infection; to interrupt this cycle, carnivores should be excluded from animal houses and from feed, water and bedding for livestock. Uncooked meat or offal should never be fed to carnivores. Because freezing can drastically decrease or eliminate infectious sarcocysts, meat should be frozen if not cooked. Exposure to heat at 55°C for 20 minutes kills sarcocysts.[64] Dead livestock should be buried or incinerated. Dead animals should never be left in the field for vultures and carnivores to eat.

SUMMARY

Much needs to be learned about preventing *N caninum*, *T gondii*, and *Sarcocystis* spp. infections in ruminants. Additional research on inducing immunity to congenital transmission of *N caninum* is needed but few laboratories are exploring this difficult area of study. In addition, research is needed regarding the pathogenesis of *N caninum* abortion, life cycle of the parasite in cattle, and sources of infection. *T gondii* abortions in sheep and goats remain a production challenge to the industry. The effects of *Sarcocystis* infections in ruminants are difficult to evaluate because nearly all ruminants raised on pasture contain sarcocysts in their muscles.

DISCLOSURE

The authors have nothing to disclose.

REFERENCES

1. Dubey JP, Hemphill A, Calero-Bernal R, et al. Neosporosis in animals. 1st edition. Boca Raton (FL): CRC Press, Taylor & Francis Group; 2017. p. 1–529. ISBN: 9781498752541.
2. Bjerkås I, Mohn SF, Presthus J. Unidentified cyst-forming sporozoon causing encephalomyelitis and myositis in dogs. Z Parasitenkd 1984;70:271–4.
3. Dubey JP, Carpenter JL, Speer CA, et al. Newly recognized fatal protozoan disease of dogs. J Am Vet Med Assoc 1988;192:1269–85.
4. Dubey JP, Hattel AL, Lindsay DS, et al. Neonatal *Neospora caninum* infections in dogs: isolation of the causative agent and experimental transmission. J Am Vet Med Assoc 1988;193:1259–63.
5. Lindsay DS, Dubey JP. Immunohistochemical diagnosis of *Neospora caninum* in tissue sections. Am J Vet Res 1989;50:1981–3.
6. McAllister MM, Dubey JP, Lindsay DS, et al. Dogs are definitive hosts of *Neospora caninum*. Int J Parasitol 1998;28:1473–8.
7. Lindsay DS, Dubey JP, Duncan RB. Confirmation that the dog is a definitive host for *Neospora caninum*. Vet Parasitol 1999;82:327–33.
8. Gondim LFP, McAllister MM, Pitt WC, et al. Coyotes (*Canis latrans*) are definitive hosts of *Neospora caninum*. Int J Parasitol 2004;34:159–61.
9. Dubey JP, Jenkins MC, Rajendran C, et al. Gray wolf (*Canis lupus*) is a natural definitive host for *Neospora caninum*. Vet Parasitol 2017;181:382–7.
10. Rosypal AC, Lindsay DS. The sylvatic cycle of *Neospora caninum*: where do we go from here? Trends Parasitol 2005;25:439–40.
11. Dubey JP, Lindsay DS. A review of *Neospora caninum* and neosporosis. Vet Parasitol 1996;67:1–59.
12. Ortega-Mora LM, Ferre I, del Pozo I, et al. Detection of *Neospora caninum* in semen of bulls. Vet Parasitol 2003;117:301–8.
13. Baillargeon P, Fecteau G, Paré J, et al. Evaluation of the embryo transfer procedure proposed by the International Embryo Transfer Society as a method of controlling vertical transmission of *Neospora caninum* in cattle. J Am Vet Med Assoc 2001;218:1803–6.
14. Davison HC, Guy CS, McGarry JW, et al. Experimental studies on the transmission of *Neospora caninum* between cattle. Res Vet Sci 2001;70:163–8.
15. Uggla A, Stenlund S, Holmdahl OJM, et al. Oral *Neospora caninum* inoculation of neonatal calves. Int J Parasitol 1998;28:1467–72.
16. Dijkstra T, Eysker M, Schares G, et al. Dogs shed *Neospora caninum* oocysts after ingestion of naturally infected bovine placenta but not after ingestion of colostrum spiked with *Neospora caninum* tachyzoites. Int J Parasitol 2001;31:747–52.
17. Thilsted JP, Dubey JP. Neosporosis-like abortions in a herd of dairy cattle. J Vet Diagn Invest 1989;1:205–9.
18. Anderson ML, Blanchard PC, Barr BC, et al. *Neospora*-like protozoan infection as a major cause of abortion in California dairy cattle. J Am Vet Med Assoc 1991; 198:241–4.
19. McAllister M, Huffman EM, Hietala SK, et al. Evidence suggesting a point source exposure in an outbreak of bovine abortion due to neosporosis. J Vet Diagn Invest 1996;8:355–7.
20. McAllister MM, Björkman C, Anderson-Sprecher R, et al. Evidence of point-source exposure to *Neospora caninum* and protective immunity in a herd of beef cows. J Am Vet Med Assoc 2000;217:881–7.

21. Anderson ML, Palmer CW, Thurmond MC, et al. Evaluation of abortions in cattle attributable to neosporosis in selected dairy herds in California. J Am Vet Med Assoc 1995;207:1206–10.

22. Okeoma CM, Williamson NB, Pomroy WE, et al. Isolation and molecular characterization of Neospora caninum in cattle in New Zealand. N Z Vet J 2004;52: 364–70.

23. Sawada M, Kondo H, Tomioka Y, et al. Isolation of Neospora caninum from the brain of a naturally infected adult dairy cow. Vet Parasitol 2000;90:247–52.

24. Okeoma CM, Williamson NB, Pomroy WE, et al. The use of PCR to detect Neospora caninum DNA in the blood of naturally infected cows. Vet Parasitol 2004; 122:307–15.

25. Dubey JP, Schares G. Diagnosis of bovine neosporosis. Vet Parasitol 2006; 140:1–34.

26. Dubey JP, Buxton D, Wouda W. Pathogenensis of bovine neosporosis. J Comp Pathol 2006;134:267–89.

27. Álvarez-García G, Collantes-Fernández E, Costas E, et al. Influence of age and purpose for testing on the cut-off selection of serological methods in bovine neosporosis. Vet Res 2003;34:341–52.

28. Baszler TV, Gay LJC, Long MT, et al. Detection by PCR of Neospora caninum in fetal tissues from spontaneous bovine abortions. J Clin Microbiol 1999;37: 4059–64.

29. von Blumröder D, Schares G, Norton R, et al. Comparison and standardisation of serological methods for the diagnosis of Neospora caninum infection in bovines. Vet Parasitol 2004;120:11–22.

30. Schares G, Conraths FJ, Reichel MP. Bovine neosporosis: comparison of serological methods using outbreak sera from a dairy herd in New Zealand. Int J Parasitol 1999;29:1659–67.

31. Trees AJ, Williams DJL. Endogenous and exogenous transplacental infection in Neospora caninum and Toxoplasma gondii. Trends Parasitol 2005;21:558–61.

32. Björkman C, McAllister MM, Frössling J, et al. Application of the Neospora caninum IgG avidity ELISA in assessment of chronic reproductive losses after an outbreak of neosporosis in a herd of beef cattle. J Vet Diagn Invest 2003;15:3–7.

33. Baszler TV, Adams S, Vander-Schalie J, et al. Validation of a commercially available monoclonal antibody-based competitive-inhibition enzyme-linked immunosorbent assay for detection of serum antibodies to Neospora caninum in cattle. J Clin Microbiol 2001;39:3851–7.

34. Reichel MP, Ellis JT. Control options for Neospora caninum infections in cattle - current state of knowledge. N Z Vet J 2002;50:86–92.

35. Dijkstra T, Barkema HW, Hesselink JW, et al. Point source exposure of cattle to Neospora caninum consistent with periods of common housing and feeding and related to the introduction of a dog. Vet Parasitol 2002;105:89–98.

36. Schares G, Bärwald A, Staubach C, et al. Potential risk factors for bovine Neospora caninum infection in Germany are not under the control of the farmers. Parasitology 2004;129:301–9.

37. Innes EA, Andrianarivo AG, Björkman C, et al. Immune responses to Neospora caninum and prospects for vaccination. Trends Parasitol 2002;18:497–504.

38. Marugan-Hernandez V. Neospora caninum and bovine neosporosis: current vaccine research. J Comp Pathol 2017;157:193–200.

39. Barling KS, Lunt DK, Graham SL, et al. Evaluation of an inactivated Neospora caninum vaccine in beef feedlot steers. J Am Vet Med Assoc 2003;222:624–7.

40. Romero JJ, Pérez E, Frankena K. Effect of a killed whole *Neospora caninum* tachyzoite vaccine on the crude abortion rate of Costa Rican dairy cows under field conditions. Vet Parasitol 2004;23:149–59.
41. Marsh AE, Barr BC, Packham AE, et al. Description of a new *Neospora* species (Protozoa: Apicomplexa: Sarcocystidae). J Parasitol 1998;84:983–91.
42. Marsh AE, Howe DK, Wang G, et al. Differentiation of *Neospora hughesi* from *Neospora caninum* based on their immunodominant surface antigen, SAG1 and SRS2. Int J Parasitol 1999;29:1575–82.
43. Walsh CP, Vemulapalli R, Sriranganathan N, et al. Molecular comparison of the dense granule proteins GRA6 and GRA7 of *Neospora hughesi* and *Neospora caninum*. Int J Parasitol 2001;31:253–8.
44. Walsh CP, Duncan RB, Zajac AM, et al. *Neospora hughesi*: experimental infections in mice, gerbils, and dogs. Vet Parasitol 2000;92:119–28.
45. Dubey JP. Toxoplasmosis of animals and man. 2nd edition. Boca Raton (FL): CRC Press; 2010.
46. Dubey JP, Lindsay DS, Speer CA. Structure of *Toxoplasma gondii* tachyzoites, bradyzoite, and sporozoites, and biology and development of tissue cysts. Clin Microbiol Rev 1998;11:267–99.
47. Dubey JP, Frenkel JK. Cyst-induced toxoplasmosis in cats. J Protozool 1972;19: 155–77.
48. Speer CA, Dubey JP. Ultrastructural differentiation of *Toxoplasma gondii* schizonts (types B to E) and gamonts in the intestines of cats fed bradyzoites. Int J Parasitol 2005;35:193–206.
49. Dubey JP. Unexpected oocyst shedding by cats fed *Toxoplasma gondii* tachyzoites: in vivo stage conversion and strain variation. Vet Parasitol 2005;133: 289–98.
50. Dubey JP. Comparative infectivity of oocysts and bradyzoites of *Toxoplasma gondii* for intermediate (mice) and definitive (cats) hosts. Vet Parasitol 2006;40: 69–75.
51. Wallace GD. Serologic and epidemiologic observations on toxoplasmosis on three Pacific Atolls. Am J Epidemiol 1969;90:103–11.
52. Munday B. Serologic evidence for *Toxoplasma* infection in isolated groups of sheep. Res Vet Sci 1972;13:100–2.
53. Dubey JP, Rollor EA, Smith K, et al. Low seroprevalence of *Toxoplasma gondii* in feral pigs from a remote island lacking cats. J Parasitol 1997;83:839–41.
54. Dubey JP. Toxoplasmosis - a waterborne zoonosis. Vet Parasitol 2004;26:57–72.
55. Tenter AM, Heckeroth AR, Weiss LM. *Toxoplasma gondii*: from animals to humans. Int J Parasitol 2000;30:1217–58.
56. Desmonts G, Couvreur J. Congenital toxoplasmosis. A prospective study of 378 pregnancies. N Engl J Med 1974;290:1110–6.
57. Remington JS, McLeod R, Thulliez P, et al. Toxoplasmosis. In: Remington JS, Klein JO, editors. Infectious diseases of the fetus and newborn infant. Philadelphia: W. B. Saunders; 2001. p. 205–346.
58. Lindsay DS, Dubey JP. *Toxoplasma gondii*: the changing paradigm of congenital toxoplasmosis. Parasitology 2011;138:1829–31.
59. Buxton D. Toxoplasmosis: the first commercial vaccine. Parasitol Today 1993;9: 335–7.
60. Dubey JP, Calero-Bernal R, Rosenthal BM, et al. Sarcocystosis of animals and man. 2nd edition. Boca Raton (FL): CRC Press; 2016.
61. Wouda W, Snoep JJ, Dubey JP. Eosinophilic myositis due to *Sarcocystis hominis* in a beef cow. J Comp Pathol 2006;135:249–53.

62. Dubey JP, Udtujan RM, Cannon L, et al. Condemnation of beef because of *Sarcocystis hirsuta* infection. J Am Vet Med Assoc 1990;196:1095–6.

63. Tenter AM. Current research on *Sarcocystis* species of domestic animals. Int J Parasitol 1995;25:1311–30.

64. Fayer R. Effects of refrigeration, cooking, and freezing on *Sarcocystis* in beef from retail food stores. Proc Helminthol Soc Wash 1975;42:138–40.

Cryptosporidium and Giardia in Ruminants

Monica Santin, DVM, PhD

KEYWORDS

- *Cryptosporidium* • *Giardia* • Ruminants • Cattle • Sheep • Goat

KEY POINTS

- Giardiasis and cryptosporidiosis have been documented in ruminants worldwide regardless of the husbandry system.
- Infections with *Cryptosporidium* and *Giardia* are an animal health concern because of the direct economic losses associated with the infection.
- There is also a public health concern because *Cryptosporidium* and *Giardia* are highly prevalent in ruminants and humans, indicating potential for human exposure from environmental contamination.
- The application of molecular techniques has resulted in expanded knowledge regarding the taxonomy and epidemiology of *Giardia* and *Cryptosporidium*.

INTRODUCTION

Cryptosporidium and *Giardia* are two common enteric pathogens of animals and humans with global distribution. They are transmitted by the fecal-oral route via direct contact with an infected host or through consumption of contaminated water or food with infective stages (oocysts or cysts). *Cryptosporidium* and *Giardia* infections can be asymptomatic or cause mild to severe gastrointestinal illness in both animals and humans. Both parasites are an animal health concern because of the direct economic losses associated with infection, but there is also a public health concern because of the potential for human exposure to environmental contamination of *Cryptosporidium* oocyst and *Giardia* cysts from animals.[1,2] The application of molecular approaches for the diagnosis of these two parasites has led to significantly improved knowledge regarding the epidemiology of these protozoans.

CRYPTOSPORIDIOSIS

Cryptosporidiosis is caused by the protozoan *Cryptosporidium*. The genus *Cryptosporidium* includes ubiquitous protozoan parasites that infect many vertebrate hosts,

Environmental Microbial and Food Safety Laboratory, Beltsville Agricultural Research Center, Agricultural Research Service, US Department of Agriculture, BARC-East, Building 173, 10300 Baltimore Avenue, Beltsville, MD 20705, USA
E-mail address: monica.santin-duran@ars.usda.gov

Vet Clin Food Anim 36 (2020) 223–238
https://doi.org/10.1016/j.cvfa.2019.11.005
0749-0720/20/Published by Elsevier Inc.

including humans. In ruminants, cryptosporidiosis has been reported worldwide regardless of husbandry system.[3,4] The most common symptom associated with *Cryptosporidium* is diarrhea, but lack of appetite, fever, or malabsorption could also be observed.[4] Infections with *Cryptosporidium* are a significant problem for animal health, mostly in neonatal livestock, causing economic losses associated with decreased growth rate and mortality in the infected animals. In addition, cryptosporidiosis increases the cost of animal health care and veterinary services. In humans, cryptosporidium infections usually produce self-limited profuse, watery diarrhea that can last up to 3 weeks in persons with healthy immune systems but can lead to life-threatening malnutrition and wasting in immunocompromised individuals.

Life Cycle and Transmission

Cryptosporidium has a complex life cycle that involves both sexual and asexual replication in a single host[5] (**Fig. 1**). After ingestion of the infective stage (sporulated oocyst) by a suitable host, excystation occurs in the gastrointestinal tract and 4 sporozoites are released. Then, the sporozoites invade the gastric or intestinal epithelium depending on the *Cryptosporidium* species. Although the parasites are intracellular, they are extracytoplasmatic, so there is no contact with the host-cell cytoplasm. Sporozoites undergo asexual reproduction (merogony) and then sexual reproduction (gametogony) upon differentiating into either macrogamonts (female) or microgamonts (male). After fusion of a microgamont with a macrogamont, a zygote is formed, which then develops into an oocyst. Oocysts sporulate in situ and, when mature, contain 4 naked sporozoites. Because oocysts sporulate in situ, autoinfection is possible when sporozoites are released from the oocysts within the same host.

 Cryptosporidium is transmitted via the fecal-oral route by both direct and indirect transmission. Direct transmission occurs through ingestion of oocysts present in feces of the infected hosts, whereas indirect transmission occurs by ingestion of water or food contaminated with oocysts. There are several factors that contribute to the transmissibility of *Cryptosporidium*. These factors include (1) simple fecal-oral transmission route with oocysts excreted fully sporulated and immediately infective to other suitable hosts; (2) oocysts can persist in harsh conditions for long periods of time; (3) oocysts are resistant to many conventional disinfectants, including chlorine; (4) ability of infected hosts to shed very large quantities of oocysts (eg, a neonatal calf can shed up to 30 billion oocysts over a 1–2 weeks); and (5) the low infectious dose (10–30 oocysts).[5,6]

Epidemiology, Zoonotic Potential, and Public Health

Cryptosporidium infections have been documented in ruminants worldwide. Point prevalence studies indicate a wide range of infection rates, whereas longitudinal studies indicate that morbidity rates often reach 100%.[3] Variations in the reported prevalence among studies are related to many different factors, including study design, sample size, geographic region, climate, season, age, breed, management practices, or detection methods used. A recent systematic review and meta-analysis of *Cryptosporidium* in livestock found that prevalence in farmed animals was higher in the Americas and Europe than in other continents, which was attributed to the intensive farm animal production in those regions.[7]

 Infections are most commonly diagnosed in neonatal animals. Young animals can become infected and begin shedding *Cryptosporidium* oocysts shortly after birth,[8] with the highest rates of infection reported in animals between 1 and 3 weeks of age.[9–14] A potential source of infection for neonatal lambs and kids could be the presence of adults with subclinical infections, especially during the periparturient period,

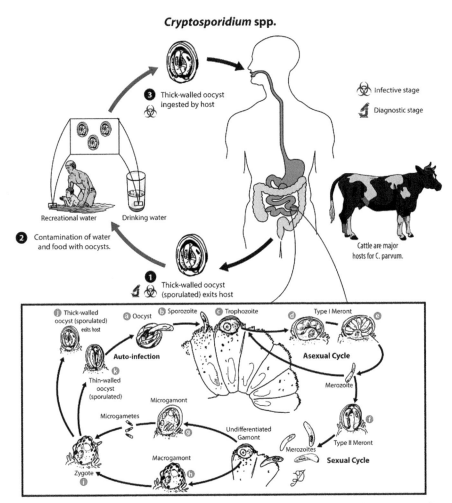

Fig. 1. Life cycle of *Cryptosporidium* species. Sporulated oocysts, containing 4 sporozoites, are excreted by the infected host through feces (1). Transmission of *Cryptosporidium* species occurs by the fecal-oral route (2). Following ingestion by a suitable host (3), excystation (a) occurs. The sporozoites are released and parasitize the epithelial cells of the gastrointestinal tract (b, c). In these cells, the parasites undergo asexual multiplication (merogony) (d, e, f) and then sexual multiplication (gametogony) producing microgamonts (male) (g) and macrogamonts (female) (h). Fertilization of the macrogamonts by the microgametes (i). After fusion of a microgamont with a macrogamont, a zygote is formed, which then develops into an oocyst and sporulates in the infected host. There are 2 different types of oocysts (thick walled and thin walled). Thick-walled oocysts are excreted with feces into the environment (j), whereas thin-walled oocysts are involved in an autoinfective cycle (k). (Image courtesy of DPDx, Centers for Disease Control and Prevention (https://www.cdc.gov/dpdx.)

when increased oocyst shedding has been shown.[15–18] In beef cattle, no periparturient increase in *Cryptosporidium parvum* oocysts excretion was observed, but oocysts were frequently detected in asymptomatic cows, suggesting that they may play a role in calf infections.[19] In contrast, no clear connection has been found between the presence of oocyst-excreting adults and the infections in neonate calves, suggesting there are additional factors contributing to infections in newborn calves, such as the presence of wildlife (small rodents or birds) or environmental contamination (dirty water and manure sources).[20] In addition, in longitudinal studies performed on a Scottish dairy farm, adult cows were not considered the source of infection for newborn calves, because different subtypes of *C parvum* were identified in the calves and adults.[8]

In the last 2 decades, substantial progress has been made in identifying *Cryptosporidium* species present in ruminants. Before the application of molecular tools, most studies reported the presence of oocysts of *Cryptosporidium* species in ruminants. Until the early 2000s, most studies, reported only *C parvum* and "*Cryptosporidium muris*" in ruminants, because of the morphologic similarity of *Cryptosporidium* oocysts from different species. Later, molecular studies and cross-species transmission studies identified "*C muris*" from cattle as a new species, namely *Cryptosporidium andersoni*.[21] Subsequently, with the assistance of molecular techniques, additional species of *Cryptosporidium* have been described in ruminants.[22–25]

There are 4 main *Cryptosporidium* species responsible for infections in cattle: *C parvum*, *Cryptosporidium bovis*, *Cryptosporidium ryanae*, and *C andersoni*.[9,21–23] Other species have also been sporadically reported in cattle, including *Cryptosporidium hominis*, *Cryptosporidium suis*, *Cryptosporidium canis*, and *Cryptosporidium felis*.[3] However, it is likely these species are not maintained within cattle populations but result from occasional contact with their respective primary hosts. *C andersoni*, one of the largest species of *Cryptosporidium*, infects the abomasum, whereas *C parvum*, *C ryanae*, and *C bovis*, which are of similar size and smaller than *C andersoni*, infect the small intestine. Most studies worldwide suggest an age-related distribution of *Cryptosporidium* species in cattle, with *C parvum* being the predominant species in preweaned calves, *C bovis* and *C ryanae* as the predominant species in postweaned calves, and *C andersoni* as the predominant species in juvenile and adult cattle.[9,11,26,27] However, this is not the case in China, where *C parvum* is less common and *C bovis* is the dominant species in preweaned dairy calves.[14,28] This finding could indicate differences in the transmission of *Cryptosporidium* species in preweaned dairy calves in China.

Molecular epidemiologic studies have identified different species and genotypes of *Cryptosporidium* in sheep. The most common species identified are *Cryptosporidium ubiquitum*, *Cryptosporidium xiaoi*, and *C parvum*, although others, such *C andersoni*, *C bovis*, *C ryanae*, *C hominis*, *Cryptosporidium fayeri*, and *C suis*, have been identified sporadically in sheep.[18,24,25,29–34] Although most studies in sheep showed a predominance of *C ubiquitum* and *C xiaoi* worldwide,[10,18] studies from European countries have reported that *C parvum* predominates.[13,33,35–37] The distribution of *Cryptosporidium* species in sheep is not as clearly associated with age as it is in cattle. Some studies reported *C ubiquitum* as the most common species in older animals, whereas *C parvum* or *C xiaoi* were the predominant species in lambs younger than 1 month of age.[18,35,36] However, other studies have found *C ubiquitum* in similar numbers in lambs and adults.[10,38]

In goats, the most common *Cryptosporidium* species identified are *C ubiquitum*, *C xiaoi*, and *C parvum*, whereas other species and genotypes, such *C hominis*, *Cryptosporidium baileyi*, *C andersoni*, and rat genotype II, have only been identified sporadically.[12,13,39,40]

Animals can be reservoirs of zoonotic *Cryptosporidium* species.[1] Ruminants have been implicated as a source of zoonotic *Cryptosporidium* outbreaks originating from direct contact with infected animals.[41,42] Zoonotic species of *Cryptosporidium* in ruminants include *C parvum* and *C ubiquitum*. *C parvum* is the second most common species that infects humans[1] and *C ubiquitum* is considered an emerging human pathogen.[43] Both species have a broad host range and are responsible for zoonotic infections with a wide geographic distribution. Although other *Cryptosporidium* species commonly reported in ruminants have been sporadically found in humans, they are not considered major zoonotic species. *C andersoni* has been reported in humans in China, France, Malawi, Iran, the United Kingdom, and Australia.[44–49] *C bovis* has also been reported in farm workers in India and Australia,[50,51] and *C xiaoi* was reported in 2 patients with human immunodeficiency virus/acquired immunodeficiency syndrome in Ethiopia.[52]

Before the use of molecular subtyping tools to characterize the transmission dynamics of *Cryptosporidium* infections in humans and animals, it was presumed that infections caused by *C parvum* were from zoonotic transmission. At present, sequencing a portion of the hypervariable 60-kDa glycoprotein gene (*gp60*) allows further characterization into subtypes that are grouped within families. The use of *gp60* subtyping has identified human-specific, animal-specific, and zoonotic subtypes for *C parvum* and *C ubiquitum*.[1,43,53] Host adaptation for *C ubiquitum* subtypes is apparent with subtypes in XIIa found in ruminants, XIIb to XIIf in rodents, and XIIa (ruminant adapted) and XIIb to XIId (rodent adapted) in humans.[33,43] Similarly, *C parvum* subtypes within families IIb, IIc, and IIe are found only in humans, whereas subtypes within families IIa and IId are found in both humans and animals.[1] Subtyping of *C parvum* from preweaned calves has identified almost exclusively IIa and IId subtypes with differences in subtypes across geographic locations or host age.[1,3,28,53–56] There are still few data available on *C parvum* subtypes in small ruminants, and there are inconsistencies on the distribution of IIa and IId subtypes among different studies with respect to most common subtypes in goat kids or lambs.[9,35,57] These discrepancies could be associated with different management strategies and the ability of small ruminants to get in contact with other livestock such as cattle, the main reservoir of IIa subtypes.

Pathogenesis, Clinical Features, and Impact in Production

Cryptosporidium infections are frequently reported as a cause of diarrhea in neonatal ruminants. Neonatal diarrhea in ruminants can involve multiple pathogens (parasites, bacteria, and viruses) in addition to management and nutritional factors, but *Cryptosporidium* infection is unequivocally recognized by veterinarians as a major cause of diarrhea in neonatal ruminants.[4] A wide range of clinical signs can be observed in infected animals and can range from asymptomatic to death.[3,4] Differences in the severity of cryptosporidiosis are likely multifactorial and associated, among other factors, with host immune status, coinfections with other pathogens, and with different species/genotypes of *Cryptosporidium*. In cattle, most reports of disease are associated with *C parvum* and are characterized by an acute onset of profuse watery diarrhea, often associated with loss of appetite, depression, and weakness.[53,58,59] Mortality from dehydration has been reported in neonatal calves, but it is rare in endemic herds with high morbidity rates.[11,60] *C parvum* is mostly found in the epithelium of the lower small intestine causing enteritis, decreased villous length, villous atrophy, and fusion of villi.[61] A recent study that evaluated management practice and environmental factors associated with average daily gain in preweaned dairy calves in US dairy operations showed a significantly lower average daily gain in calves infected with *Cryptosporidium*.[62] Infections in cattle with the host-adapted cattle species *C bovis* and *C ryanae* have not been associated with illness.[22,23] Infections with *C andersoni* follow a more chronic course and do not cause diarrhea.[63] Although cattle infected with *C andersoni* have no clinical signs, it has been suggested that infections may interfere with milk production in dairy cows[64] and may cause significant reduction in rate of weight gain in beef cattle.[65] In addition, increased plasma pepsinogen levels, pale and thickened gastric mucosa, and dilated gastric glands have been associated with *C andersoni* infections.[63,66]

In small ruminants, the major clinical signs of cryptosporidiosis are diarrhea and weight loss. Different clinical manifestations have been associated with age and the species of *Cryptosporidium*. Although molecular information on cryptosporidiosis in small ruminants is still limited, clinically ill lambs and kids seem to be more often infected with *C parvum*, whereas *C xiaoi* and *C ubiquitum* are mostly reported in healthy lambs.[10,13,35,36,67] No clinical signs were observed in lambs experimentally infected with *C xiaoi* and *C ubiquitum*.[24,25] However, there are reports of *C parvum* in healthy animals, which could perhaps serve as asymptomatic carriers, and the presence of *C xiaoi* and *C ubiquitum* in diarrheic animals.[33,34,68,69] In addition, *C andersoni* has been identified in sheep without clinical signs.[29] In general, there is limited information on the impact of cryptosporidiosis in small ruminant production, and future studies should investigate the potential impacts of infection, including studies of asymptomatic animals. In Australia, *Cryptosporidium* infection in lambs had a negative impact on carcass profit indicators (carcass weight and dressing percentage) as well as reduced live weight, and an increase in fecal consistency scores.[70] In goats, *Cryptosporidium* infection was associated with lower growth rate with and without diarrhea beyond preweaning.[69]

Diagnosis

Cryptosporidiosis should be included in the differential diagnosis in all cases of neonatal diarrhea in ruminants (intestinal cryptosporidiosis) and in cases in which dairy and feedlot cattle are not performing well (abomasal cryptosporidiosis associated with *C andersoni*). Detection and identification protocols for *Cryptosporidium* oocysts can be used directly on fecal specimens, but generally feces should be subjected to concentration methods to increase sensitivity.[71] Flotation with saturated sugar solution is the most common method to concentrate oocysts in ruminants.[72] For decades microscopic examination was the only method for detecting *Cryptosporidium* using the modified acid-fast protocol and later immunofluorescent antibody techniques to visualize oocysts. Under the microscope, oocysts are colorless, spherical or slightly ovoid, smooth, thick walled, and contain 4 elongated sporozoites. The size of *Cryptosporidium* oocysts reported in ruminants range from 3.7 × 3.2 μm (*C ryanae*) to 7.4 × 5.5 μm (*C andersoni*). However, differentiating *Cryptosporidium* species/genotypes using microscopy is not possible because oocysts are similar in shape and overlap in size. Oocyst size is helpful to differentiate gastric and intestinal *Cryptosporidium* species because oocysts from species infecting the stomach (eg, *C andersoni*) are larger than those from intestinal species (eg, *C parvum*, *C xiaoi*, or *C ryanae*).

Antigen detection kits based on enzyme-labeled antibodies to detect *Cryptosporidium* oocysts are commercially available.[73] Because there is wide variability in sensitivity of the different coproantigen detection immunoassays, they do not seem to increase sensitivity compared with microscopy,[72] but they are less time consuming and easier to perform. However, a disadvantage is that not all commercial antibody kits recognize all *Cryptosporidium* species or genotypes.[71]

Molecular methods that use polymerase chain reaction (PCR) and DNA sequencing, PCR restriction fragment polymorphism, real-time PCR assays, or multiplex PCR are more sensitive than microscopy and immunologic assays for the detection of *Cryptosporidium* in feces.[71,72] The small subunit ribosomal RNA (rRNA) gene is currently considered the most reliable locus for detection and identification of *Cryptosporidium* species and genotypes.[1] In addition, subtyping using the *gp60* gene is essential to better understand the dynamics of *Cryptosporidium* transmission. A major advantage of molecular methods is that they allow genetic characterization to identify species, genotypes, and subtypes, a requirement for epidemiologic studies designed to understand *Cryptosporidium* transmission routes.[1] However, molecular methods are mostly restricted to research and specialized laboratories.

Treatment and Prevention

Although vaccine trials to prevent cryptosporidiosis have been conducted in calves, currently there is no vaccine available.[74] However, it is unclear whether vaccination is justified because cryptosporidiosis is usually self-limiting and infected animals with normal immune systems improve without treatment.[58] In severe cases, clinical symptoms such as watery diarrhea or dehydration can be managed by supportive treatment with electrolytes.[75] Several drugs have been tested to treat *Cryptosporidium* in ruminants, but with limited success. Only the halofuginone lactate (which is not available in the United States) has been licensed for treatment of *Cryptosporidium* in ruminants, but its efficacy is controversial.[76] In newborn calves, treatment with halofuginone lactate is recommended orally (after colostrum or milk/milk replacer feeding) for the first 7 days of life at a dose of 100 μg of halofuginone base per kilogram of body weight (https://www.ema.europa.eu/en/medicines/veterinary/EPAR/halocur). A recent study indicated that administration of the correct prophylactic treatment with halofuginone (based on the calf's age and duration of treatment) is critical and that incorrect dosing has minimal impact on mortality and is equivalent to not treating, regarding the proportion of calves shedding oocysts.[77] A delay in *Cryptosporidium* oocyst shedding was also shown coupled with improved neonatal survival, but there was a negative effect on weight gain also reported.[77] Similarly, other studies showed efficacy in reducing *Cryptosporidium* oocyst shedding compared with placebo groups, but with no clear differences in the occurrence of diarrhea.[76,78] A study evaluating the effect of halofuginone in goat kids experimentally infected with *C parvum* reported a reduction in oocyst shedding, diarrhea, and mortality in kids that received the treatment.[79]

Cryptosporidium oocysts are resistant to most common commercial disinfectants.[5] To successfully control *Cryptosporidium*, proper management strategies to prevent transmission among animals are necessary. The use of good husbandry practices are needed, including decreased stocking density on farms, separating young and adult animals, ensuring that neonatal animals have received adequate colostrum, and keeping animals with diarrhea in isolation. In addition, adequate sanitation practices should include cleaning stalls before the introduction of new animals, especially neonatal animals, to destroy oocysts using either heat or chemical disinfection (hydrogen peroxide), sterilization processes using steam, or ultraviolet light. From a public health perspective, manure must be properly managed to minimize fecal contamination of food and water with oocysts of zoonotic *Cryptosporidium* species, and good hygiene practices among those handing animals, especially young ruminants, should include frequent hand washing.

GIARDIASIS

The protozoan flagellate *Giardia* is the causal agent of giardiasis. *Giardia* species can infect multiple hosts, ranging from mammals to birds and amphibians. At present, 8 species of *Giardia* are considered valid: *Giardia microti*, *Giardia cricetidarum*, and *Giardia muris* infect rodents; *Giardia ardeae* and *Giardia psittaci* birds; *Giardia agilis* amphibians; *Giardia peramelis* marsupials; and *G duodenalis* (syns. *Giardia intestinalis* and *Giardia lamblia*) infects most vertebrates, including humans.[80] *Giardia duodenalis* is one of the most common enteric parasites in humans and mammals worldwide, causing an estimated 280 million human cases of gastroenteritis annually, with higher infection rates in developing countries.[2,81] *G duodenalis* is considered a species complex consisting of 8 assemblages (designated A to H) based on genetic analysis but with little variation in morphology.[82,83] Assemblages A and B have low host specificity, infecting humans and a wide range of animals. In contrast, assemblages C to H are host adapted,[2] with C and D reported mainly in canines, E in artiodactyls, F in felines, G in rodents, and H in seals. It has been proposed to recover previously used *Giardia* species names based on host occurrence[84]; however, to accept this proposal, proper redescription that includes morphologic, biological, and genetic data will be necessary.

Life Cycle and Transmission

The life cycle of *Giardia* is simple and comprises only 2 stages: the cyst and the trophozoite (**Fig. 2**). When infective stages (cysts) are ingested by the host, they excyst in the duodenum, releasing 2 trophozoites. Trophozoites are not invasive and undergo repeated mitotic division on the mucosal surface of the small intestine. Later, in response to bile salt and other conditions present in the gut, trophozoites develop to cysts (the environmentally resistant form) that are passed in the feces.

Transmission is fecal-oral and occurs via direct contact with infected humans (anthroponotic transmission) or animals (zoonotic) and indirectly by ingestion of water or food contaminated with cysts (water-borne and food-borne transmission).[83,85] Factors that contribute to the successful spread of giardiasis include (1) large numbers of cysts released into the environment by infected hosts; (2) cysts that are immediately infectious after excretion and that remain viable for extended times under the right conditions (cool temperatures and moisture); and (3) low infectious dose.[83,86,87]

Epidemiology, Zoonotic Potential, and Public Health

Reports of *G duodenalis* are frequent in ruminants worldwide.[10,70,88–91] Infection rates vary greatly among studies and range from ~1% to as much as ~60% in cattle, sheep, and goats.[2] However, in longitudinal studies the cumulative incidence increases to 100% in ruminants.[60,92–94] Differences in prevalence among studies are most likely associated with different management practices, age of the animals examined, and detection methods used.[10,95] A higher prevalence is consistently observed in younger animals compared with adults,[10,92,95,96] with the highest occurrence reported around 2 months of age.[34,60,92,95] Among the different methods used to detect infections, higher prevalences are reported by PCR and enzyme-linked immunosorbent assay than by microscopy.[10]

Molecular epidemiologic surveys in ruminants worldwide have reported E as the predominant assemblage followed by lower frequencies of assemblage A, and sporadic reports of assemblage B.[2,29,88,92,97,98] There are also rare reports of canine assemblages C and D in ruminants, but it is unclear whether they represent true infections.[34,99] Assemblage E is not usually identified in humans and thus its zoonotic risk is minimal.[2] In contrast, assemblages A and B are common in humans and can be transmitted zoonotically, indicating a significant public health impact,[2] and there are reports of farmers infected with those assemblages.[31]

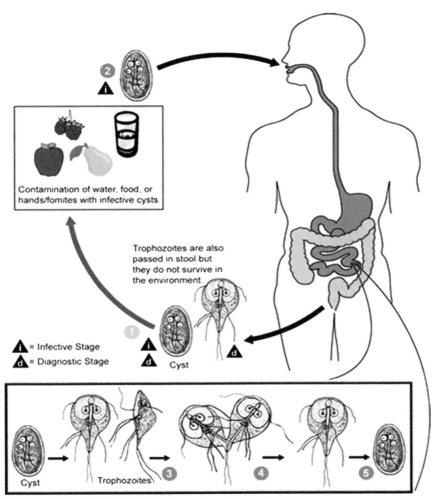

Fig. 2. Life cycle of *G duodenalis*. Cyst is the infective responsible for transmission of giardiasis (1). Infection occurs by the ingestion of cysts by the fecal-oral route (2). In the small intestine, excystation releases trophozoites (each cyst produces 2 trophozoites) (3). Trophozoites multiply by repeated mitotic division, remaining in the lumen of small intestine (4). Encystation occurs as the parasites transit toward the colon (5). (Image courtesy of DPDx, Centers for Disease Control and Prevention (https://www.cdc.gov/dpdx.)

Pathogenesis, Clinical Features, and Impact in Production

Giardiasis is a common disease in ruminants, characterized by diarrhea, weight loss, and malabsorption, but asymptomatic infections are also common.[60,92,100,101] The importance of *Giardia* as a cause of diarrhea in ruminants is still unclear, because diarrhea in ruminants is associated with a combination of other host factors, including infections with other pathogens and husbandry practices. In addition, field studies have suggested that even asymptomatic infections can have a negative impact in production and growth performance in livestock.[100,101] A recent study evaluating average daily gain in preweaned dairy calves in the United States reported that calves negative for *Giardia* gained more weight than calves positive for *Giardia*.[62]

Diagnosis

Microscopic examination of fecal samples remains the cornerstone of diagnostic testing for *Giardia*. During *Giardia* infections, cysts are shed sporadically, and the detection of cysts may require the examination of several fecal samples.[10] To increase sensitivity, concentration techniques are recommended.[102] Both cysts and trophozoites can be observed in fecal samples, but trophozoites are only present when watery diarrhea occurs. Under the microscope, cysts have an ovoid shape (8–15 μm long) with 2 to 4 nuclei and fibrils and median bodies, and trophozoites (10–20 μm long) have a pyriform shape with ventral sucking disk, 2 nuclei, 2 median bodies, and 8 flagella (4 lateral, 2 ventral, and 2 posterior).[103] Microscopy is rapid and inexpensive but requires a skilled parasitologist for proper identification and has decreased sensitivity when low numbers of cysts are present.[102] The use of immunofluorescent antibodies to stain and visualize the cysts using immunofluorescent microscopy assists in detection. In addition, immunologic and molecular methods are also commonly used and are reported to be highly sensitive and specific.[102,103] Antigen detection immunoassays have the advantage of being easy to standardize, requiring a short time to provide results, and showing higher sensitivity and specificity than microscopy.[102] PCR assays are becoming more common and are considered more sensitive that microscopy and immunoassays. The loci most commonly used in PCR are small subunit rRNA, triose phosphate isomerase, glutamate dehydrogenase, and β-giardin.[2] A clear advantage of molecular assays is the ability to do further sequence analysis from PCR-positive samples to allow assemblage identification. However, PCR and sequencing are used for research and are not routinely used for diagnosis.

Treatment and Prevention

There are no drugs or vaccines currently licensed for *Giardia* in ruminants. A vaccine is available for dogs (GiardiaVax), but a study that evaluated its efficacy in prevention of *Giardia* infections in calves reported lack of success in preventing giardiasis or reducing cyst excretion in this species.[104] Chemotherapy treatment is controversial. Giardiasis in ruminants is likely to be chronic and, because there are high levels of *Giardia* cysts in the farm environment, reinfections are common, requiring repeated treatments that make chemotherapy cost-prohibitive for producers. In addition, repeated treatments increase the potential for developing drug resistance. Some studies have reported that the use of fenbendazole and albendazole (currently approved as anthelmintics) and paromomycin (broad-spectrum antibiotic) were effective and reduced cyst excretion, improved fecal consistency, and resulted higher weight gains.[105–108] However, another study found conflicting evidence and reported a higher risk of *Giardia* infection in calves associated with the administration of anthelmintics.[109]

Limiting the spread of *Giardia* among ruminants is difficult, and longitudinal studies indicate that most animals eventually become infected. However, improved husbandry and good management can be beneficial and can decrease cyst numbers in the farm environment, thus reducing the risk of transmission. These practices should include regular cleaning and disinfection, the use of floor surfaces that are easy to clean in barns, prompt removal of feces from animal housing, use of single-cow calving areas, and adequate intake of colostrum by neonatal animals to ensure adequate transfer of passive immunity.[89,109]

SUMMARY

Infections with *G duodenalis* and *Cryptosporidium* species are common in ruminants, and most animals become infected within the first months of life. Both parasites are causal agents of diarrhea in neonatal ruminants and have also been proved to have a negative impact on growth and performance, even in subclinical infections. In addition to potential production losses, some *G duodenalis* assemblages and *Cryptosporidium* species frequently identified in ruminants are zoonotic, indicating that ruminants may serve as a potential source for human infections either through direct contact with infected animals or through ingestion of cysts or oocysts via contaminated food or water. Control measures based on good husbandry management practices would be beneficial for both animal health and public health.

DISCLOSURE

The author has nothing to disclose.

REFERENCES

1. Xiao L. Molecular epidemiology of cryptosporidiosis: an update. Exp Parasitol 2010;124:80–9.
2. Feng Y, Xiao L. Zoonotic potential and molecular epidemiology of *Giardia* species and giardiasis. Clin Microbiol Rev 2011;24:110–40.
3. Santín M, Trout JM. Livestock. In: Fayer R, Xiao L, editors. *Cryptosporidium* and cryptosporidiosis. Boca Raton (FL): CRC Press; 2008. p. 451–83.
4. Santín M. Clinical and subclinical infections with *Cryptosporidium* in animals. N Z Vet J 2013;61:1–10.
5. Fayer R. General biology. In: Fayer R, Xiao L, editors. *Cryptosporidium* and cryptosporidiosis. Boca Raton (FL): CRC Press; 2008. p. 1–42.
6. Messner MJ, Berger P. *Cryptosporidium* infection risk: results of new dose-response modeling. Risk Anal 2016;36:1969–82.
7. Hatam-Nahavandi K, Ahmadpour E, Carmena D, et al. *Cryptosporidium* infections in terrestrial ungulates with focus on livestock: a systematic review and meta-analysis. Parasit Vectors 2019;12:453.
8. Thomson S, Innes EA, Jonsson NN, et al. Shedding of cryptosporidium in calves and dams: evidence of re-infection and shedding of different gp60 subtypes. Parasitology 2019;146:1404–13.
9. Santín M, Trout JM, Xiao L, et al. Prevalence and age-related variation of *Cryptosporidium* species and genotypes in dairy calves. Vet Parasitol 2004;122: 103–17.
10. Santín M, Trout JM, Fayer R. Prevalence and molecular characterization of *Cryptosporidium* and *Giardia* species and genotypes in sheep in Maryland. Vet Parasitol 2007;146:17–24.
11. Santín M, Trout JM, Fayer R. A longitudinal study of cryptosporidiosis in dairy cattle from birth to 2 years of age. Vet Parasitol 2008;155:15–23.
12. Majeed QAH, El-Azazy OME, Abdou NMI, et al. Epidemiological observations on cryptosporidiosis and molecular characterization of *Cryptosporidium* spp. in sheep and goats in Kuwait. Parasitol Res 2018;117:1631–6.
13. Papanikolopoulou V, Baroudi D, Guo Y, et al. Genotypes and subtypes of *Cryptosporidium* spp. in diarrheic lambs and goat kids in northern Greece. Parasitol Int 2018;67:472–5.
14. Cai M, Guo Y, Pan B, et al. Longitudinal monitoring of *Cryptosporidium* species in pre-weaned dairy calves on five farms in Shanghai, China. Vet Parasitol 2017; 241:14–9.

15. Ortega-Mora LM, Requejo-Fernández JA, Pilar-Izquierdo M, et al. Role of adult sheep in transmission of infection by *Cryptosporidium parvum* to lambs: confirmation of periparturient rise. Int J Parasitol 1999;29:1261–8.

16. Castro-Hermida JA, Delafosse A, Pors I, et al. *Giardia duodenalis* and *Cryptosporidium parvum* infections in adult goats and their implications for neonatal kids. Vet Rec 2005;157:623–7.

17. Xiao L, Herd RP, McClure KE. Periparturient rise in the excretion of *Giardia* sp. cysts and *Cryptosporidium parvum* oocysts as a source of infection for lambs. J Parasitol 1994;80(1):55–9.

18. Ye J, Xiao L, Wang Y, et al. Periparturient transmission of *Cryptosporidium xiaoi* from ewes to lambs. Vet Parasitol 2013;197:627–33.

19. Scott CA, Smith HV, Mtambo MM, et al. An epidemiological study of *Cryptosporidium parvum* in two herds of adult beef cattle. Vet Parasitol 1995;57:277–88.

20. Smith RP, Clifton-Hadley FA, Cheney T, et al. Prevalence and molecular typing of *Cryptosporidium* in dairy cattle in England and Wales and examination of potential on-farm transmission routes. Vet Parasitol 2014;204:111–9.

21. Lindsay DS, Upton SJ, Owens DS, et al. *Cryptosporidium andersoni* n. sp. (Apicomplexa: Cryptosporiidae) from cattle, *Bos taurus*. J Eukaryot Microbiol 2000; 47:91–5.

22. Fayer R, Santín M, Xiao L. *Cryptosporidium bovis* n. sp. (Apicomplexa: Cryptosporidiidae) in cattle (*Bos taurus*). J Parasitol 2005;91:624–9.

23. Fayer R, Santín M, Trout JM. *Cryptosporidium ryanae* n. sp. (Apicomplexa: Cryptosporidiidae) in cattle (*Bos taurus*). Vet Parasitol 2008;156:191–8.

24. Fayer R, Santín M. *Cryptosporidium xiaoi* n. sp. (Apicomplexa: Cryptosporidiidae) in sheep (*Ovis aries*). Vet Parasitol 2009;164:192–200.

25. Fayer R, Santín M, Macarisin D. *Cryptosporidium ubiquitum* n. sp. in animals and humans. Vet Parasitol 2010;172:23–32.

26. Brook EJ, Anthony Hart C, French NP, et al. Molecular epidemiology of *Cryptosporidium* subtypes in cattle in England. Vet J 2009;179:378–82.

27. Ouakli N, Belkhiri A, de Lucio A, et al. *Cryptosporidium*-associated diarrhoea in neonatal calves in Algeria. Vet Parasitol Reg Stud Reports 2018;12:78–84.

28. Feng Y, Gong X, Zhu K, et al. Prevalence and genotypic identification of *Cryptosporidium* spp., *Giardia duodenalis* and *Enterocytozoon bieneusi* in pre-weaned dairy calves in Guangdong, China. Parasit Vectors 2019;12:41.

29. Ryan UM, Bath C, Robertson I, et al. Sheep may not be an important zoonotic reservoir for *Cryptosporidium* and *Giardia* parasites. Appl Environ Microbiol 2005;71:4992–7.

30. Yang R, Jacobson C, Gardner G, et al. Longitudinal prevalence, oocyst shedding and molecular characterisation of *Cryptosporidium* species in sheep across four states in Australia. Vet Parasitol 2014;200:50–8.

31. Squire SA, Yang R, Robertson I, et al. Molecular characterization of *Cryptosporidium* and *Giardia* in farmers and their ruminant livestock from the Coastal Savannah zone of Ghana. Infect Genet Evol 2017;55:236–43.

32. Baroudi D, Hakem A, Adamu H, et al. Zoonotic *Cryptosporidium* species and subtypes in lambs and goat kids in Algeria. Parasit Vectors 2018;11:582.

33. Díaz P, Navarro E, Prieto A, et al. *Cryptosporidium* species in post-weaned and adult sheep and goats from N.W. Spain: public and animal health significance. Vet Parasitol 2018;254:1–5.

34. Sahraoui L, Thomas M, Chevillot A, et al. Molecular characterization of zoonotic *Cryptosporidium* spp. and *Giardia duodenalis* pathogens in Algerian sheep. Vet Parasitol Reg Stud Rep 2019;16:100280.

35. Quílez J, Torres E, Chalmers RM, et al. Cryptosporidium genotypes and sub-types in lambs and goat kids in Spain. Appl Environ Microbiol 2008;74:6026–31.
36. Mueller-Doblies D, Giles M, Elwin K, et al. Distribution of *Cryptosporidium* species in sheep in the UK. Vet Parasitol 2008;154:214–9.
37. Drumo R, Widmer G, Morrison LJ, et al. Evidence of host-associated populations of *Cryptosporidium parvum* in Italy. Appl Environ Microbiol 2012;78:3523–9.
38. Wang Y, Feng Y, Cui B, et al. Cervine genotype is the major *Cryptosporidium* genotype in sheep in China. Parasitol Res 2010;106:341–7.
39. Koinari M, Lymbery AJ, Ryan UM. *Cryptosporidium* species in sheep and goats from Papua New Guinea. Exp Parasitol 2014;141:134–7.
40. Kaupke A, Michalski MM, Rzeżutka A. Diversity of *Cryptosporidium* species occurring in sheep and goat breeds reared in Poland. Parasitol Res 2017;116:871–9.
41. Chalmers RM, Robinson G, Elwin K, et al. Analysis of the *Cryptosporidium* spp. and *gp60* subtypes linked to human outbreaks of cryptosporidiosis in England and Wales, 2009 to 2017. Parasit Vectors 2019;12:95.
42. Gharpure R, Perez A, Miller AD, et al. Cryptosporidiosis outbreaks - United States, 2009-2017. MMWR Morb Mortal Wkly Rep 2019;68:568–72.
43. Li N, Xiao L, Alderisio K, et al. Subtyping *Cryptosporidium ubiquitum*, a zoonotic pathogen emerging in humans. Emerg Infect Dis 2014;20:217–24.
44. Guyot K, Follet-Dumoulin A, Lelièvre E, et al. Molecular characterization of *Cryptosporidium* isolates obtained from humans in France. J Clin Microbiol 2001;39:3472–80.
45. Leoni F, Amar C, Nichols G, et al. Genetic analysis of *Cryptosporidium* from 2414 humans with diarrhoea in England between 1985 and 2000. J Med Microbiol 2006;55:703–7.
46. Morse TD, Nichols RA, Grimason AM, et al. Incidence of cryptosporidiosis species in pediatric patients in Malawi. Epidemiol Infect 2007;135:1307–15.
47. Waldron LS, Dimeski B, Beggs PJ, et al. Molecular epidemiology, spatiotemporal analysis, and ecology of sporadic human cryptosporidiosis in Australia. Appl Environ Microbiol 2011;77:7757–65.
48. Agholi M, Hatam GR, Motazedian MH. HIV/AIDS-associated opportunistic protozoal diarrhea. AIDS Res Hum Retroviruses 2013;29:35–41.
49. Jiang Y, Ren J, Yuan Z, et al. *Cryptosporidium andersoni* as a novel predominant *Cryptosporidium* species in outpatients with diarrhea in Jiangsu Province, China. BMC Infect Dis 2014;14:555.
50. Khan SM, Debnath C, Pramanik AK, et al. Molecular characterization and assessment of zoonotic transmission of *Cryptosporidium* from dairy cattle in West Bengal, India. Vet Parasitol 2010;171:41–7.
51. Ng JS, Eastwood K, Walker B, et al. Evidence of *Cryptosporidium* transmission between cattle and humans in northern New South Wales. Exp Parasitol 2012;130:437–41.
52. Adamu H, Petros B, Zhang G, et al. Distribution and clinical manifestations of *Cryptosporidium* species and subtypes in HIV/AIDS patients in Ethiopia. PLoS Negl Trop Dis 2014;8:e2831.
53. Li N, Wang R, Cai M, et al. Outbreak of cryptosporidiosis due to *Cryptosporidium parvum* subtype IIdA19G1 in neonatal calves on a dairy farm in China. Int J Parasitol 2019;49:569–77.
54. Feng Y, Xiao L. Molecular epidemiology of cryptosporidiosis in China. Front Microbiol 2017;8:1701.

55. Muhid A, Robertson I, Ng J, et al. Prevalence of and management factors contributing to *Cryptosporidium* sp. infection in pre-weaned and post-weaned calves in Johor, Malaysia. Exp Parasitol 2011;127:534–8.

56. Silverlås C, Näslund K, Björkman C, et al. Molecular characterisation of *Cryptosporidium* isolates from Swedish dairy cattle in relation to age, diarrhoea and region. Vet Parasitol 2010;169:289–95.

57. Díaz P, Quílez J, Prieto A, et al. *Cryptosporidium* species and subtype analysis in diarrhoeic pre-weaned lambs and goat kids from north-western Spain. Parasitol Res 2015;114:4099–105.

58. Fayer R, Gasbarre L, Pasquali P, et al. *Cryptosporidium parvum* infection in bovine neonates: dynamic clinical, parasitic and immunologic patterns. Int J Parasitol 1998;28:49–56.

59. Trotz-Williams LA, Jarvie BD, Martin SW, et al. Prevalence of *Cryptosporidium parvum* infection in southwestern Ontario and its association with diarrhea in neonatal dairy calves. Can Vet J 2005;46:349–51.

60. O'Handley RM, Cockwill C, McAllister TA, et al. Duration of naturally acquired giardiosis and cryptosporidiosis in dairy calves and their association with diarrhoea. J Am Vet Med Assoc 1999;214:391–6.

61. Tzipori S, Smith M, Halpin C, et al. Experimental cryptosporidiosis in calves: clinical manifestations and pathological findings. Vet Rec 1983;112:116–20.

62. Shivley CB, Lombard JE, Urie NJ, et al. Preweaned heifer management on US dairy operations: part VI. Factors associated with average daily gain in preweaned dairy heifer calves. J Dairy Sci 2018;101:9245–58.

63. Kvác M, Vítovec J. Prevalence and pathogenicity of *Cryptosporidium andersoni* in one herd of beef cattle. J Vet Med B Infect Dis Vet Public Health 2003;50:451–7.

64. Esteban E, Anderson BC. *Cryptosporidium muris*: prevalence, persistency, and detrimental effect on milk production in a drylot dairy. J Dairy Sci 1995;78:1068–72.

65. Ralston B, Thompson RC, Pethick D, et al. *Cryptosporidium andersoni* in Western Australian feedlot cattle. Aust Vet J 2010;88:458–60.

66. Anderson BC. Cryptosporidiosis in bovine and human health. J Dairy Sci 1998;81:3036–41.

67. Chalmers RM, Elwin K, Reilly WJ, et al. *Cryptosporidium* in farmed animals: the detection of a novel isolate in sheep. Int J Parasitol 2002;32:21–6.

68. Navarro-i-Martinez L, da Silva AJ, Bornay-Llinares FJ, et al. Detection and molecular characterization of *Cryptosporidium bovis*-like isolate from a newborn lamb in Spain. J Parasitol 2007;93:1536–8.

69. Jacobson C, Al-Habsi K, Ryan U, et al. *Cryptosporidium* infection is associated with reduced growth and diarrhoea in goats beyond weaning. Vet Parasitol 2018;260:30–7.

70. Sweeny JP, Ryan UM, Robertson ID, et al. *Cryptosporidium* and *Giardia* associated with reduced lamb carcase productivity. Vet Parasitol 2011;182:127–39.

71. Ryan U, Zahedi A, Paparini A. *Cryptosporidium* in humans and animals-a one health approach to prophylaxis. Parasite Immunol 2016;38:535–47.

72. Ahmed SA, Karanis P. Comparison of current methods used to detect *Cryptosporidium* oocysts in stools. Int J Hyg Environ Health 2018;221:743–63.

73. Smith. Livestock. In: Fayer R, Xiao L, editors. *Cryptosporidium* and cryptosporidiosis. Boca Raton (FL): CRC Press; 2008. p. 173–207.

74. Innes EA, Bartley PM, Rocchi M, et al. Developing vaccines to control protozoan parasites in ruminants: dead or alive? Vet Parasitol 2011;180:155–63.

75. Foster DM, Smith GW. Pathophysiology of diarrhea in calves. Vet Clin North Am Food Anim Pract 2009;25:13–36, xi.

76. Williams LA, Jarvie BD, Peregrine AS, et al. Efficacy of halofuginone lactate in the prevention of cryptosporidiosis in dairy calves. Vet Rec 2011;168:509.

77. Niine T, Dorbek-Kolin E, Lassen B, et al. *Cryptosporidium* outbreak in calves on a large dairy farm: effect of treatment and the association with the inflammatory response and short-term weight gain. Res Vet Sci 2018;117:200–8.

78. Meganck V, Hoflack G, Piepers S, et al. Evaluation of a protocol to reduce the incidence of neonatal calf diarrhoea on dairy herds. Prev Vet Med 2015;118: 64–70.

79. Petermann J, Paraud C, Pors I, et al. Efficacy of halofuginone lactate against experimental cryptosporidiosis in goat neonates. Vet Parasitol 2014;202:326–9.

80. Lyu Z, Shao J, Xue M, et al. A new species of *Giardia* Künstler, 1882 (Sarcomastigophora: Hexamitidae) in hamsters. Parasit Vectors 2018;11:202.

81. Einarsson E, Ma'ayeh S, Svärd SG. An up-date on *Giardia* and giardiasis. Curr Opin Microbiol 2016;34:47–52.

82. Xiao L, Feng Y. Molecular epidemiologic tools for waterborne pathogens *Cryptosporidium* spp. and *Giardia duodenalis*. Food and Waterborne Parasitology 2017;8–9:14–32. Available at: https://doi.org/10.1016/j.fawpar.2017.09.002.

83. Ryan U, Hijjawi N, Feng Y, et al. *Giardia*: an under-reported foodborne parasite. Int J Parasitol 2019;49:1–11.

84. Thompson RCA, Ash A. Molecular epidemiology of *Giardia* and *Cryptosporidium* infections - What's new? Infect Genet Evol 2019;75:103951.

85. Benedict KM, Collier SA, Marder EP, et al. Case-case analyses of cryptosporidiosis and giardiasis using routine national surveillance data in the United States - 2005-2015. Epidemiol Infect 2019;147:e178.

86. Teunis PFM, van der Heijden OG, van der Giessen JWB, et al. The dose-response relation in human volunteers for gastro-intestinal pathogens. Report 2845500002. Bilthoven (The Netherlands): RIVM; 1996. Available at: http://hdl.handle.net/10029/9966.

87. Erickson MC, Ortega YR. Inactivation of protozoan parasites in food, water, and environmental systems. J Food Prot 2006;69:2786–808.

88. Gómez-Muñoz MT, Cámara-Badenes C, Martínez-Herrero Mdel C, et al. Multilocus genotyping of *Giardia duodenalis* in lambs from Spain reveals a high heterogeneity. Res Vet Sci 2012;93:836–42.

89. Urie NJ, Lombard JE, Shivley CB, et al. Preweaned heifer management on US dairy operations: part III. Factors associated with *Cryptosporidium* and *Giardia* in preweaned dairy heifer calves. J Dairy Sci 2018;101:9199–213.

90. Utaaker KS, Myhr N, Bajwa RS, et al. Goats in the city: prevalence of *Giardia duodenalis* and *Cryptosporidium* spp. in extensively reared goats in northern India. Acta Vet Scand 2017;59:86.

91. Wang G, Wang G, Li X, et al. Prevalence and molecular characterization of *Cryptosporidium* spp. and *Giardia duodenalis* in 1-2-month-old highland yaks in Qinghai Province, China. Parasitol Res 2018;117:1793–800.

92. Santín M, Trout JM, Fayer R. A longitudinal study of *Giardia duodenalis* genotypes in dairy cows from birth to 2 years of age. Vet Parasitol 2009;162:40–5.

93. Sweeny JP, Ryan UM, Robertson ID, et al. Longitudinal investigation of protozoan parasites in meat lamb farms in southern Western Australia. Prev Vet Med 2011;101:192–203.

94. Al-Habsi K, Yang R, Williams A, et al. Zoonotic *Cryptosporidium* and *Giardia* shedding by captured rangeland goats. Vet Parasitol Reg Stud Rep 2017; 7:32–5.

95. Naguib D, El-Gohary AH, Mohamed AA, et al. Age patterns of *Cryptosporidium* species and *Giardia duodenalis* in dairy calves in Egypt. Parasitol Int 2018;67: 736–41.

96. Mahato MK, Singh DK, Rana HB, et al. Prevalence and risk factors associated with *Giardia duodenalis* infection in dairy cattle of Chitwan, Nepal. J Parasit Dis 2018;42:122–6.

97. Geurden T, Thomas P, Casaert S, et al. Prevalence and molecular characterisation of *Cryptosporidium* and *Giardia* in lambs and goat kids in Belgium. Vet Parasitol 2008;155:142–5.

98. Wang R, Li N, Jiang W, et al. Infection patterns, clinical significance, and genetic characteristics of *Enterocytozoon bieneusi* and *Giardia duodenalis* in dairy cattle in Jiangsu, China. Parasitol Res 2019;118:3053–60.

99. Ng J, Yang R, Whiffin V, et al. Identification of zoonotic *Cryptosporidium* and *Giardia* genotypes infecting animals in Sydney's water catchments. Exp Parasitol 2011;128:138–44.

100. Olson ME, McAllister TA, Deselliers L, et al. Effects of giardiasis on production in a domestic ruminant (lamb) model. Am J Vet Res 1995;56:1470–4.

101. Geurden T, Vandenhoute E, Pohle H, et al. The effect of a fenbendazole treatment on cyst excretion and weight gain in calves experimentally infected with *Giardia duodenalis*. Vet Parasitol 2010;169:18–23.

102. Soares R, Tasca T. Giardiasis: an update review on sensitivity and specificity of methods for laboratorial diagnosis. J Microbiol Methods 2016;129:98–102.

103. Cama VA, Mathison BA. Infections by intestinal coccidia and *Giardia duodenalis*. Clin Lab Med 2015;35:423–44.

104. Uehlinger FD, O'Handley RM, Greenwood SJ, et al. Efficacy of vaccination in preventing giardiasis in calves. Vet Parasitol 2007;146:182–8.

105. Xiao L, Saeed K, Herd RP. Efficacy of albendazole and fenbendazole against *Giardia* infection in cattle. Vet Parasitol 1996;61:165–70.

106. O'Handley RM, Cockwill C, Jelinski M, et al. Effects of repeat fenbendazole treatment in dairy calves with giardiosis on cyst excretion, clinical signs and production. Vet Parasitol 2000;89:209–18.

107. O'Handley RM, Buret AG, McAllister TA, et al. Giardiasis in dairy calves: effects of fenbendazole treatment on intestinal structure and function. Int J Parasitol 2001;31:73–9.

108. Geurden T, Claerebout E, Dursin L, et al. The efficacy of an oral treatment with paromomycin against an experimental infection with *Giardia* in calves. Vet Parasitol 2006;135:241–7.

109. Muhid A, Robertson I, Ng J, et al. Prevalence of *Giardia* spp. infection in preweaned and weaned calves in relation to management factors. Vet J 2012; 191:135–7.

Moving?

Make sure your subscription moves with you!

To notify us of your new address, find your **Clinics Account Number** (located on your mailing label above your name), and contact customer service at:

Email: journalscustomerservice-usa@elsevier.com

800-654-2452 (subscribers in the U.S. & Canada)
314-447-8871 (subscribers outside of the U.S. & Canada)

Fax number: 314-447-8029

Elsevier Health Sciences Division
Subscription Customer Service
3251 Riverport Lane
Maryland Heights, MO 63043

*To ensure uninterrupted delivery of your subscription, please notify us at least 4 weeks in advance of move.

Printed and bound by CPI Group (UK) Ltd, Croydon, CR0 4YY

03/10/2024

01040484-0005